STRUCTURAL EQUATION MODELING WITH EQS

Basic Concepts, Applications, and Programming

Second Edition

Multivariate Applications Series

Sponsored by the Society of Multivariate Psychology, the goal of this series is to apply complex statistical methods to significant social or behavioral issues, in such a way so as to be accessible to a nontechnical-oriented readership (e.g., nonmethodological researchers, teachers, students, government personnel, practitioners, and other professionals). Applications from a variety of disciplines such as psychology, public health, sociology, education, and business are welcome. Books can be single- or multiple-authored or edited volumes that (1) demonstrate the application of a variety of multivariate methods to a single, major area of research; (2) describe a multivariate procedure or framework that could be applied to a number of research areas; or (3) present a variety of perspectives on a controversial topic of interest to applied multivariate researchers.

There are currently 11 books in the series:

- *What if there were no significance tests?* co-edited by Lisa L. Harlow, Stanley A. Mulaik, and James H. Steiger (1997).
- *Structural Equation Modeling with LISREL, PRELIS, and SIMPLIS: Basic Concepts, Applications, and Programming* written by Barbara M. Byrne (1998).
- *Multivariate Applications in Substance Use Research: New Methods for New Questions,* co-edited by Jennifer S. Roe, Laurie Chassin, Clark C. Presson, and Steven J. Sherman (2000).
- *Item Response Theory for Psychologists,* co-authored by Susan E. Embretson and Steven P. Reise (2000).
- *Structural Equation Modeling with AMOS: Basic Concepts, Applications, and Programming,* written by Barbara M. Byrne (2001).
- *Conducting Meta-Analysis Using SAS,* written by Winfred Arthur, Jr., Winston Bennett, Jr., and Allen I. Huffcutt (2001).
- *Modeling Intraindividual Variability with Repeated Measures Data: Methods and Applications,* co-edited by D. S. Moskowitz and Scott L. Hershberger (2002).
- *Multilevel Modeling: Methodological Advances, Issues, and Applications,* co-edited by Steven P. Reise and Naihua Duan (2003).
- *The Essence of Multivariate Thinking: Basic Themes and Methods,* written by Lisa Harlow (2005).
- *Contemporary Psychometrics:* A Festschrift for Roderick P. McDonald, co-edited by Albert Maydeu-Olivares and John J. McArdle (2005).
- *Structural Equation Modeling with EQS: Basic Concepts, Applications, and Programming, Second Edition,* written by Barbara M. Byrne (2006).

Anyone wishing to submit a book proposal should send the following; (1) author/title; (2) timeline including completion date; (3) brief overview of the book's focus, including table of contents, and ideally a sample chapter (or more); (4) a brief description competing publications; and (5) targeted audiences.

For more information, please contact the series editor, Lisa Harlow, at Department of Psychology, University of Rhode Island, 10 Chafee Road, Suite 8, Kingston, RI 02881–0808; Phone (401) 874–4242; Fax (401) 874–5562; or e-mail LHarlow@uri.edu. Information may also be obtained from members of the advisory board: Leona Aiken (Arizona State University), Gwyneth Boodoo (Educational Testing Services), Barbara M. Byrne (University of Ottawa), Patrick Curran (University of North Carolina), Scott E. Maxwell (University of Notre Dame), David Rindskopf (City University of New York), Liora Schmelkin (Hofstra University), and Stephen West (Arizona State University).

STRUCTURAL EQUATION MODELING WITH EQS
Basic Concepts, Applications, and Programming

Second Edition

Barbara M. Byrne
University of Ottawa

LEA

LAWRENCE ERLBAUM ASSOCIATES, PUBLISHERS

2006   Mahwah, New Jersey   London

Senior Editor: Debra Riegert
Editorial Assistant: Rebecca Larsen
Cover Design: Kathryn Houghtaling Lacey
Full Service Compositor: TechBooks

This book was typeset in 10/12 pt. Times, Italic, Bold, and Bold Italic.
The heads were typeset in Americana, Americana Italic, Americana Bold, Futura, and Futura Italic.

Lawrence Erlbaum Associates, Inc., Publishers
10 Industrial Avenue
Mahwah, New Jersey 07430
www.erlbaum.com

Library of Congress Cataloging-in-Publication Data

Byrne, Barbara M.
Structural equation modeling with EQS : basic concepts, applications, and programming /
    Barbara M. Byrne. — 2nd ed.
        p.   cm.
    Includes bibliographical references and index.
        ISBN 0-8058-4125-3 (cloth : alk. paper) — ISBN 0-8058-4126-1 (pbk. : alk. paper)
        1. EQS (Computer file)   2. Structural equation modeling–Data processing.
    3. Social sciences—Statistical methods—Data processing.
    I. Title.

    QA278.3.B97   2006
    519.5'35—dc22   2005031008

Contents

v

Preface

As with the first edition of this book, my overall goal is to provide readers with a nonmathematical introduction to basic concepts associated with structural equation modeling (SEM) and to illustrate basic applications of SEM using the EQS program. All applications in this volume are based on EQS 6.1, the most up-to-date version of the program at this time. Although there is always the possibility of newer versions of the program appearing at a later date, the basic principles covered in the book remain intact.

This book is specifically designed and written for readers who may have little or no knowledge of either SEM or the EQS program. It is intended neither as a text on the topic of SEM nor as a comprehensive review of the many statistical and graphical functions available in the EQS program. Rather, my primary aim is to provide a practical guide to SEM using the EQS approach. As such, readers are "walked through" a diversity of SEM applications that include confirmatory factor analytic (CFA) and full latent variable models tested on a wide variety of data (i.e., single/multigroup, normal/non-normal, complete/incomplete, continuous/categorical) and are based on either the analysis of covariance structures or the analysis of mean and covariance structures. Throughout the book, each application is accompanied by numerous illustrative "how-to" examples related to particular procedural aspects of the program. In summary, each application is accompanied by the following:

- statement of the hypothesis to be tested
- schematic representation of the model under study
- full explanation of related EQS input files
- full explanation and interpretation of related EQS output files
- published reference from which the application is drawn
- illustrated use and function associated with a wide variety of drop-down menus and graphical icons used in building, testing, and evaluating models, as well as for other important data management tasks
- data file on which the application is based

This second edition differs in several important ways from the initial volume. First, the number of applications has been expanded to include the testing of a latent growth model, a multilevel model, a second-order model based on categorical data, a missing data model based on the EM (expectation maximization) algorithm, and latent mean differences based on a higher order factor model. Second, most applications are based on different data. Third, given that EQS 6.1 is structured within a Windows™ interface, each application is accompanied by illustrative vignettes detailing how to perform particular procedural and/or data management tasks. Fourth, the EQS DIAGRAMMER has undergone substantial improvement since earlier versions and is now a state-of-the-art feature that makes modeling with EQS easy, intriguing, and fun. I demonstrate how to use the DIAGRAMMER to build various models and, throughout the book, illustrate many of its various capabilities. Finally, all data files used for the applications of this book are included on a disk, located in a pocket inside the back cover.

The book is divided into four major parts: Part I comprises two introductory chapters. In chapter 1, I introduce you to the fundamental concepts underlying SEM methodology. I also present a general overview of model specification within the framework of EQS and, in the process, introduce you to basic EQS notation. Chapter 2 focuses solely on the EQS 6.1 program. Here, the key elements associated with building and executing model files are described. Indeed, EQS provides you with a choice of three methods by which to specify a model: depending on your preference, you can do so manually, interactively, or graphically. In this chapter, I walk you through each of these model specification techniques.

Part II is devoted to applications involving single-group analyses; these include two first-order CFA models, one second-order CFA model, and one full latent variable model. The first-order CFA applications demonstrate testing for the validity of the theoretical structure of a construct (chap. 3) and the factorial structure of a measuring instrument (chap. 4). The second-order CFA model bears on the factorial structure of a measuring instrument (chap. 5). The final single-group application tests for the validity of an empirically derived causal structure (chap. 6).

In Part III, I present applications related to multigroup analyses based on the analysis of covariance, as well as on covariance and mean structures. Based on the analysis of only covariance structures, I show how to test for measurement and structural invariance across groups as they relate to a measuring instrument (chap. 7) and a causal structure (chap. 8). Working from a somewhat different perspective, and based on the analysis of covariance and mean structures, I first outline the basic concepts associated with latent mean structures. I then demonstrate how to test for measurement invariance related to a first-order factor model (chap. 9) and a second-order factor model (chap. 10). In addition, I further illustrate how to test for latent mean differences related to both of these first- and second-order models.

Part IV comprises the final three chapters of the book and presents models that are increasingly becoming of substantial interest to practitioners of SEM. In addressing the issue of construct validity, chapter 11 illustrates the specification and testing of a multitrait–multimethod (MTMM) model. Chapter 12 focuses on longitudinal data and presents a latent growth curve (LGC) model that is tested with and without a predictor variable included. Finally, in chapter 13, I illustrate the specification and testing of a simple multilevel model.

Although there are now several SEM texts available, this book is distinct from the rest in a number of ways. First, it is the only book to demonstrate—by application to actual data—a wide range of CFA and full latent variable models drawn from published studies, along with a detailed explanation of each input and output file. Second, it is the only book to incorporate applications based solely on the EQS 6.1 program. Third, it is the first and only book to illustrate a unified approach to use of the most state-of-the-art and appropriate goodness-of-fit indexes for a variety of problematic data types likely to be encountered in practice, including complete and incomplete non-normal data, categorical data, and multilevel data. Fourth, it is the only book to literally "walk" readers through (a) model specification, estimation, evaluation, and post hoc modification decisions and processes associated with a variety of applications; (b) three approaches (i.e., manual, interactive, and graphical) to building EQS model files; and (c) the use of numerous drop-down menus to initiate a variety of analytic, data management, editorial, and visual EQS procedures. Overall, this volume serves well as a companion book to the EQS manual (Bentler, 2005) and user's guide (Bentler & Wu, 2002), as well as to any statistics textbook devoted to the topic of SEM.

In writing a book of this nature, it is essential to have access to a number of different data sets that lend themselves to various applications. To facilitate this need, all examples presented throughout the book, with the exception of chapter 13, are drawn from my own research. Related journal references are cited for readers who may be interested in a more detailed discussion of theoretical frameworks, aspects of the methodology, and/or substantive issues and findings. It is important to emphasize that although all applications are based on data of a social/psychological nature, they could just as easily have been based on data representative of the health sciences, leisure studies, marketing, or a multitude of other disciplines; my data, then, serve only as one example of each application. Indeed, I urge readers to seek out and examine similar examples as they relate to other subject areas.

Having now written four introductory books on the application of SEM with respect to particular programs (Byrne, 1989, 1994a, 1998, 2001), I must say that the writing of this second edition of the EQS book was by far the most enjoyable! Admittedly, such a project demands eons of time and is certainly not without its frustrations, but thanks to the ongoing support of Peter Bentler and Eric Wu and the superb technical support provided by Multivariate Software, such difficulties were always quickly resolved and transformed into important learning experiences. In weaving together the textual, graphical, and statistical threads that form the fabric of this book, I hope that I have provided my readers with a comprehensive understanding of basic concepts and applications of SEM as well as an extensive working knowledge of the EQS 6.1 program. Achievement of this goal has necessarily meant the concomitant juggling of word-processing, "grabber," and statistical programs to produce the end result. It has been an incredible editorial journey but one that has left me feeling truly enriched for having had this wonderful learning experience. I can only hope that as my readers wend their way through the chapters of this book, the journey will be equally exciting and fulfilling. EQS is a wonderful program—its graphical interface is fantastic, its analytic capability is state-of-the-art, its help menu and technical support are awesome, and best of all, it's so easy to use! I hope this book helps you enjoy it to the fullest!

ACKNOWLEDGMENTS

As with the writing of each of my other books, there are many people to whom I owe a great deal of thanks. First and foremost, I am indebted in so many ways to Peter Bentler, author of the EQS 6.1 program, and truly a very special person. Although I have never been one of Peter's students in a formal sense, I am fortunate to have benefited from his informal mentoring over a period of about 20 years. As a doctoral student in the early 1980s, I quickly discovered that Peter Bentler was the only person who spoke about SEM in a language that I could understand. Furthermore, he always took the time to answer my many questions—fortunately for me, he continues to answer my seemingly endless questions, to advise me on particular application difficulties, and to keep me updated on new additions and/or modifications to the EQS program. Thanks, Peter, for always being there whenever I needed answers.

I am also grateful to Eric Wu, programmer of the EQS program and mastermind behind the DIAGRAMMER, its amazing graphical interface. Not only has Eric been quick to help me resolve any graphical difficulties whenever I encountered them, but he has also built in particular features that addressed my needs along the way. Many thanks are due as well to Kevin Kim, Multivariate Software's technical-support guru. I haven't found a question yet that Kevin was not able to answer—and I've kept him busy with a lot of them! Thanks also, Kevin, for your super-fast (almost instantaneous) replies to my emails; I am most appreciative! Finally, I wish to thank Elizabeth Houck, Multivariate Software's Special Projects Director, for her warm and caring support during the span of this project and for her continued enthusiasm, optimism, and absolutely wonderful sense of humor.

Special thanks are extended to my incomparable LEA editor, Debra Riegert, whom I consider to be a paragon of patience. Although this book has been in the works for two or three years, Debra has never once applied pressure regarding its completion. Rather, she has always been encouraging, supportive, helpful, and, overall, a very good friend. Thanks so much Debra, for just letting me do my own thing.

Last, but certainly not least, I am so grateful to my husband, Alex, for his continued patience, support, and understanding of the incredible number of hours that my computer and I necessarily spend together on a project of this sort. I consider myself to be fortunate indeed!

STRUCTURAL EQUATION MODELING WITH EQS

Basic Concepts, Applications, and Programming

Second Edition

I

Introduction

1

Structural Equation Models: The Basics

Structural equation modeling (SEM) is a statistical methodology that takes a confirmatory (i.e., hypothesis-testing) approach to the analysis of a structural theory bearing on some phenomenon. Typically, this theory represents "causal" processes that generate observations on multiple variables (Bentler, 1988). The term *structural equation modeling* conveys two important aspects of the procedure: (a) that the causal processes under study are represented by a series of structural (i.e., regression) equations, and (b) that these structural relations can be modeled pictorially to enable a clearer conceptualization of the theory under study. The hypothesized model can then be tested statistically in a simultaneous analysis of the entire system of variables to determine the extent to which it is consistent with the data. If goodness-of-fit is adequate, the model argues for the plausibility of postulated relations among variables; if it is inadequate, the tenability of such relations is rejected.

Several aspects of SEM set it apart from the older generation of multivariate procedures. First, as noted previously, it takes a confirmatory rather than an exploratory approach to the data analysis (although aspects of the latter can be addressed). Furthermore, by demanding that the pattern of intervariable relations be specified a priori, SEM lends itself well to the analysis of data for inferential purposes. By contrast, most other multivariate procedures are essentially descriptive by nature (e.g., exploratory factor analysis [EFA]) so that hypothesis-testing is difficult if not impossible. Second, whereas traditional multivariate procedures are

3

incapable of either assessing or correcting for measurement error, SEM provides explicit estimates of these error variance parameters. Indeed, alternative methods (e.g., those rooted in regression or the general linear model) assume that error in the explanatory (i.e., independent) variables vanishes. Thus, applying those methods when there is error in the explanatory variables is tantamount to ignoring error that may lead, ultimately, to serious inaccuracies—especially when the errors are sizeable. Such mistakes are avoided when corresponding SEM analyses (in simple terms) are used (T. Raykov, personal communication, March 30, 2000). Third, whereas data analyses using the former methods are based on observed measurements only, those using SEM procedures can incorporate both unobserved (i.e., latent) and observed variables. Finally, there are no widely and easily applied alternative methods for modeling multivariate relations or for estimating point and/or interval indirect effects; these important features are available using SEM methodology.

Given these highly desirable characteristics, SEM has become a popular methodology for nonexperimental research in which methods for testing theories are not well developed and ethical considerations make experimental design unfeasible (Bentler, 1980). SEM can be utilized effectively to address numerous research problems involving nonexperimental research; in this book, I illustrate the most common applications (e.g., chaps. 3, 4, 6, 7, and 8) as well as some that are less frequently found in the substantive literature (e.g., chaps. 5, 9, 10, 11, 12, and 13). In each chapter, I walk you through the entire analytic process, from specification of the hypothesized model for the input file to interpretation of findings in the output file. Throughout the book, we work with EQS 6.1, the most recent version of the EQS program (Bentler, 2005; Bentler & Wu, 2002). Before showing you how to use EQS in testing SEM models, however, it is essential that I first review key concepts associated with the methodology. We turn now to their brief explanation.

BASIC CONCEPTS

Latent Versus Observed Variables

In the behavioral sciences, researchers are often interested in studying theoretical constructs that cannot be observed directly. These abstract phenomena are termed *latent variables, or factors*. Examples of latent variables in psychology are self-concept and motivation; in sociology, powerlessness and anomie; in education, verbal ability and teacher expectancy; and in economics, capitalism and social class.

Because latent variables are not observed directly, it follows that they cannot be measured directly. Thus, the researcher must operationally define the latent variable of interest in terms of behavior believed to represent it. As such, the unobserved variable is linked to one that is observable, thereby making its measurement possible. Assessment of the behavior, then, constitutes the direct measurement of an observed variable albeit the indirect measurement of an unobserved variable (i.e., the underlying construct). The term *behavior* is used here in the very broadest sense to include scores on a particular measuring instrument. Thus, observation may include, for example, self-report responses to an attitudinal scale, scores on an achievement test, *in vivo* observation scores representing some physical task or activity, coded responses to interview questions, and the like. These measured scores (i.e., measurements) are termed *observed* or *manifest variables*; within the context of SEM methodology, they serve as indicators of the underlying construct that they are presumed to represent. Given this necessary bridging process between observed variables and unobserved latent variables, it should now be clear why methodologists urge researchers to be circumspect in their selection of assessment measures. Whereas the choice of psychometrically sound instruments bears importantly on the credibility of all study findings, such selection becomes even more critical when the observed measure is presumed to represent an underlying construct.[1]

Exogenous Versus Endogenous Latent Variables

In working with SEM models, it is helpful to distinguish between latent variables that are exogenous and those that are endogenous. *Exogenous latent variables* are synonymous with independent variables; they "cause" fluctuations in the values of other latent variables in the model. Changes in the values of exogenous variables are not explained by the model; rather, they are considered to be influenced by other factors external to it. Background variables, such as gender, age, and socioeconomic status, are examples of such external factors. *Endogenous latent variables* are synonymous with dependent variables and, as such, are influenced by the exogenous variables in the model, either directly or indirectly. Fluctuation in the values of endogenous variables is said to be explained by the model because all latent variables that influence them are included in the model specification. In the interest of both simplicity and consistency throughout the remainder of the book, the terms *independent* and *dependent* rather than exogenous and endogenous variables, respectively, are used in the various SEM models described.

The Factor Analytic Model

The oldest and best known statistical procedure for investigating relations between sets of observed and latent variables is that of factor analysis. In using this approach to data analyses, the researcher examines the covariation among a set of observed variables to gather information on their underlying latent constructs (i.e., factors). There are two basic types of factor analyses: exploratory factor analysis (EFA) and

---

[1]Throughout the remainder of the book, the terms *latent*, *unobserved*, and *unmeasured* variables are used synonymously to represent a hypothetical construct or factor; the terms *observed*, *manifest*, and *measured* variables also are used interchangeably.

confirmatory factor analysis (CFA). We turn now to a brief description of each. However, for a more extensive discussion of each, see Byrne (2005a; 2005b).

EFA is designed for the situation in which links between the observed and latent variables are unknown or uncertain. The analysis thus proceeds in an exploratory mode to determine how and to what extent the observed variables are linked to their underlying factors. Typically, the researcher wishes to identify the minimal number of factors that underlie (or account for) covariation among the observed variables. For example, suppose a researcher develops a new instrument designed to measure five facets of physical self-concept (i.e., Health, Sport Competence, Physical Appearance, Coordination, and Body Strength). Following the formulation of questionnaire items designed to measure these five latent constructs, the researcher would then conduct an EFA to determine the extent to which the item measurements (the observed variables) were related to the five latent constructs. In factor analysis, these relations are represented by *factor loadings*. The researcher would hope that items designed to measure health, for example, exhibited high loadings on that factor albeit low or negligible loadings on the other four factors. This factor analytic approach is considered exploratory in the sense that the researcher has no prior knowledge that the items do indeed measure the intended factors. (For texts that discuss EFA, see Comrey, 1992; Gorsuch, 1983; McDonald, 1985; and Mulaik, 1972. For informative articles on EFA, see Fabrigar, Wegener, MacCallum, & Strahan, 1999; MacCallum, Widaman, Zhang, & Hong, 1999; Preacher & MacCallum, 2003; and Wood, Tataryn, & Gorsuch, 1996.)

In contrast to EFA, CFA is appropriately used when the researcher has some knowledge of the underlying latent variable structure. Based on knowledge of the theory, empirical research, or both, the researcher postulates relations between the observed measures and the underlying factors a priori and then tests this hypothesized structure statistically. For instance, based on the previous example, the researcher would argue for the loading of items designed to measure sport-competence self-concept on that specific factor and not on the health, physical appearance, coordination, or body-strength self-concept dimensions. Accordingly, a priori specification of the CFA model would allow all sport-competence self-concept items to be free to load on that factor but restricted to have zero loadings on the remaining factors. The model would then be evaluated by statistical means to determine the adequacy of its goodness-of-fit to the sample data. (For more detailed discussions of CFA, see, e.g., Bollen, 1989a; Long, 1983a; and Raykov & Marcoulides, 2000.)

In summary, the factor analytic model (i.e., EFA or CFA) focuses solely on how and the extent to which the observed variables are linked to their underlying latent factors. More specifically, it is concerned with the extent to which the observed variables are generated by the underlying latent constructs and, thus, strength of the regression paths from the factors to the observed variables (i.e., the factor loadings) are of primary interest. Although interfactor relations are also of interest, any regression structure among them is not considered in the factor analytic model.

Because the CFA model focuses solely on the link between factors and their measured variables, within the framework of SEM, it represents what is termed a *measurement model*.

The Full Latent Variable Model Meas. and Struct.

In contrast to the factor analytic model, the full latent variable model allows for the specification of regression structure among the latent variables. That is, the researcher can hypothesize the impact of one latent construct on another in the modeling of causal direction. This model is termed *full* (or *complete*) because it comprises both a measurement model and a structural model: the measurement model depicts the links between the latent variables and their observed measures (i.e., the CFA model), and the structural model depicts the links among the latent variables themselves.

A full latent variable model that specifies direction of cause from one direction only is termed a *recursive model*; one that allows for reciprocal or feedback effects is termed a *nonrecursive model*. Only applications of recursive models are considered in this book.

General Purpose and Process of Statistical Modeling

Statistical models provide an efficient and convenient way to describe the latent structure underlying a set of observed variables. Expressed either diagrammatically, or mathematically via a set of equations, such models explain how the observed and latent variables are related to one another.

Typically, researchers postulate a statistical model based on their knowledge of the related theory, on empirical research in the area of study, or on some combination of both. Once the model is specified, the researcher then tests its plausibility based on sample data that comprise all observed variables in the model. The primary task in this model-testing procedure is to determine the goodness-of-fit between the hypothesized model and the sample data. As such, the researcher imposes the structure of the hypothesized model on the sample data and then tests how well the observed data fit this restricted structure. Because it is highly unlikely that a perfect fit will exist between the observed data and the hypothesized model, there is necessarily a differential between the two; this differential is termed the *residual*. The model-fitting process can therefore be summarized as follows:

$$\text{Data} = \text{Model} + \text{Residual}$$

where

Data represent score measurements related to the observed variables as derived from persons comprising the sample.

Model represents the hypothesized structure linking the observed variables to the latent variables and, in some models, linking particular latent variables to one another.

Residual represents the discrepancy between the hypothesized model and the observed data.

In summarizing the general strategic framework for testing structural equation models, Jöreskog (1993) distinguished among three scenarios that he termed *strictly confirmatory*, *alternative models*, and *model-generating*. In the strictly confirmatory scenario, the researcher postulates a single model based on theory, collects the appropriate data, and tests the fit of the hypothesized model to the sample data. From the results of this test, the researcher either rejects or fails to reject the model; no further modifications to the model are made. In the alternative models scenario, the researcher proposes several alternative (i.e., competing) models, all of which are grounded in theory. Following analysis of a single set of empirical data, the researcher selects one model as most appropriate in representing the sample data. Finally, the model generating scenario represents the case in which the researcher, having postulated and rejected a theoretically derived model on the basis of its poor fit to the sample data, proceeds in an exploratory (rather than confirmatory) manner to modify and reestimate the model. The primary focus in this instance is to locate the source of misfit in the model and to determine a model that better describes the sample data. Jöreskog (1993) notes that although respecification may be either theory- or data-driven, the ultimate objective is to find a model that is both substantively meaningful and statistically well fitting. He further posits that despite the fact that "a model is tested in each round, the whole approach is model generating, rather than model testing" (Jöreskog, 1993, p. 295).

Of course, even a cursory review of the empirical literature clearly shows the model generating scenario to be the most common of the three—and for good reason. Given the many costs associated with the collection of data, it would be a rare researcher indeed who could afford to terminate his or her research on the basis of a rejected hypothesized model! As a consequence, the strictly confirmatory scenario is not commonly found in practice. Although the alternative models approach to modeling has also been a relatively uncommon practice, at least two important papers on the topic (i.e., MacCallum, Roznowski, & Necowitz, 1992; and MacCallum, Wegener, Uchino, & Fabrigar, 1993) recently precipitated more activity with respect to this analytic strategy.

Statistical theory related to these model-fitting processes is found in (a) texts devoted to the topic of SEM (e.g., Bollen, 1989a; Kaplan, 2000; Kline, 1998; Loehlin, 1992; Long, 1983b; Maruyama, 1998; Raykov & Marcoulides, 2000; and Schumacker & Lomax, 1996); (b) edited books devoted to the topic (e.g., Bollen & Long, 1993; Hoyle, 1995a; Marcoulides & Moustaki, 2002; and Marcoulides & Schumacker, 1996); and (c) methodologically oriented journals (e.g., *British*

Journal of Mathematical and Statistical Psychology, Journal of Educational and Behavioral Statistics, Multivariate Behavioral Research, Psychological Methods, Psychometrika, Sociological Methodology, Sociological Methods & Research, and *Structural Equation Modeling: A Multidisciplinary Journal*).

THE GENERAL STRUCTURAL EQUATION MODEL

Symbol Notation

Structural equation models are schematically portrayed using particular configurations of four geometric symbols: a circle (or ellipse), a square (or rectangle), a single-headed arrow, and a double-headed arrow. By convention, circles (or ellipses, ⬭) represent unobserved latent factors; squares (or rectangles, ▭) represent observed variables; single-headed arrows (⟶) represent the impact of one variable on another; and double-headed arrows (⟷) represent covariances or correlations between pairs of variables. In building a model of a particular structure under study, researchers use these symbols within the framework of four basic configurations, each of which represents an important component in the analytic process. These configurations are briefly described as follows:

- ⬭⟶▭ • Path coefficient for regression of an observed variable onto an unobserved latent variable (or factor).
- ⬭⟶⬭ • Path coefficient for regression of one factor onto another factor.
- ⟶▭ • Measurement error associated with an observed variable.
- ⬂⬭ • Residual error in the prediction of an unobserved factor.

The Path Diagram

Schematic representations of models are termed *path diagrams* because they provide a visual portrayal of relations assumed to hold among the variables under study. Essentially, as discussed later, a path diagram depicting a particular SEM model is actually the graphical equivalent of its mathematical representation whereby a set of equations relates dependent variables to their explanatory variables. As a means of illustrating how the above four symbol configurations may represent a particular causal process let me now walk you through the simple model shown in Fig. 1.1.

In reviewing this model, we see that there are two *unobserved latent factors*—math self-concept (MSC) and math achievement (MATH)—and five *observed variables*—three are considered to measure MSC (SDQ5; SDQ11; SDQ18) and two to measure MATH (MATHGR; MATHACH). These five observed variables function as indicators of their respective underlying latent factors.

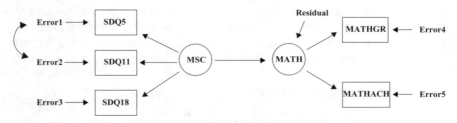

FIG. 1.1.   A general structural equation model.

Associated with each observed variable is an error term (Error1–Error5) and, with the factor being predicted (MATH), a residual term (*Residual*). There is an important distinction between these two error terms. Error associated with observed variables represents *measurement error* which reflects on their adequacy in measuring the related underlying factors (MSC; MATH). Measurement error derives from two sources: *random measurement error* (in the psychometric sense) and *error uniqueness*, a term used to describe error variance arising from some characteristic considered specific (or unique) to a particular indicator variable. Such error often represents nonrandom measurement error. Residual terms represent error in the prediction of dependent factors from independent factors. For example, the residual term shown in Fig. 1.1 represents error in the prediction of MATH (the dependent factor) from MSC (the independent factor).

In essence, both measurement and residual error terms represent unobserved variables. Thus, it would seem perfectly reasonable that, consistent with the representation of factors, they too could be modeled as ellipse (or circle) enclosures. In fact, this is the modeling approach implemented in at least one SEM program: AMOS (Arbuckle, 2003).

In addition to symbols that represent variables, certain others are used in path diagrams to denote hypothesized processes involving the entire system of variables. In particular, one-way arrows represent structural regression coefficients, thus indicating the impact of one variable on another. In Fig. 1.1, for example, the unidirectional arrow pointing toward the dependent factor, MATH, implies that the independent factor MSC "causes" math achievement (MATH).[2] Likewise, the three unidirectional arrows leading from MSC to each of the three observed variables (SDQ5, SDQ11, SDQ18) and those leading from MATH to each of its indicators (MATHGR and MATHACH) suggest that these score values are each

---

[2]In this book, a "cause" is a direct effect of a variable on another within the context of a complete model. Its magnitude and direction are given by the partial regression coefficient. If the complete model contains all relevant influences on a given dependent variable, its causal precursors are correctly specified. In practice, however, models may omit key predictors and may be misspecified so that it may be inadequate as a "causal model" in the philosophical sense.

influenced by their respective underlying factors. As such, these path coefficients represent the magnitude of expected change in the observed variables for every change in the related latent variable (or factor). It is important to note that, typically, these observed variables represent subscale scores (see, e.g., chaps. 11 and 12), item scores (see, e.g., chaps. 4, 5, 7, 9, 10, and 13), item pairs (see, e.g., chap. 3), and/or carefully selected item bundles (see, e.g., chaps. 6 and 8).

The one-way arrows pointing from the five error terms indicate the impact of measurement error (random and unique) on the observed variables and, from the residual, the impact of error in the prediction of MATH. Finally, as noted previously, curved two-way arrows represent covariances or correlations between pairs of variables. Thus, the bidirectional arrow linking Error1 and Error2, as shown in Fig. 1.1, implies that measurement error associated with SDQ5 correlates with that associated with SDQ11.

Structural Equations

As noted at the beginning of this chapter, in addition to lending themselves to pictorial description via a schematic presentation of the causal processes under study, structural equation models can also be represented by a series of regression (i.e., structural) equations. Because (a) regression equations represent the influence of one or more variables on another, and (b) this influence, conventionally in SEM, is symbolized by a single-headed arrow pointing from the variable of influence to the variable of interest, we can think of each equation as summarizing the impact of all relevant variables in the model (observed and unobserved) on one specific variable (observed or unobserved). Thus, one relatively simple approach to formulating these equations is to note each variable that has one or more arrows pointing toward it and then record the summation of all such influences for each of these dependent variables.

To illustrate this translation of regression processes into structural equations, let's turn again to Fig. 1.1. We can see that there are six variables with arrows pointing toward them; five represent observed variables (SDQ5, SDQ11, SDQ18; MATHGR, MATHACH) and one represents an unobserved variable (or factor; MATH). Thus, we know that the regression functions symbolized in the model shown in Fig. 1.1 can be summarized in terms of six separate equation-like representations of linear dependencies, as follows:

$$MATH = MSC + Residual$$
$$SDQ5 = MSC + Error1$$
$$SDQ11 = MSC + Error2$$
$$SDQ18 = MSC + Error3$$
$$MATHGR = MATH + Error4$$
$$MATHACH = MATH + Error5$$

Nonvisible Components of a Model   HELP

Although in principle there is a one-to-one correspondence between the schematic presentation of a model and its translation into a set of structural equations, neither one of these model representations tells the whole story. Some parameters critical to the estimation of the model are not explicitly shown and thus may not be obvious to the novice structural-equation modeler. For example, in both the path diagram and the previous equations, there is no indication that the variances of the independent variables are parameters in the model; indeed, such parameters are essential to all structural equation models.

Likewise, it is equally important to notice the specified nonexistence of certain parameters in a model. For example, in Fig. 1.1, there is no curved arrow between Error4 and Error5, which suggests the lack of covariance between the error terms associated with the observed variables MATHGR and MATHACH. Similarly, there is no hypothesized covariance between MSC and the residual. Absence of this path addresses the common and most often necessary assumption that the predictor (or independent) variable is in no way associated with any error arising from the prediction of the criterion (or dependent) variable.

Basic Composition

The general SEM model can be decomposed into two submodels: a measurement model and a structural model. The measurement model defines relations between the observed and unobserved variables. In other words, it provides the link between scores on a measuring instrument (i.e., the observed indicator variables) and the underlying constructs they are designed to measure (i.e., the unobserved latent variables). The measurement model, then, represents the CFA model described earlier in that it specifies the pattern by which each measure loads on a particular factor. In contrast, the structural model defines relations among the unobserved variables. Accordingly, it specifies the manner by which particular latent variables directly or indirectly influence (i.e., "cause") changes in the values of certain other latent variables in the model.

For didactic purposes in clarifying this important aspect of SEM composition, let's now examine Fig. 1.2, in which the same model presented in Fig. 1.1 has been demarcated into measurement and structural components.

Considered separately, the elements modeled within each rectangle in Fig. 1.2 represent two CFA models. The enclosure of the two factors within the ellipse represents a full latent variable model and thus would not be of interest in CFA research. The CFA model to the left of the diagram represents a one-factor model (MSC) measured by three observed variables (SDQ5 – SDQ18), whereas the CFA model on the right represents a one-factor model (MATH) measured by two observed variables (MATHGR–MATHACH). In both cases, the regression of the observed variables on each factor and the variances of both the factor and the

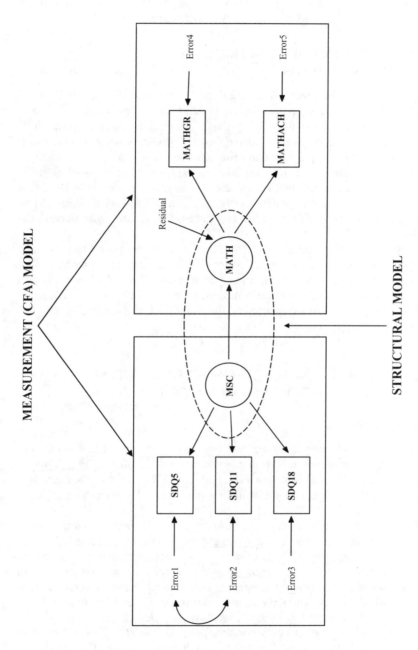

FIG. 1.2. A general structural equation model demarcated into measurement and structural components.

errors of measurement are of primary interest; the error covariance would be of interest only in analyses related to the CFA model bearing on MSC.

The Formulation of Covariance and Mean Structures

The core parameters in structural equation models that focus on the analysis of covariance structures are the regression coefficients and the variances and covariances of the independent variables. When the focus extends to the analysis of mean structures, the means and intercepts also become central parameters in the model. However, given that sample data comprise observed scores only, there needs to be an internal mechanism whereby the data are transposed into parameters of the model. This task is accomplished via a mathematical model representing the entire system of variables. Such representation systems can and do vary with each SEM computer program; the mechanism used by the EQS program is discussed in the next chapter.

As with any form of communication, one must first understand the language before being able to understand the message conveyed; so it is in comprehending the specification of SEM models. Now that you are familiar with the basic concepts underlying SEM, let's take a second look at the models just presented—albeit this time with the specifications recast within the framework and lexicon of the EQS program.

THE GENERAL EQS STRUCTURAL EQUATION MODEL

EQS Notation

EQS regards all variables as falling into one of two categories: measured (observed) variables or unmeasured (unobserved) variables. All measured variables are designated as V's and constitute the actual data of a study. All other variables are hypothetical and represent the structural network of the phenomenon under investigation.

Although conceptually unnecessary, it makes sense in practice to differentiate among the unmeasured variables: (a) the latent construct itself (regarded generally as a factor in EQS), designated as F; (b) a residual associated with the measurement of each observed variable (V), designated as E; and (c) a residual associated with the prediction of each factor, designated as D. Residual terms are often referred to as "disturbances," which is the terminology used in the EQS program. For consistency with EQS, the term *disturbance* is used in lieu of *residual* throughout the remainder of this book. Finally, for simplicity, all E's and D's are numbered to correspond with the V's and F's with which they are associated, respectively.

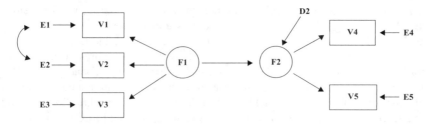

FIG. 1.3.   A general EQS structural equation model.

The EQS Path Diagram

To comprehend more fully how this labeling system works, let's turn to Fig. 1.3, which you will readily note is a replication of Fig. 1.1 albeit recast as an EQS–specified model. Given the detailed description of this path diagram presented earlier, no further explanation is provided here. Nonetheless, comments bearing on the number accompanying each labeled variable in the model are noteworthy. First, EQS automatically numbers each observed variable in accordance with its data-entry placement. As such, the first variable in the data set would be designated V1, the second V2, and so on. Second, the numeric value associated with each error (E) and disturbance (D) term is consistent with its related observed (V) and unobserved (F) variables, respectively. Thus, although there is only one disturbance term in this model, it is labeled D2 rather than D1.

The Bentler–Weeks Representation System

As discussed earlier, given that sample data constitute observed scores only, every SEM program requires some means of transposing these scores into parameters of the model. This is accomplished via a mathematical model representing the entire system of variables. In EQS, the mathematical model derives from the work of Bentler and Weeks (1979, 1980). (For a comparative review of the representation systems for EQS and LISREL; see, e.g., Bentler, 1988.)

The thrust of the Bentler–Weeks model is that all variables in a model can be categorized as either *dependent* or *independent* variables. Any variable that has a unidirectional arrow aimed at it represents a dependent variable; if there is no unidirectional arrow aimed at it, a variable is considered independent. As is customary, dependent variables are explained in terms of other variables in the model, whereas independent variables serve as the explanatory variables. Not so customary, however, is the Bentler–Weeks conceptualization of that which constitutes a dependent or independent variable. Indeed, their interpretation of this concept is much broader than is typical. According to Bentler and Weeks, any variable that is not a dependent variable is automatically considered an independent variable, regardless of whether it is an observed score, an unobserved factor, or a disturbance term. For example, in Fig. 1.3, the dependent variables are V_1, V_2, V_3, V_4, V_5, and F_2; the independent variables are E_1, E_2, E_3, E_4, E_5, F_1, and D_2.

A dependent variable, then, is any variable that can be expressed as a structural regression function of other variables. Thus, for every dependent variable, this regression function can be summarized in the form of an equation. As with the equations based on the variables shown in Fig. 1.1, each regression function modeled in Fig. 1.3 can be translated into equations specific to EQS. As will become evident in the applications illustrated later, these equations essentially serve to define the model for the program. The related equations are as follows:

$$F_2 = F_1 + D_2$$
$$V_1 = F_1 + E_1$$
$$V_2 = F_1 + E_2$$
$$V_3 = F_1 + E_3$$
$$V_4 = F_2 + E_4$$
$$V_5 = F_2 + E_5$$

It is clear that the one-way arrows linking the factors to the observed variables and Factor 1 to Factor 2 represent regression coefficients. However, explanation regarding the linkage of disturbance terms to their associated variables via one-way arrows may be somewhat less obvious. Although these arrows also symbolize regression coefficients, their paths are implicit in the prediction of one variable from another; they are considered to be known and are therefore fixed to 1.0. For example, in the language of simple regression, the prediction of V_1 from F_1 can be written as $V_1 = b_{11}F_1 + E_1$, where b_{11} represents the unknown beta weight associated with the predictor F_1 and E_1 represents error in this prediction. Note that there is no beta weight associated with the error term, thereby indicating that it is not to be estimated. By implication then, the beta weight for E_1 is considered known and fixed arbitrarily to 1.0.[3] Similarly, the prediction of F_2 from F_1 can be written as $F_2 = b_{12}F_1 + D_2$, where D_2 represents error in the prediction—albeit this prediction involves the prediction of one factor from another—whereas the former prediction equation involved the prediction of an observed variable from a factor (hence, the distinction between the terms E and D).

Finally, an important corollary of the Bentler–Weeks model is that the variances of dependent variables or their covariances with other variables are never parameters of the model; rather, they remain to be explained by those parameters.

---

[3] If, on the other hand, it were of interest to estimate the regression path, this can certainly be done. However, in this case, the variance of E_1 would need to be fixed to 1.0 because both the regression coefficient and the variance cannot be estimated simultaneously. This fact is linked to the concept of model identification, which is addressed in chapter 2.

In contrast, the variances and covariances of independent variables are important parameters that need to be estimated.

In this chapter, I have presented you with a few of the basic concepts associated with SEM and with a general overview of model specification within the framework of EQS. In chapter 2, however, I provide you with substantially greater detail regarding the specification of models within the context of the manual, interactive, and graphical choices available in the EQS program. Throughout the chapter, I show you how to use the DIAGRAMMER feature in building models, review many of the drop-down menus, and detail specified and illustrated components of three basic SEM models. As you work your way through the applications included in this book, you will become increasingly more confident in both your understanding of SEM and in using the EQS program—and I know that you will absolutely love what the much-improved DIAGRAMMER feature can do! So, let's move on to chapter 2 and a more comprehensive look at SEM modeling with EQS 6.1.

2

Using the EQS Program

Now that the basic EQS notation is understood, it's time to see (a) how these symbols can be linked together to form admissible program statements and paragraphs used in the building of an SEM input file, and (b) how to execute these input files so that the model specified can be tested. My primary aim here is to present a multi-faceted albeit thorough overview of these program capabilities; consequently, this chapter is necessarily extensive. However, after working, through this material, I am hopeful that you will have a better "feel" for the program and a substantially better appreciation of the rich bank of model-building and model-testing resources that await you in using EQS.

We begin this guided tour of EQS programming by first inspecting all required and most optional components of the input file. For a more comprehensive view of how these components blend together, I then review their application with respect to three different models (i.e., first-order CFA, second-order CFA, and full SEM). Along the way, I introduce you to the important concept of model (or statistical) identification. At the next stop in our tour, the question of how to create an EQS input file is addressed. Here, I present you with three different approaches to the task—manual; interactive, using the BUILD_EQS option; and graphic, using the DIAGRAMMER option. Based on the same three models demonstrated at the previous stop, I walk you through the building process as it relates to both the interactive and graphic methods. Continuing on to the next stop on the tour, we visit the output section of this process. Here, a brief albeit general overview of

EQS output resulting from an executed input file is presented. Finally, at the last stop on the tour, I present you with a summary of possible error messages that can occur when using the EQS program.

COMPONENTS OF THE EQS INPUT FILE

An EQS input file describes the model under study. It is composed of several statements clustered within paragraphs according to certain rules. In this subsection, we look at the basic dicta governing the construction of EQS input files, then examine the basic components of an EQS input file, and, finally, review three methods to formulate and execute EQS input files related to three different SEM models.

Basic Rules and Caveats in Creating EQS Input Files

Keywords

As in most computer programs, EQS uses a system of keywords that are interpreted by the program as basic commands. Primary key words in EQS are the names used to identify particular paragraphs comprising the input file (e.g., the /SPECIFICATIONS paragraph). Secondary keywords represent each statement within a paragraph; they operate as subcommands. As such, they refer to one particular aspect of the paragraph, thereby allowing the user to choose one of several options pertinent to this component. For example, one aspect of the /SPECIFICATIONS paragraph involves the method of estimation. Of the available choices, the user may wish to employ generalized least squares estimation, which would be stated as ME=GLS, where ME is the abbreviated form of the keyword METHOD, a subcommand indicating the method of estimation to be used, and GLS is the three-letter keyword indicating that generalized least squares is the estimation method to be used.

Two major rules govern the use of paragraph keywords: (a) they must always be preceded by a slash (e.g., /SPECIFICATIONS), and (b) the line in which the keyword appears must contain no other input information. One optional use of paragraph keywords is that they may be abbreviated to the first three characters (e.g., /SPE). However, the user may prefer more than three letters because it results in a more meaningful keyword, and this choice is quite acceptable. For example, abbreviating /SPECIFICATIONS to /SPEC appears to be a better choice.

Descriptive Statements

All information describing the model and data must be expressed as specific statements written within the appropriate paragraph. A semicolon (;) must separate each statement. Although not necessary, it is often helpful to construct input files in such a way that renders them easy to read. One way to do this is to start paragraph keywords in column 1, with all other statements within the paragraph indented a few characters. Finally, all input statements should be specified in no more than 80 columns per line.

At times, you may wish to insert a reminder comment in the input file regarding some aspect of the data or analysis. EQS allows you to include such in-line comments in any line of the input file by means of an exclamation mark (!), which must precede the comment. The program then ignores all material to the right of the exclamation symbol.

File Editors

For EQS to run, the input file must be a plain file that contains no hidden control characters. Because most word processors (e.g., Word™, Wordperfect™) use such symbols in the formulation of text, the invisible characters must first be stripped before they can be read by EQS. However, this constraint is easily addressed by saving the input file in ASCII format, which can be read by EQS.

Data Input

Data in the form of a covariance or correlation matrix can be embedded within the input file or reside in an external file. Raw data must always reside in a separate file. Specific details regarding the integration of data files with the EQS input file are addressed in the following subsection.

Basic Components of the EQS Input File

As discussed earlier, the basic structure of an EQS input file comprises a series of statements grouped within paragraphs, each of which is introduced by means of a keyword preceded by a slash. However, not all paragraphs are needed in any particular input file. At this time, important features related to six basic paragraphs are reviewed; other paragraphs are examined in subsequent chapters as they bear on particular model applications. For greater elaboration on each subsection, readers are referred to the manual (Bentler, 2005) or the user's guide (Bentler & Wu, 2002), both available via the Help window of the program.

/TITLE (Optional)

Although this paragraph is optional (i.e., not required to run an EQS job), it is not only highly recommended to use it but also that a generous amount of information is included in the title. Not uncommon is the situation in which what might have seemed obvious when the initial analysis of a model was conducted may not seem quite so obvious several months later when, for whatever reason, the user reexamines the data using the same input files. Liberal use of title information is particularly helpful when numerous EQS runs were implemented for a given data set. EQS allows as many lines as desired in this title section.

An example of a /TITLE paragraph is as follows:

> **/TITLE**
> CFA of BDI-French Version
> Initial Model

/SPECIFICATIONS (SPEC; Required)

This paragraph defines both the data to be analyzed and the method of analysis to be used. In particular, it details (a) information related to the data (location, matrix form); (b) the number of cases and input variables; (c) the desired method of estimation; and (c) other information that may be needed to guide the EQS run.

There are three important factors with respect to the /SPEC paragraph: (1) although input information can be placed in any order, a semicolon must delineate each operand; (2) information related to sample size and number of variables must always be provided; and (3) subcommand keywords can be abbreviated to three- and two-letter format. We now take a general look at a few aspects of this paragraph.

Data (DA).   Use of this keyword is governed by two conditions: (1) the data to be analyzed exists in some external file, and (2) the computing environment involves an interactive system. As such, the statement would read DA = 'C:\EQS61\Files\FRBDI.dat';, where C:EQS61\Files represents the location of the data and FRBDI.dat represents the name of the data file, both of which are enclosed within single quotes. As explained earlier, these data can be in raw, correlation, or covariance matrix form.

Variables (VAR).   The number stated here should represent the total number of variables in the data set; it does not represent the number of variables to be analyzed in any specific EQS run. The program automatically sorts out which variables to include in the analyses by its subsequent reading of the /EQUATIONS and /VARIANCES paragraphs.

Cases (CAS).   This term defines the number of subjects comprising the sample data. The number should represent all cases regardless of any that may be deleted later. Such deletions, as specified by the user and considered by EQS in the analytic procedures, never actually alter the original data set; thus, the number of cases always stays the same. If the input data are in the form of a correlation or covariance matrix, it is critical that the number of cases be correct because EQS has no way of checking its accuracy; an incorrect number will lead to incorrect statistics. However, if the input data comprise raw scores, this number does not need to be specific; EQS automatically tallies the number of cases in the file, which is used in all computations. Any discrepancy between the specified and actual number of cases is noted in the output.

Method (ME).   The EQS user can now select from nine methods of estimation: maximum likelihood (ML), least squares (LS), generalized least squares (GLS), elliptical LS (ELS), elliptical GLS (EGLS), elliptical reweighted LS (ERLS), heterogeneous kurtosis GLS (HKGLS), heterogeneous kurtosis RLS (HKRLS), and arbitrary distribution GLS (AGLS). If no method is specified, the program automatically uses ML estimation; in other words, ML represents the default method. For details related to these estimation methods, see the manual (Bentler, 2005).

A special feature of the EQS program is that it also allows for the specification of several estimation methods in a single job submission (e.g., ME=ML, AGLS;). A maximum of two methods can be specified when AGLS is included and a maximum of three methods otherwise. The elliptical and arbitrary distribution methods are always automatically preceded by their normal theory counterparts. More specifically, the ELS, EGLS, and ERLS methods are preceded by the normal theory methods of LS, GLS, and ML, respectively; AGLS is preceded by LS. Nonetheless, the user can override these default prior methods by simply specifying another valid method. (For more details regarding both the specification and appropriate use of these methods, see Bentler, 2005).

Finally, an extremely valuable feature unique to the EQS program is the availability of robust statistics associated with any selected method of estimation except AGLS. For example, by specifying ME=ML,ROBUST, the output provides a robust chi square statistic (χ^2) called the Satorra–Bentler scaled statistic (S-Bχ^2; Satorra & Bentler, 1988, 1994) and robust standard errors (Bentler & Dijkstra, 1985), both of which have been corrected for non-normality in large samples. The S-Bχ^2 has been shown to more closely approximate χ^2 than the usual test statistic and the robust standard errors to be correct in large samples despite the fact that the distributional assumptions regarding the variables are wrong (Bentler, 2005). Although these robust statistics are computationally demanding, they have been shown to perform better than uncorrected statistics where the assumption of normality fails to hold and better than asymptotic distribution-free GLS (AGLS) in all but the largest samples (Chou, Bentler, & Satorra, 1991; Hu, Bentler, & Kano, 1992). One important caveat regarding the use of robust statistics, however, is that they can be computed only from raw data.

Analysis (ANAL).   This keyword describes the type of matrix to be analyzed if it is something other than a covariance matrix, which is default. If the analyses are to be based on the covariance matrix but the data were input as a correlation matrix, then the standard deviations must be added to the input. This is accomplished by providing a separate paragraph introduced with the keyword /STANDARD DEVIATIONS (or /STA) and then listing the standard deviations on the next line, leaving one blank between each; more than one line can be used if necessary. Three instructions must be remembered when using the /STA paragraph: (1) there must be exactly the same number of standard deviations as there are variables in the correlation matrix being read, (2) the standard deviations must be in the same order as the variables in the input matrix, and (3) no semicolon is used to end this input section.

Matrix (MA). This keyword describes the form of the input data—that is, whether it is a correlation, covariance, or raw data matrix. As noted earlier, raw data are always presumed to reside in an external file; covariance or correlation data matrices can either be embedded within the input file (i.e., as an internal file) or reside in a separate (external) file. When covariance (or correlation) matrices reside as an internal file, the data are specified within a separate paragraph, labeled /MATRIX (MAT). If, on the other hand, they reside in an external file, their location is noted via the DATA (DA) keyword. Once EQS has located the data file, it then needs to know how to read the data. If the data are in free format, which is default, EQS can read the file as long as each element in the matrix is separated by at least one blank space. If the data are not in free format, this information is provided by means of a Fortran statement, which must be immediately preceded by the FORMAT (FO) keyword. Finally, if the user wishes the analysis to not be based on the covariance matrix (which is default), the matrix to be analyzed must be noted using the ANALYSIS (ANAL) keyword.

Now, let's pull this all together and look at two specification paragraphs describing an input data matrix.

(i) The data matrix as an internal file:

```
/SPECIFICATIONS
  CASE=250; VAR=4; ME=ML; MA=COR;
/MATRIX
  1.00
   .34 1.00
   .55  .27 1.00
   .48  .33  .63 1.00
/STANDARD DEVIATIONS
  1.09  .59  .98 1.10
```

NOTE:
- The input of data never requires a semicolon. Thus, there is no ";" in the /MATRIX and /STANDARD DEVIATIONS paragraphs.
- Although the input data are in correlation matrix form, specification of the standard deviations enables analyses to be based on the covariance matrix.

(ii) The data matrix as an external file:

```
/SPECIFICATIONS
   CASE=250; VAR=4; ME=ML, ROBUST; MA=COV;
   DA='C:\EQS61\Files\FRBDI.dat'; FO=(4F2.0);
```

In addition to the subcommands of the /SPEC paragraph shown here, others are either optional or used with particular applications. Because many such applications are described in this book, they are not discussed until their appearance in subsequent chapters.

/LABELS (Optional)

This paragraph can be used to identify the names of observed (V's) and/or latent (F's) variables in the model. Labels may be one to eight characters in length and are assigned to only V- and F-type variables. Observed variables should be numbered according to their position in the data set. Thus, the specification that V5 = MATH indicates that the fifth variable in the data matrix is to be labeled "MATH." Although the numbering of latent variables is arbitrary, it should be logically sequenced within the context of the model.

Because EQS automatically assigns V1 to the first observed variable, V2 to the second variable, and so on, these designations are used as labels if the user does not provide names for the variables; likewise the latent variables are automatically assigned the labels F1, F2, and so forth. If the user provides labels for only some of the variables, these names override the default labels (e.g., V1).

/EQUATIONS (EQU; Required)[1]

This keyword signals specification information regarding the model under study. Specifically, the paragraph defines every regression path in the model. By means of a series of equation statements, the /EQU paragraph specifies all linkages among the independent and dependent variables, as well as among dependent and dependent variables, and identifies those parameters to be constrained (i.e., to zero, 1.0, or some other value) and those to be freely estimated.

Before completing this part of the input file, it is critical to construct a path diagram of your model in which (a) all observed and latent variables are clearly labeled; (b) all structural regression paths are specified; (c) all error and disturbance terms are specified, along with their related regression paths; (d) all hypothesized

---

[1]With EQS, there is now a newly established /MODEL paragraph that allows the user to express model specifications in a more simplified and concise manner. In addition, the E and D variables are generated automatically by the program. When this paragraph is used, it replaces the /EQU keyword as well as the /VAR and /COV keywords.

covariances (among independent variables) are specified; and (e) all parameters to be estimated (including factor variances) are identified by means of an asterisk. Once you have this visual representation of your model, it is easy to complete all equations in the /EQU paragraph by simply reading off the path diagram.

How to Write Equations. As noted in chapter 1, the completion of these equations is carried out as follows. For each *dependent* variable (i.e., any variable having an arrow pointing toward it), write one equation summarizing the direct impact on it from other variables in the model. Thus, there will always be as many equations in the /EQUATIONS paragraph as there are dependent variables in the model being tested. The dependent variable will always be on the left-hand side of the equation, with all *independent* (i.e., explanatory) variables appearing on the right. (Recall from Chap. 1 that in EQS, the terms *dependent* and *independent* variables are defined within the context of the Bentler–Weeks model.) Finally, once the equations have been formed, be sure to insert asterisks next to all parameters to be estimated. EQS provides estimates for only the asterisked parameters; all others are regarded as fixed.

The Use of Start Values. Start values refer to the point at which a program begins an iterative process to establish parameter estimates. Users can either allow the program to supply these values (EQS uses default values such as 0.0 for covariances) or provide their own values. User-provided start values represent a "best guess" of what the expected value of a particular parameter estimate will be. These best-guess values are included in the equation, acting as modifiers of the parameters to be estimated; they always precede the asterisk.

Although start values need not be specified for most EQS jobs, they often facilitate the iterative process when complex models are under study; such models can generate problems of nonconvergence if the start values provided by EQS are inadequate. However, for the EQS user, the problem of trying to determine appropriate start values is gone forever as a result of an ingenious feature called the RETEST option, which automatically generates these start values and then allows the user to edit the input file accordingly. This unique time-saving tool is demonstrated in chapter 6. (For a more extensive discussion of start values, see Bollen, 1989a.)

Now, let's examine a few /Equations paragraphs.

(i) Equations without start values:

> **/EQUATIONS**
> $V1 = F1 + E1$;
> $F3 = {}^*F1 + {}^*F2 + D3$;

(ii) Equations with start values:

> **/EQUATIONS**
> V1 = .9 F1 + E1;
> F3 = .6 *F1 + −.2*F2 + D3;

NOTE:
- The start value associated with F1 is fixed at .9 by choice.
- The start values associated with E1 and D3 have no value specified; these parameters are considered to be known and are fixed to 1.00 by program default. (A more detailed explanation of this phenomenon is provided later.)

/VARIANCES (VAR; Required)

This paragraph specifies the status of variances related to independent variables in the model. As such, each variance must be identified either as a fixed parameter in the model or as one to be freely estimated. (Recall that variances for dependent variables are never specified, regardless of whether they are fixed or free.) As in the /EQUATIONS paragraph, variances to be estimated are identified with an asterisk. Although further elaboration of this paragraph is provided later in this chapter, let's look at a couple of examples of the /VAR paragraph.

(i) Variances without start values:

> **/VARIANCES**
> F1, F2 = *;
> F1 to F3 = *;
> F4-F6 = *;

NOTE:
- Consecutive lists of variables can be specified using either "to" or a dash. As such, F1 to F3 indicates that the variances of F1, F2, and F3 are to be estimated. Likewise, F4, through F6 specifies that the variances of F4, F5, and F6 are to be estimated.
- Variable labels (as defined in the /LABEL paragraph) can be used in lieu of the V- or F-labels. However, because labels with fewer than eight characters can cause an error, it is recommended that, in this case, the hyphen be used rather than the "to" convention.

(ii) Variances with start values:

> **/VARIANCES**
> F1,F2 = .3*;
> F1 to F3 = .4*;
> F4-F6 = .6*;

/COVARIANCES (COV; Optional)

For obvious reasons, this paragraph is necessary only when covariances are specified in the model. As such, it is used to specify both fixed nonzero and free covariances among the independent variables. However, any variable involved in a covariance must also have its variance specified in the /VAR paragraph; consequently, covariances also cannot be specified for dependent variables.[2] In specifying a covariance, the pair of variables is stated and separated by a comma, as exemplified in the following:

> **/COVARIANCES**
> E1,E3 = *;
> F1 to F3 = *;
> F4-F6 = *;

NOTE:
- Use of "to" and "-" indicate that the covariances related to all possible pairs of variables are to be estimated. For example, the specification of "F1 to F3 = *;" indicates that estimated parameters are F1,F2; F1,F3; F2,F3.

The final paragraph in all EQS input files must be /END. This keyword marks the termination of program input.

Input File Examples

To provide a more comprehensive view of how the various sections of the EQS input file relate to the path diagram of a particular model, we now review three simple albeit different models: (a) a first-order CFA model (Fig. 2.1), (b) a second-order CFA model (Fig. 2.2), and (c) a full SEM model (Fig. 2.3). However, due to space limitations, a complete input file is shown only for Fig. 2.1; the /SPECIFICATIONS and /LABELS paragraphs are absent for the two remaining models. Although

---

[2]If a user wishes to have two dependent variables covary, one option is to specify a covariance between their disturbance terms because these residuals are always independent variables in a model.

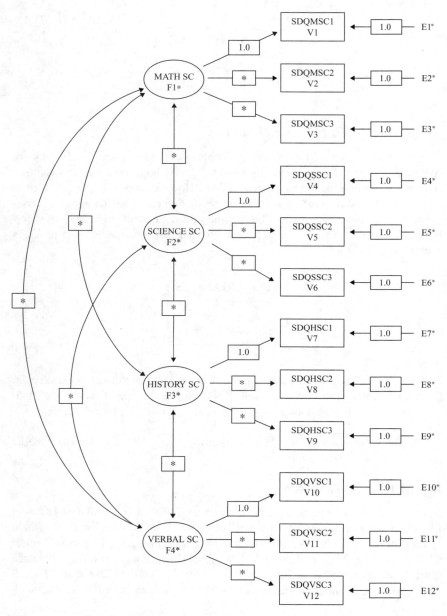

FIG. 2.1. Hypothesized first-order CFA model with EQS notation
and assigned start values.

portions of the same input files appear later in the chapter, they are presented in their original form as structured by the BUILD_EQS option. Thus, the files presented in this subsection provide an idea of how to make the file more concise if so desired. To derive maximum benefit from this subsection, study each figure while referring to its respective input statement.

First-Order CFA Model

```
/TITLE
  Example 1st-order CFA Input File (Figure 2.1)
  Initial Model
/SPECIFICATIONS
DA='C:\EQS61\FILES\CFASC.DAT'; FO=(12F1.0);
CASE=361; VAR=12; ME=ML; MA=RAW;
/LABELS
  V1=SDQMSC1;   V2=SDQMSC2;   V3=SDQMSC3;
  V4=SDQSSC1;   V5=SDQSSC2;   V6=SDQSSC3;
  V7=SDQHSC1;   V8=SDQHSC3;   V9=SDQHSC3;
  V10=SDQVSC1;  V11=SDQVSC2;  V12=SDQVSC3;
  F1=MSC;  F2=SSC;  F3=HSC;  F4=VSC;
/EQUATIONS
  V1 =  F1 + E1;
  V2 = *F1 + E2;
  V3 = *F1 + E3;
          V4 =  F2 + E4;
          V5 = *F2 + E5;
          V6 = *F2 + E6;
                  V7 =  F3 + E7;
                  V8 = *F3 + E8;
                  V9 = *F3 + E9;
                          V10 =  F4 + E10;
                          V11 = *F4 + E11;
                          V12 = *F4 + E12;
/VARIANCES
  F1 to F4 = *;
  E1 to E12 = *;
/COVARIANCES
  F1 to F4 = *;
/END
```

Although this input file appears to be fairly straightforward, three features are worthy of elaboration. First, the "to" convention has been used in both the /VARIANCES and /COVARIANCES paragraphs, thereby indicating that the variances of all the independent variables (F1-F4) are to be freely estimated as well as their covariances. Second, recall that an independent variable can have either its path or its variance estimated but not both. Thus, because we are only interested in the variances of the error terms, note that in the /EQUATIONS paragraph, their related beta weights are automatically assigned by the program a fixed value of 1.0. Although these values are not shown in the input file (see E1-E12), they are visible in Fig. 2.1. Finally, note that the first measurement indicator for each factor (V1, V4, V7, V10) has been specified as fixed (i.e., there is no asterisk next to these parameters). As shown in Fig. 2.1, these parameters are constrained to equal a value of 1.0; EQS automatically assigns this value to these fixed parameters—thus, the value of 1.0 does not appear in the input file. Two points need to be made in this regard: (a) the value assigned to these parameters need not be 1.0—although any numeric may be assigned to these parameters, a value of 1.0 has typically been the assignment of choice; and (b) the constrained parameter need not be limited to the first indicator variable; any one of a congeneric set[3] of parameters may be chosen. Beyond these technical notations, however, the most important point regarding the fixed factor loadings is that they address the issue of *model identification* (also termed *statistical identification*), a topic to which we turn shortly.

Critical to knowing whether a model is statistically identified is understanding the number of estimable parameters in the model. Thus, one extremely important caveat in working with structural equation models is to always tally the number of freely estimated parameters prior to running the analyses. As a prerequisite to the discussion of model identification, then, let's count the number of parameters to be estimated for the model portrayed in Fig. 2.1. Reviewing the figure, we ascertain that there are 12 regression coefficients (factor loadings) and 16 variances (12 error variances, 4 factor variances), and 6 factor covariances. The 1's assigned to one of each set of regression-path parameters represent a fixed value of 1.00; as such, these parameters are *not* to be estimated. In total, then, there are 30 parameters to be estimated for the CFA model depicted in Fig. 2.1. A brief discussion of the important concept of model identification follows.

The Concept of Model Identification. Model identification is a complex topic that is difficult to explain in nontechnical terms. Although a thorough

---

[3] A set of measures is said to be "congeneric" if each measure in the set purports to assess the same construct, except for errors of measurement (Jöreskog, 1971a). For example, as shown in Fig. 2.1, SDQMSC1, SDQMSC2, and SDQMSC3 all serve as measures of math SC (self-concept); therefore, they represent a congeneric set of indicator variables.

explanation of the identification principle exceeds the scope of this book, it is not critical to the reader's understanding and use of the book. Nonetheless, because some insight into the general concept of the identification issue undoubtedly helps to better understand why, for example, particular parameters are specified as having certain fixed values, what follows is a brief nonmathematical explanation of the basic idea underlying this concept. Essentially, only the so-called "t-rule" is addressed, one of several tests associated with identification. The reader is encouraged to consult the following texts for a more comprehensive treatment of the topic: Bollen, 1989a; Kline, 1998; Long, 1983a, 1983b; and Saris & Stronkhorst, 1984. I also recommend a clear and readable description of this topic in a book chapter by MacCallum (1995).

In broad terms, the issue of identification focuses on whether there is a unique set of parameters consistent with the data. This question bears directly on the transposition of the variance–covariance matrix of observed variables (the data) into the structural parameters of the model under study. If a unique solution for the values of the structural parameters can be found, the model is considered identified. As a consequence, the parameters are considered estimable and the model therefore testable. On the other hand if a model cannot be identified, it indicates that the parameters are subject to arbitrariness, thereby implying that different parameter values define the same model. Such being the case, attainment of consistent estimates for all parameters is not possible and, thus, the model cannot be evaluated empirically. By way of a simple example, the process would be conceptually akin to trying to determine unique values for X and Y when the only information available is that $X + Y = 15$. Generalizing this example to covariance-structure analysis, the model identification issue focuses on the extent to which a unique set of values can be inferred for the unknown parameters from a given covariance matrix of analyzed variables reproduced by the model.

Structural models may be *just-identified*, *overidentified*, or *underidentified*. A just-identified model is one in which there is a one-to-one correspondence between the data and the structural parameters. That is, the number of data variances and covariances equals the number of parameters to be estimated. However, despite the capability of the model to yield a unique solution for all parameters, the just-identified model is not scientifically interesting because it has no degrees of freedom and therefore can never be rejected. An overidentified model is one in which the number of estimable parameters is less than the number of data points (i.e., variances and covariances of the observed variables). This situation results in positive degrees of freedom that allow for rejection of the model, thereby rendering it of scientific use. The aim in SEM is to specify a model such that it meets the criterion of overidentification. Finally, an underidentified model is one in which the number of parameters to be estimated exceeds the number of variances and covariances (i.e., data points). As such, the model contains insufficient information (from the input data) to attain a determinate solution of parameter estimation; that is, an infinite number of solutions are possible for an underidentified model.

Reviewing the CFA model in Fig. 2.1, let's determine how many data points there are to work with (i.e., How much information do we have with respect to our data?). As noted previously, these data points constitute the variances and covariances of the observed variables; with p variables, there are $p(p + 1)/2$ such elements. Given that there are 12 observed variables, this means there are $12(12 + 1)/2 = 78$ data points. Before this discussion of identification, we determined a total of 30 unknown parameters. Thus, with 78 data points and 30 parameters to be estimated, we have an overidentified model with 48 degrees of freedom.

However, it is important to note that the specification of an overidentified model is a necessary but not sufficient condition to resolve the identification problem. Indeed, the imposition of constraints on particular parameters can sometimes be beneficial in helping the researcher to attain an overidentified model. Examples of such a constraint are illustrated in chapters 5 and 10 with the application of a second-order CFA model.

Linked to the issue of identification is the requirement that every latent variable must have its scale determined. This requirement arises because latent variables are unobserved and, therefore, have no definite metric scale. This requirement can be accomplished in one of two ways. The first approach is tied to specification of the measurement model, whereby the unmeasured latent variable is mapped onto its related observed indicator variable. This scaling requisite is satisfied by constraining to some nonzero value (typically 1.0), one factor loading parameter in each congeneric set of loadings. This constraint holds for both independent and dependent latent variables. In reviewing Fig. 2.1, this means that for one of the three regression paths leading from each self-concept (SC) factor to a set of observed indicators, some fixed value should be specified; this fixed parameter is termed a *reference* variable. With respect to the model in Fig. 2.1, for example, the scale was established by constraining to a value of 1.0, the first parameter in each set of observed variables.

With a better idea of important aspects of the specification of a CFA model in general, specification using the EQS program in particular, and the basic notions associated with model identification, we continue on our walk-through of the two remaining models reviewed in this chapter.

Second-Order CFA Model

```
/TITLE
  Example 2nd-order CFA Input File (Figure 2.2)
  Initial Model
      ⋮
      ▾
/EQUATIONS
  V1 =  F1 + E1;
  V2 = *F1 + E2;
  V3 = *F1 + E3;
              V4 =  F2 + E4;
              V5 = *F2 + E5;
              V6 = *F2 + E6;
                      V7 =  F3 + E7;
                      V8 = *F3 + E8;
                      V9 = *F3 + E9;
                              V10 =  F4 + E10;
                              V11 = *F4 + E11;
                              V12 = *F4 + E12;
  F1 = *F5 + D1;
   F2 = *F5 + D2;
    F3 = *F5 + D3;
     F4 = *F5 + D4;
/VARIANCES
  F5 = 1.0;
  D1 to D4 = *;
  E1 to E12 = *;
/END
```

This model supports the notion that math, science, history, and verbal self-concepts (SCs) are caused by some higher order global academic self-concept construct. Thus, although the first-order structure of this model remains basically the same as in Fig. 2.1, four important features must be noted. First, in contrast to the first-order CFA example in which all equations in the /EQUATIONS paragraph represented regression paths among all observed variables and their related underlying factors, the equations specified for this second-order model also include regression paths among factors. Specifically, these parameters represent the impact of F5 (an independent variable) on F1, F2, F3, and F4. Second, because the estimation of all higher order factor loadings are typically of interest in second-order models, the variance of the single higher order factor, F5, has been constrained to 1.0, as specified in the /VARIANCES paragraph.[4] This constraint, of course, addresses

[4]Alternatively, if the variance of F5 had been of interest, one of the higher order loadings would have to be constrained to 1.0 (or another nonzero value).

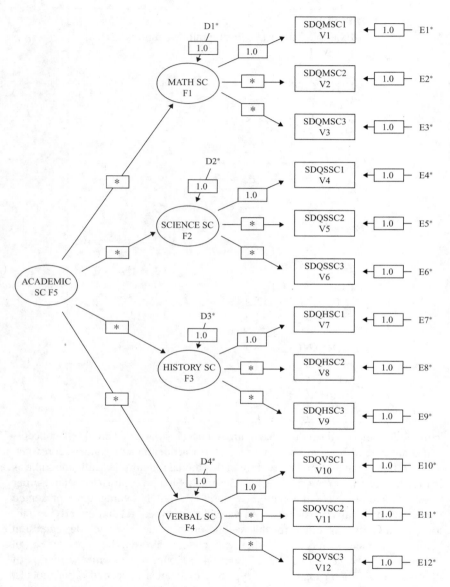

FIG. 2.2. Hypothesized second-order CFA model with EQS notation and assigned start values.

the issue of model identification discussed earlier. Third, given that academic SC is hypothesized to cause each of the four first-order factors, F1 through F4 now represent dependent variables in the Bentler–Weeks sense. As such, math, science, history, and verbal SCs are hypothesized as being predicted from academic SC but with some degree of error, which is captured by the disturbance term associated with each of these factors. Thus, in the /VARIANCES paragraph, note also that the variances of the disturbances (the D's) are designated as freely estimated. Relatedly, their paths are automatically constrained to 1.0 by the program, as shown in Fig. 2.2. Finally, in second-order models, any covariance among the first-order factors is presumed to be explained by the higher order factor(s). Accordingly, note the absence of double-headed arrows linking the four first-order factors in the path diagram and the absence of a /COVARIANCES paragraph in the input file.

Full Structural Equation Model

```
/TITLE
  Example Full SEM Input File (Figure 2.3)
  Initial Model
        ⋮
        ▼
/EQUATIONS
  V1 =  F1 + E1;
  V2 = *F1 + E2;
  V3 = *F1 + E3;
            V4 =  F2 + E4;
            V5 = *F2 + E5;
            V6 = *F2 + E6;
                      V7 =  F3 + E7;
                      V8 = *F3 + E8;
                      V9 = *F3 + E9;
                                V10 =  F4 + E10;
                                V11 = *F4 + E11;
  F3 = *F1 + *F2 + D3;
  F4 = *F3 + D4;
/VARIANCES
  F1 = *; F2 = *;
  D3 = *; D4 = *;
  E1 to E11 = *;
/COVARIANCES
  F1, F2 = *;
/END
```

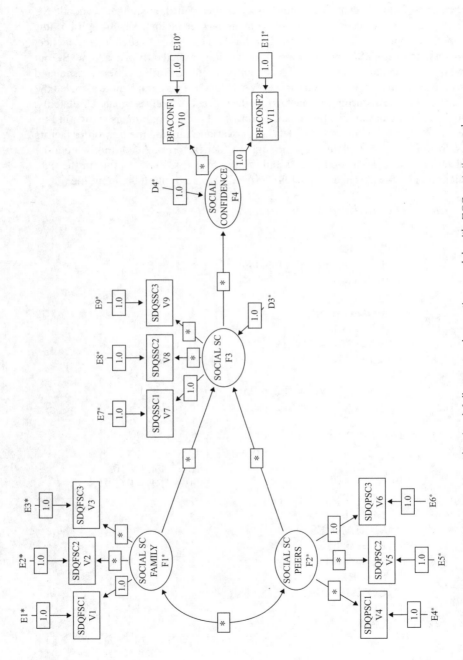

FIG. 2.3. Hypothesized full structural equation model with EQS notation and assigned start values.

36

In reviewing both the path diagram and the input file for this full SEM model, note three particular specifications. First, of the four factors composing this model, only F1 and F2 are independent variables (in the Bentler–Weeks sense); all others are dependent variables in the model. Consequently, only the variances for F1 and F2, as well as their covariances, can be estimated as specified in the input file. Second, as with the second-order model shown in Fig. 2.2, again, the regression equations involve sets of factors. In the present case, these equations are specified only for F3 and F4 because each is explained by other factors in the model. Third, given the dependent variable status of F3 and F4 in the model, note that the variance of neither is specified in the /VARIANCES paragraph; relatedly, note the specification of variances associated with their respective disturbances, D3 and D4, respectively. Finally, although Factor 3 appears to operate as both an independent and a dependent variable, this is not so. Once a variable is defined as a dependent variable in a model, it maintains that designation throughout all analyses bearing on the hypothesized model.

CREATING THE EQS INPUT FILE

With this understanding of the basic components of an EQS input file, let's proceed to the three methods used to build these files: (a) manually; (b) interactively, using the BUILD_EQS option; and (c) graphically, using the DIAGRAMMER option.

Building an Input File Manually

EQS input files can be structured manually using any word-processing program (e.g., Word™, Wordperfect™). However, because EQS files cannot interpret the hidden control-text characters inserted by these programs, any invisible symbols must be stripped from the file before an EQS run can be executed. This task is easily accomplished by saving the file in ASCII format.[5] Files created using the manual approach should be saved using the .eqs extension (e.g., bdigender.eqs). Indeed, this method was used in structuring the three input files presented previously. Although the manual approach has served us well over the past 30 years, as the modus operandi for building SEM input files, these last 10 years have rapidly catapulted us into a "New Age" of interactive computing. Keeping in sync with this important trend, EQS holds a unique position among SEM programs in that it offers users two state-of-the-art methods for building input files interactively. We now turn to these new program-building methods.

---

[5] Alternatively, use the BUILD_EQS command line editor to accomplish this task.

Building an Input File Interactively Using BUILD_EQS

When using the BUILD_EQS feature, a series of dialog boxes, each of which relates to a particular section of the input file, are presented. As each box appears, simply select from the options offered with respect to the hypothesized model. After completing each dialog box, the program automatically builds the EQS command language line by line, writing it onto the background window. Files written using BUILD_EQS are given an .eqx extension by default. Note that although the complete file is presented on screen, this .eqx window cannot be edited. Any modifications to the model must be made by either redoing the related dialog box or subsequently editing the related .eqs[6] input file.

Now, let me walk you through the building of an input file using BUILD_EQS. We start with the first-order CFA model shown in Fig. 2.1 and then move on to the models in Figs. 2.2 and 2.3. However, because most of the details remain basically the same for the latter two models, I necessarily limit the illustrations to only those capturing an important specification feature that differs from those related to Fig. 2.1.

First-Order CFA Model (see Fig. 2.1)

To initiate the BUILD_EQS process, first open a data file and then click on its related icon, which presents its drop-down menu. Fig. 2.4 identifies the icon and shows a portion of the open data file below it; Fig. 2.5 displays the drop-down menu in which only the Title/Specifications line is highlighted (all those remaining appear faded), indicating that it is the only active selection that can be made.[7] In essence, this limitation can be a blessing in disguise because it forces the user to assign a title to the input file, a task too often skipped when manually building files. Indeed, this entry can save valuable time later in the identification of particular job runs.

Displayed next is the dialog box triggered by selecting the TITLE/SPECIFICATIONS option (Fig. 2.6). The title at the top of the box is one entered as a replacement for the EQS default. Entries for the number of variables (12) and cases (361) were entered automatically by the program. Many options are offered in specifying a model; however, they are not explained in this

---

[6]Files with the .eqx extension (i.e., EQS model files) represent binary model files created by EQS (6.1) for use in Windows™ applications, whereas those with the .eqs extension (i.e., EQS command files) represent textual input files. In addition to being created manually, *.eqs files are created automatically by the program when a model file (*eqx) is executed.

[7]Although the selection Working Array is always active, it is unrelated to model specification. This option presents a dialog box in which the user can specify the amount of memory to be used.

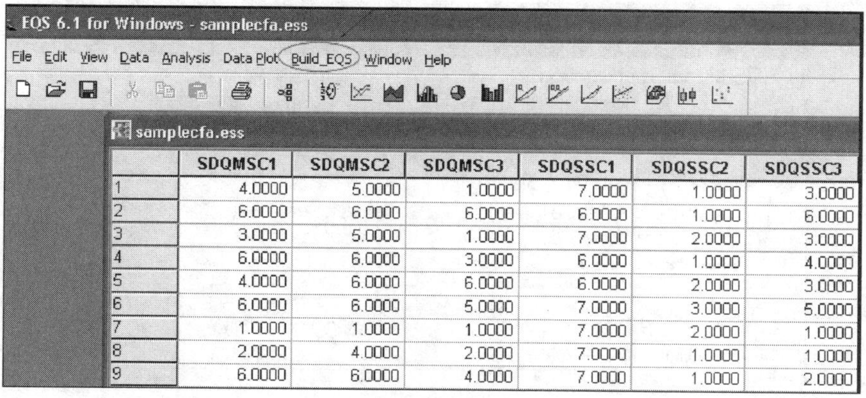

	SDQMSC1	SDQMSC2	SDQMSC3	SDQSSC1	SDQSSC2	SDQSSC3
1	4.0000	5.0000	1.0000	7.0000	1.0000	3.0000
2	6.0000	6.0000	6.0000	6.0000	1.0000	6.0000
3	3.0000	5.0000	1.0000	7.0000	2.0000	3.0000
4	6.0000	6.0000	3.0000	6.0000	1.0000	4.0000
5	4.0000	6.0000	6.0000	6.0000	2.0000	3.0000
6	6.0000	6.0000	5.0000	7.0000	3.0000	5.0000
7	1.0000	1.0000	1.0000	7.0000	2.0000	1.0000
8	2.0000	4.0000	2.0000	7.0000	1.0000	1.0000
9	6.0000	6.0000	4.0000	7.0000	1.0000	2.0000

FIG. 2.4. EQS icons displayed in the Windows™ toolbar with partial data matrix shown below.

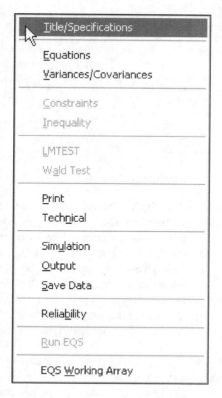

FIG. 2.5. Initial BUILD_EQS drop-down menu.

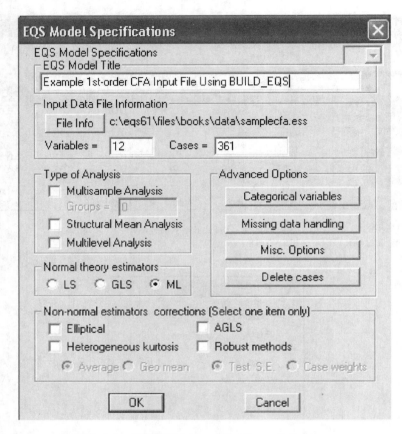

FIG. 2.6.   EQS model specifications dialog box.

introduction to the BUILD_EQS feature because they are addressed in conjunction
with particular applications throughout the book. The only additional information
of note is the selection of ML (maximum likelihood) as the normal theory estimator,
which is default and thus automatically pinpointed by EQS.

Clicking on "OK" for the Model Specification dialog box yields the partial input
file shown in Fig. 2.7. As you will readily see, this file has been completed as far
down as the /LABELS paragraph. The faded print results from a preselected light
blue color, automatically applied by the program to highlight keywords within
each paragraph; the paragraph keywords are highlighted in a contrasting shade of
blue.

To further complete the input file, click on the BUILD_EQS tab, which presents
the drop-down menu shown in Fig. 2.8. Click on the next option, which represents
the /EQUATIONS paragraph. Clicking on this option subsequently yields the dialog box shown in Fig. 2.9. In this Build Equations' box, the program has already

```
/TITLE
Example 1st-order CFA Input Using BUILD_EQS
/SPECIFICATIONS
DATA='c:\eqs61\files\books\data\samplecfa.ess';
VARIABLES=12; CASES=361;
METHOD=ML; ANALYSIS=COVARIANCE; MATRIX=RAW;
/LABELS
V1=SDQMSC1; V2=SDQMSC2; V3=SDQMSC3; V4=SDQSSC1; V5=SDQSSC2;
V6=SDQSSC3; V7=SDQHSC1; V8=SDQHSC2; V9=SDQHSC3; V10=SDQVSC1;
V11=SDQVSC2; V12=SDQVSC3;
/END
```

FIG. 2.7. Partial input file resulting from completion of model specifications dialog box.

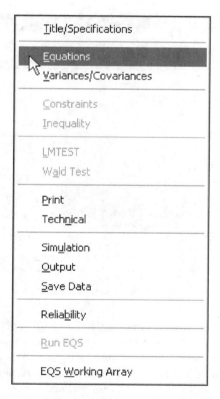

FIG. 2.8. Second (in series) BUILD_EQS drop-down menu.

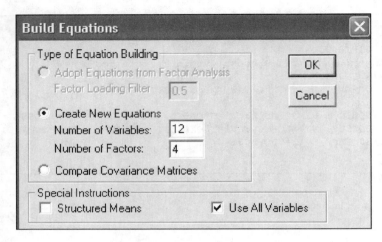

FIG. 2.9. Build equations dialog box.

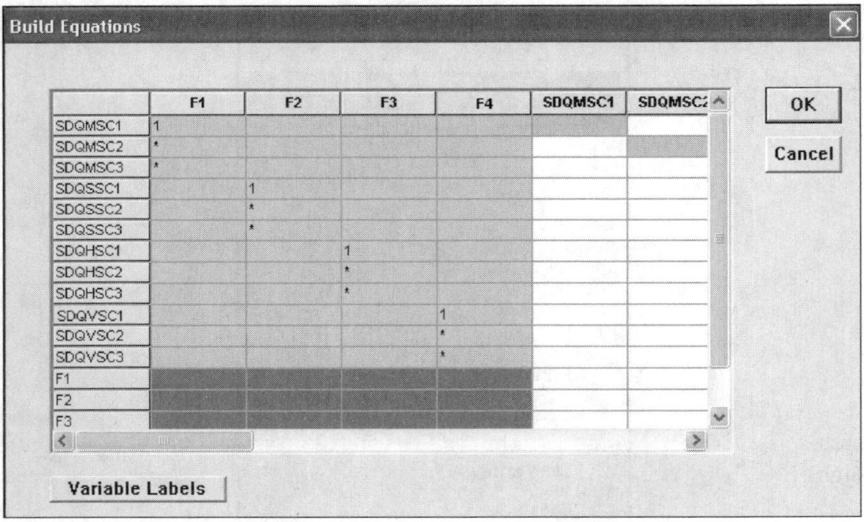

FIG. 2.10. Build equations dialog box.

included the number of variables and check-marked that all variables would be used in structuring the equations. The only manual input required is to identify the number of factors (i.e., four) on which the equations would be based.

Clicking "OK" yields the Build Equations dialog box shown in Fig. 2.10. To explain the varying levels of intensity in this printed version, the on-screen view yields a turquoise upper layer and a magenta lower layer. (F4 is hidden by the

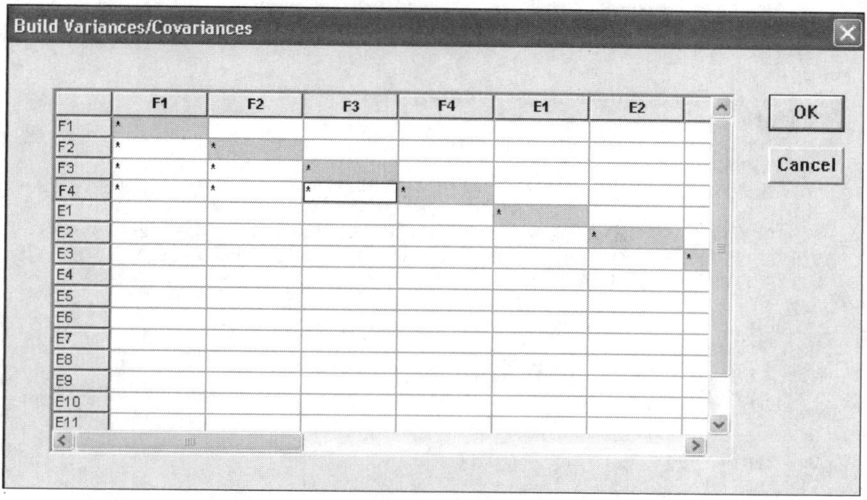

FIG. 2.11. Build variances/covariances dialog box.

slider bar at the bottom of the dialog box.) In this box, we simply identify how the observed variables load onto the four factors. This task is easily accomplished by clicking on the related slot; each click automatically produces an asterisk, thereby indicating that the parameter is to be estimated. For parameters constrained to 1.0 for purposes of identification and latent variable scaling, replace the asterisk with a "1". In this case, the first factor loading for each factor has been designated as a constrained parameter. Clicking "OK" at the top of this box subsequently yields a Build Variances/Covariances dialog box (Fig. 2.11). The estimated variances for both the factors and the error terms were already asterisked (and highlighted in turquoise) by the program. All that was left to do manually was to indicate which of the four factors were correlated with one another, which, in this case included all of them as indicated by the F-F asterisks. For example, the cell with highlighted borders indicates that the covariance between F3 and F4 (F3,F4) is to be estimated.

Clicking "OK" at the top of the last dialog box produced the completed input file, which is shown in Fig. 2.12. Because the BUILD_EQS approach creates an input file one line at a time, the resulting file is often longer than would have been the case had the file been constructed manually. However, the file can be easily made more compact by editing the related *.eqs file.

Fig. 2.13 shows the BUILD_EQS menu again. This time, except for the Reliability option, all other options are highlighted, which means that any one of them can be activated. Of particular note is the Run EQS option, which is selected when the job is to be executed.

```
/TITLE
Example 1st-order CFA Input File Using BUILD_EQS
/SPECIFICATIONS
DATA='c:\eqs61\files\books\data\samplecfa.ess';
VARIABLES=12; CASES=361;
METHOD=ML; ANALYSIS=COVARIANCE; MATRIX=RAW;
/LABELS
V1=SDQMSC1; V2=SDQMSC2; V3=SDQMSC3; V4=SDQSSC1; V5=SDQSSC2;
V6=SDQSSC3; V7=SDQHSC1; V8=SDQHSC2; V9=SDQHSC3; V10=SDQVSC1;
V11=SDQVSC2; V12=SDQVSC3;
/EQUATIONS
V1 =   1F1 + E1;
V2 =   *F1 + E2;
V3 =   *F1 + E3;
V4 =   1F2 + E4;
V5 =   *F2 + E5;
V6 =   *F2 + E6;
V7 =   1F3 + E7;
V8 =   *F3 + E8;
V9 =   *F3 + E9;
V10 =  1F4 + E10;
V11 =  *F4 + E11;
V12 =  *F4 + E12;
/VARIANCES
 F1 = *;
 F2 = *;
 F3 = *;
 F4 = *;
 E1 = *;
 E2 = *;
 E3 = *;
 E4 = *;
 E5 = *;
 E6 = *;
 E7 = *;
 E8 = *;
 E9 = *;
 E10 = *;
 E11 = *;
 E12 = *;
/COVARIANCES
F2,F1 = *;
F3,F1 = *;
F3,F2 = *;
F4,F1 = *;
F4,F2 = *;
F4,F3 = *;
/PRINT
FIT=ALL;
TABLE=EQUATION;
/END
```

FIG. 2.12.   Completed input file.

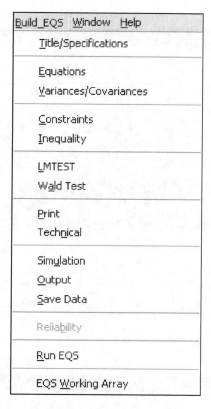

FIG. 2.13. Final BUILD_EQS drop-down menu.

Second-Order CFA Model (see Fig. 2.2)

Basically, the only significant illustrations worthy of note here are the Build Equations and Build Variances/Covariances dialog boxes; all other input file dialog boxes represent replicated specifications as shown for the first-order CFA model. The major difference with this second-order model is the hypothesized structure between F5 and the four lower order factors (F1-F4). Thus, in Fig. 2.14 (only partially visible), note the circled asterisks in the column labeled F5. Reviewing the rows in which these asterisks appear, note that the labels F1 through F4 appear to the left. In assigning asterisks to the Build Equations dialog box, it helps to know how to interpret SEM matrices that combine both the observed variables and latent factors. Following convention, one reads down from the top of the column (F5) and then left across to the factors (F1-F4). As such, the first asterisk in this column would be interpreted as F5 causes F1, which is indicative of a regression path flowing from F5 to F1.

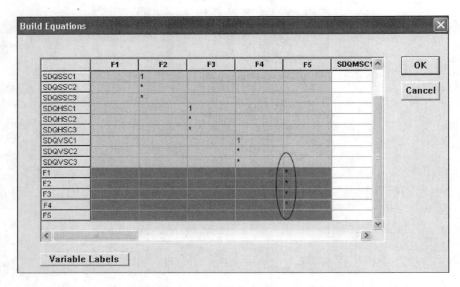

FIG. 2.14. Build equations dialog box indicating estimated second-order factor loadings.

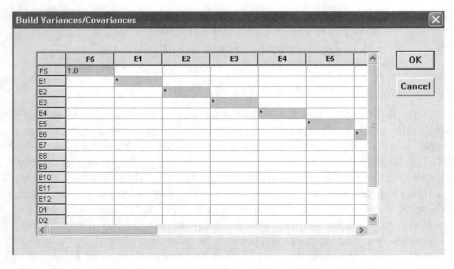

FIG. 2.15. Build variances/covariances dialog box indicating fixed variance for F5.

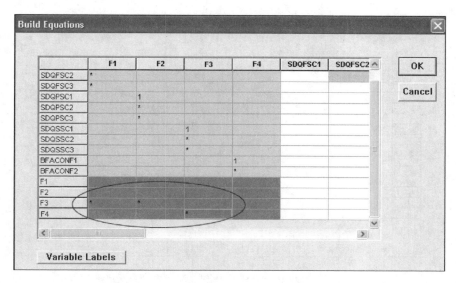

FIG. 2.16.   Build equations dialog box indicating estimated structural paths.

Turning to Fig. 2.15, only a partial representation of the Build Variances/Covariances dialog box is visible. Nonetheless, it is enough to show that, consistent with Fig. 2.2, the variance of F5 (the higher order factor) is fixed to 1.0. Although an asterisk appeared in the box for F5, it was simply replaced with the value of 1.0. However, although not all are visible in the portion of the dialog box shown in Fig. 2.15, the variances are estimated for all the error terms (E1–E12) as well as the four disturbance terms (D1–D4).

Full Structural Equation Model (see Fig. 2.3)

Again, given your familiarity with the initial construction of an input file using BUILD_EQS, there are only two significant aspects of the specification for the full model (see Fig. 2.3). The first is the Build Equations dialog box shown in Fig. 2.16, in which the structural paths are circled. Reading down from the labels listed at the top of the table, the first asterisk appearing in column 1, for example, represents the freely estimated regression path leading from F1 to F3. The second point relates to the Build Variances/Covariances dialog box illustrated in Fig. 2.17. Again, only part of this specification is visible. However, the only factor variances to be estimated are those related to F1 and F2, both of which are independent variables in the model. Likewise, the only factor covariance to be estimated is the one linking F1 and F2 (F1, F2). All remaining variances to be estimated relate to the random measurement error terms, as well as to D3 and D4, the disturbance terms associated with F3 and F4—albeit not all of the asterisks are visible in this captured Windows™ view. Being dependent variables in the model, the variance of these two factors themselves, of course, cannot be estimated.

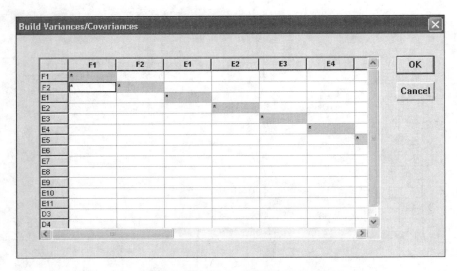

FIG. 2.17.   Build variances/covariances dialog box indicating estimated variances for F1 and F2.

Building an Input File Graphically Using the DIAGRAMMER

The graphical interface of the EQS program is embedded in its DIAGRAMMER feature. When I was writing my previous book on EQS (Byrne, 1994a), the program had just entered the world of Microsoft Windows™, and the DIAGRAMMER was in its embryonic stages of development. What a difference 11 years can make! The DIAGRAMMER has undergone continuous and rigorous development and refinement so that EQS can boast today some of the best graphical features of any SEM program. Needless to say, with a book of this type, I am necessarily limited in the number of graphical possibilities that I can illustrate. However, I hope to at least show you sufficient examples to give you a good flavor of what the DIAGRAMMER can do for you. (For thorough coverage of its myriad possibilities and descriptive details regarding their use, readers are referred to the *EQS6 Windows™ Guide* (Bentler & Wu, 2002). Let's begin the journey into the graphical world of EQS by walking through the creation of the first-order CFA model.

First-Order CFA Model (see Fig. 2.1)

To initiate operation of the DIAGRAMMER, click on its related icon, as circled in Fig. 2.18. As with BUILD_EQS, it is necessary to first open the data set on which the model will be based.

Clicking on the DIAGRAMMER icon opens the dialog box shown in Fig. 2.19. As you can see, the user is offered the choice of building three commonly specified

File Edit View Data Analysis Data Plot Build_EQS Window Help

samplecfa.ess

	SDQMSC1	SDQMSC2	SDQMSC3	SDQSSC1	SDQSSC2	SDQSSC3
1	4.0000	5.0000	1.0000	7.0000	1.0000	3.0000
2	6.0000	6.0000	6.0000	6.0000	1.0000	6.0000
3	3.0000	5.0000	1.0000	7.0000	2.0000	3.0000
4	6.0000	6.0000	3.0000	6.0000	1.0000	4.0000
5	4.0000	6.0000	6.0000	6.0000	2.0000	3.0000
6	6.0000	6.0000	5.0000	7.0000	3.0000	5.0000
7	1.0000	1.0000	1.0000	7.0000	2.0000	1.0000
8	2.0000	4.0000	2.0000	7.0000	1.0000	1.0000

FIG. 2.18. EQS Windows™ toolbar showing DIAGRAMMER Icon.

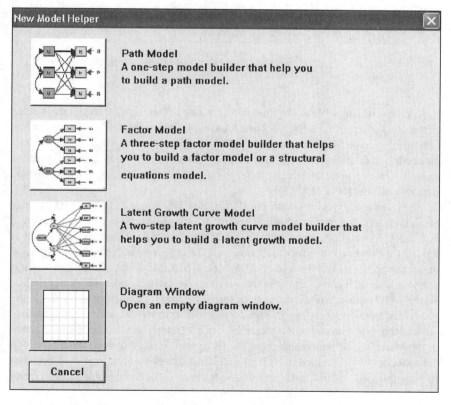

New Model Helper

Path Model
A one-step model builder that help you
to build a path model.

Factor Model
A three-step factor model builder that helps
you to build a factor model or a structural

equations model.

Latent Growth Curve Model
A two-step latent growth curve model builder that
helps you to build a latent growth model.

Diagram Window
Open an empty diagram window.

Cancel

FIG. 2.19. EQS DIAGRAMMER new model helper dialog box.

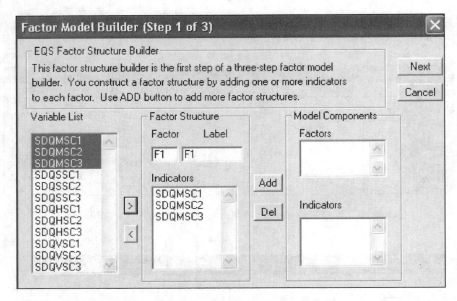

FIG. 2.20.   Factor model builder dialog box showing observed variables associated with F1.

models or selecting a blank diagram window. Each of the first three picture buttons contains a series of procedures for assistance in building the model of your choice. For straightforward and noncomplex path, factor, and latent growth curve models, proceeding with the selection of one of these icons works well. With more complex models, however, you will likely prefer to create your own model, working instead with the various DIAGRAMMER icons.

Because we are working with a fairly simple CFA model, I clicked on the Factor Model, button, which then yielded the Factor Model Builder dialog box shown in Fig. 2.20. As might be expected, Step 1 of this model-building process involves linking the observed variables to their related factors. Working from left to right, (a) select the observed variables (e.g., SDQMSC1-SDQMSC3); (b) click on the short arrow, which then copies the selected variables to the Indicators box; and (c) click on the ADD button, which moves both the factor and the indicator variables to the Model Components section. In Fig. 2.21, which provides a more comprehensive view of this process, you will observe F1, with its related observed variables, listed in the Models Components section; the three variables associated with F2 are in the process of being added to it. Figure 2.22 illustrates the final equation-building step for this CFA model, as the last three observed variables are blocked and ready to be transferred to the Model Components column.

Once the links between F4 and its related variables are added to the Model Components section, click on NEXT, which indicates to the program that the

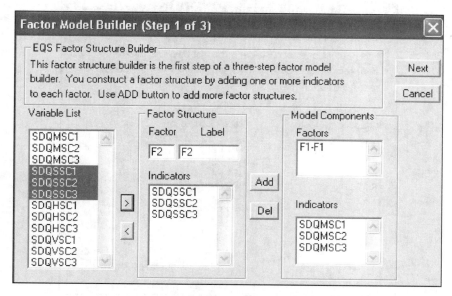

FIG. 2.21. Factor model builder dialog box showing observed variables associated with F2.

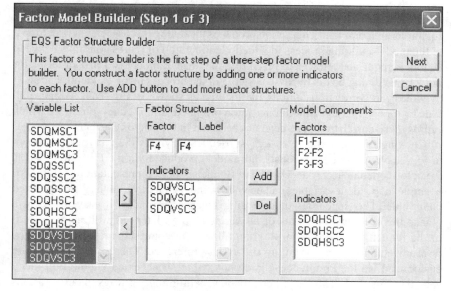

FIG. 2.22. Factor model builder dialog box showing final phase of building equations.

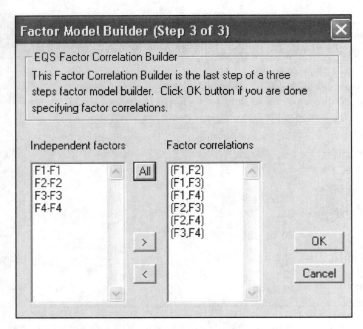

FIG. 2.23.   Factor model builder dialog box showing specification of factor correlations.

equations are complete. This action produces the dialog box associated with Step 2 of the model-building process in which identification of regression links between factors is requested. However, given that the present model is a first-order factor model, this dialog box is bypassed. Step 3 in the process involves identification of hypothesized correlations among the factors, as shown in Fig. 2.23. Because all four factors in this CFA model are intercorrelated, simply click on ALL, which causes these correlation parameters to be listed in the Factor Correlations box.

Clicking OK shown in Fig. 2.23 subsequently yields the CFA model shown in Fig. 2.24. As noted previously, all models produced via the DIAGRAMMER are color-coded in accordance with the Bentler–Weeks representation system. For example, dependent variables can be yellow, independent variables gray, and fixed paths blue. This ingenious color-coding mechanism makes it easy to see at a glance the specification status of all variables (i.e., latent as well as measured) in the model. Of course, the program allows the color schemes to be changed or removed entirely according to the user's preference. These modifications are customized via the Preferences dialog box, which is accessed via the Edit menu shown in Fig. 2.25. This dialog box displays a full range of ways to tailor various aspects of the EQS program according to individual preferences. As shown in the figure, the EQS DIAGRAMMER tab has been opened to allow modifications

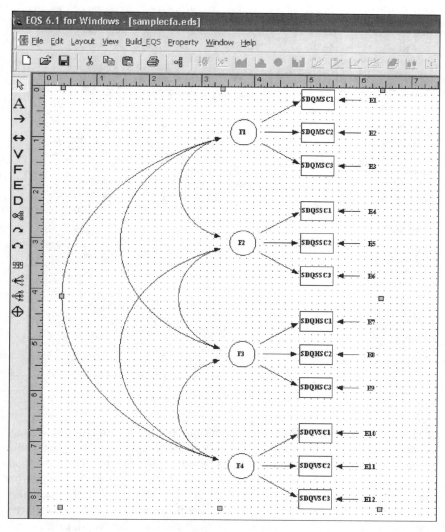

FIG. 2.24.   Completed first-order CFA model.

in addition to color, including line widths, object sizes, display orientation (i.e., portrait or landscape), and so on. As this book goes to press, I am not aware of any other SEM program that allows users such a wide range of customizing options to the program for their own use. Once again, EQS is in a class by itself.

At least three points are worthy of further explanation regarding Fig. 2.24. First, note the eight tiny empty squares encasing the model. These marks represent the

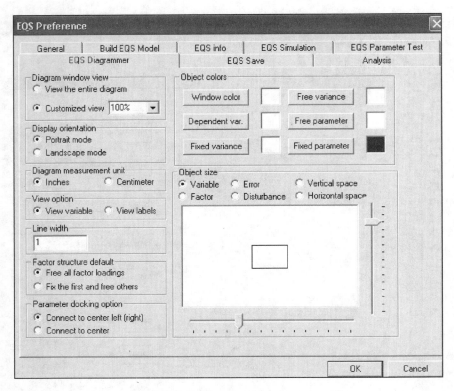

FIG. 2.25.   EQS preference dialog box.

"handles" of the figure. When they are visible, the figure can be moved intact around the page by simply clicking anywhere within them and dragging to the position desired. Second, the tiny dots on the DIAGRAMMER palette are part of its permanent wallpaper. Although EQS does have an alignment mechanism (illustrated later in this chapter; see Fig. 2.35), the dots serve to guide the placement of various model components. Third, although the indicator variables have been labeled, the factor names remain as F1 through F4. For labels (optional), simply double-click on a factor and the dialog box shown in Fig. 2.26 will appear. This Variance Specification box summarizes information related to Factor 1 and also allows the user to add a variable label and alter the start value, if you so wish. For labels in which each set of letters resides on a separate line, simply separate each set by a semicolon, as illustrated in Fig. 2.26. The end product of this action is shown in Fig. 2.27.

Building the model has been completed and the user is now ready to execute the job. To initiate this process, click the BUILD_EQS tab on the tool bar, which produces the drop-down menu shown in Fig. 2.5. The tab labeled Run EQS is

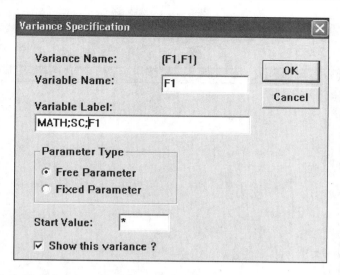

FIG. 2.26. Variance specification dialog box showing labeling of F1.

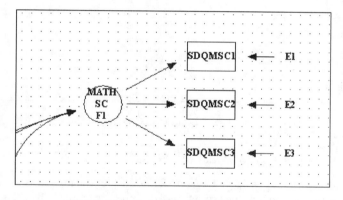

FIG. 2.27. Completed labeling or F1.

needed to run the job. However, note that this option is faded out, which indicates that it is inactive. To activate this option, first provide a title by clicking on the top tab, which yields the Model Specifications dialog box shown in Fig. 2.6. Clicking OK creates a text window within which is a parallel version of the first-order CFA input file shown previously. This file of model commands was created from the DIAGRAMMER and automatically assigned an .eqs extension by the program; it is now ready to be executed. Drop down the BUILD_EQS menu again and click Run EQS.

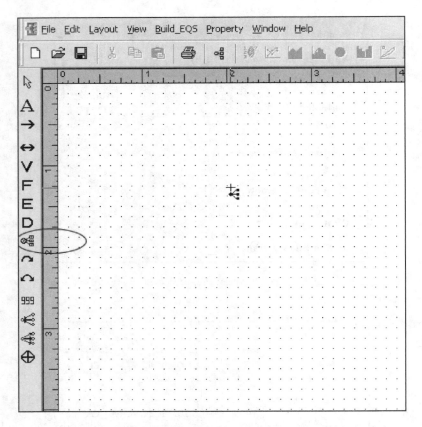

FIG. 2.28.   Toolbar icon and activation of the regression tool.

Second-Order CFA Model (see Fig. 2.2)

In building the higher order CFA model, a different approach is needed as a consequence of the second-level structure. This time, the model will be built section by section, which provides me the opportunity to demonstrate many other aspects of the DIAGRAMMER. To initiate this process, click on the DIAGRAMMER icon as before but, this time, instead of selecting the CFA model option in the Model Helper dialog box (see Fig. 2.19), click on the Empty Diagram option. This action results in a totally blank working area, as partially shown in Fig. 2.28. Next, click on the Regression icon (circled in Fig. 2.28), which activates this tool as shown in the blank space. A single left click of the mouse yields the Factor Structure Specification dialog box in which the user specifies which variables load on which factors (Fig. 2.29). Moving from left to right and holding down the Control key,[8]

---

[8]The user can also drag down the cursor to include the selected variables.

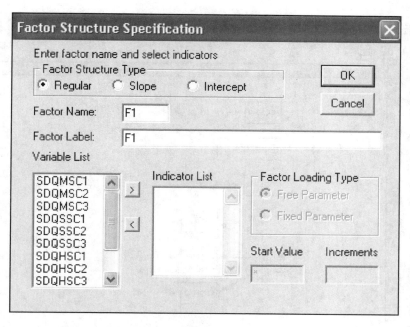

FIG. 2.29. Factor structure specification dialog box.

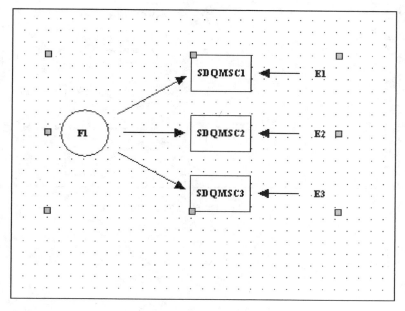

FIG. 2.30. Completed factor structure resulting from single activation of the regression tool.

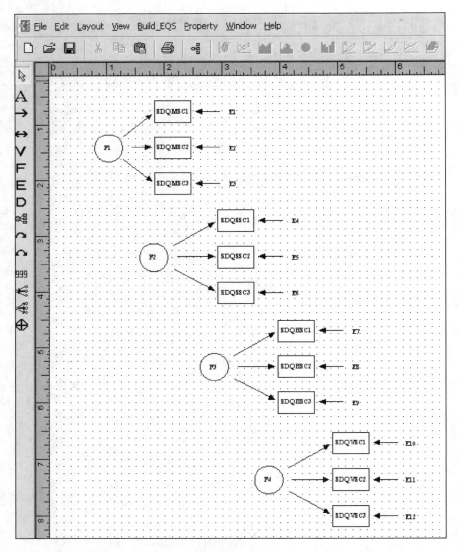

FIG. 2.31.   Completed factor structures for F1 through F4.

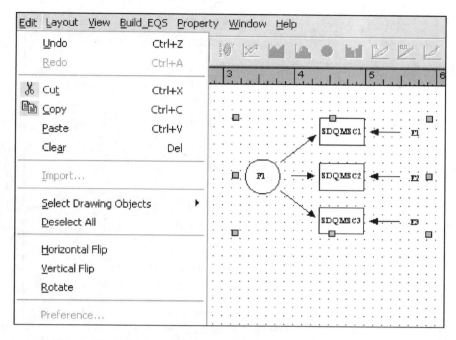

FIG. 2.32. Edit drop-down menu showing Horizontal Flip option.

first click on the three observed variables hypothesized to load on F1. Next, click on the > button, which transfers these variables to the second column. The program automatically takes care of the information in the rest of the box as the various components of the model are linked together. Finally click on OK, which presents the Factor 1 structure as shown in Fig. 2.30. Again, notice the handles surrounding the figure. Clicking anywhere on the figure activates these handles and enables the user to move the figure to different locations in the blank space.

In the case of the CFA model, this process would be repeated three more times. With each activation of the Factor Structure Specification dialog box, the program automatically specified the next factor (e.g., F2) along with all variables that have not yet been assigned to a factor. With these specifications completed, there are now four separate factor clusters, as shown in Fig. 2.31.

It is time to introduce another DIAGRAMMER feature that is useful should you prefer to build the model in reverse (i.e., with the factors on the right rather than the left). This task is easily accomplished through use of the Horizontal Flip option, that can be activated from the Edit drop-down menu, as shown in Fig. 2.32. The factor structure must be activated (as indicated by the surrounding handles) before the flip action can be implemented. For illustration purposes, only Factor 1

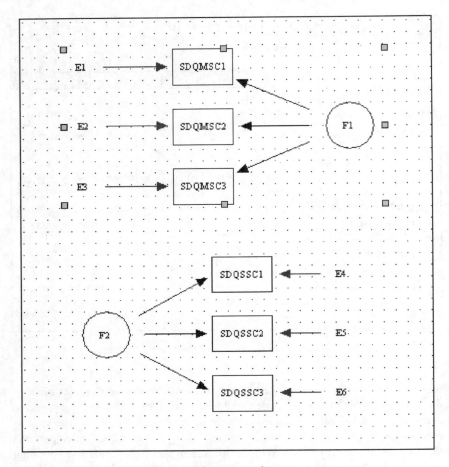

FIG. 2.33.　Reversed version of Factor 1 structure.

was reversed as shown in Fig. 2.33. However, grouping all four factor structures together before conducting the Horizontal Flip action eliminates several interim steps.

Before proceeding further, these four structures need to be aligned, and nothing could be easier than working with the DIAGRAMMER to do this job! However, to expedite this action, it is best to have all four factor structures within the viewing area. In this case, the size had to be reduced to 75%; this action was selected from the Zoom option listed on the View drop-down menu, as shown in Fig. 2.34. Once the factor structures are all in full view, and starting at the upper left-hand corner of the first factor structure, hold down the left mouse button and drag the cursor diagonally across all objects to the point where it is in Fig. 2.35. This action works

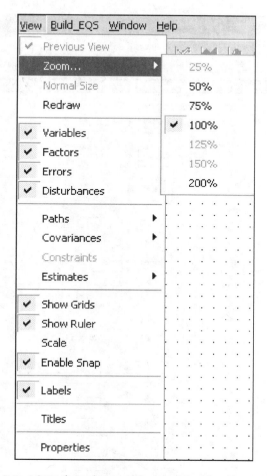

FIG. 2.34. View drop-down menu showing the Zoom option.

like an elastic band that has been pinned down at the upper left-hand corner. Once the entire structure is encased, simply release the mouse button. At the toolbar window, drop down the Layout menu (Fig. 2.36). In this case, click on Align Left, which snaps all four factor structures into perfect alignment, as shown in Fig. 2.37.

Now we're ready to build the second-order structure. Begin by clicking on the Factor (F) icon, which is circled in the toolbar shown in Fig. 2.37. This action activates the F tool and allows the user to draw a circle or an ellipse. Once the F icon has been activated, it remains so until deactivated, which is accomplished by right-clicking, the mouse or clicking on the Reset tool, the top-most icon on

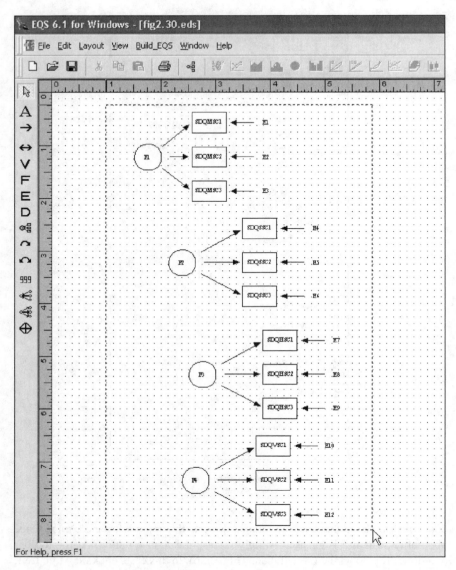

FIG. 2.35.   Capturing of separate factor structures in preparation for alignment.

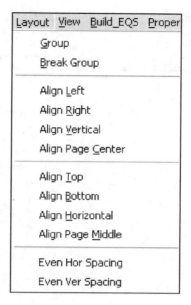

FIG. 2.36.   Layout drop-down menu showing Align Right option.

the toolbar. Thus, if the user is building a model that requires several of the same type of components (i.e., factors [Fs], indicator variables [Vs], error [E] terms or, disturbance [D] terms), simply left-clicking the mouse produces as many duplicates as desired.

The final step in building a second-order model involves drawing the regression paths from the higher order model (F5) to each of the lower order factors. This is accomplished by activating the Arrow ($\rightarrow$) tool and, with the left mouse button depressed, drawing a line from F5 to each of the four first-order factors. Figure 2.38 illustrates this action with respect to F1. An extremely valuable and unique feature of the EQS program is that it literally adapts the drawn model to comply with the Bentler–Weeks system as you work. For example, if you have elected to work in color mode, as soon as the regression path leading from F5 to F1 is completed, the color of the F1 circle changes to the color assigned to dependent variables (in the Bentler–Weeks sense), and the disturbance term, D1, is added;[9] the short regression path associated with the D is colored blue, indicating that its path is fixed to 1. Another interesting feature of working with the arrow tool is that, no matter where you begin drawing and finalize the path (e.g., perhaps slightly within the perimeter of the circle or rectangle, respectively), the program automatically

_____

[9]Depending on the model, sometimes these added disturbance components can attach themselves to another part of its immediate factor structure. To correct this situation, click on the D term, which encases it in handles by which it can be relocated to its proper position.

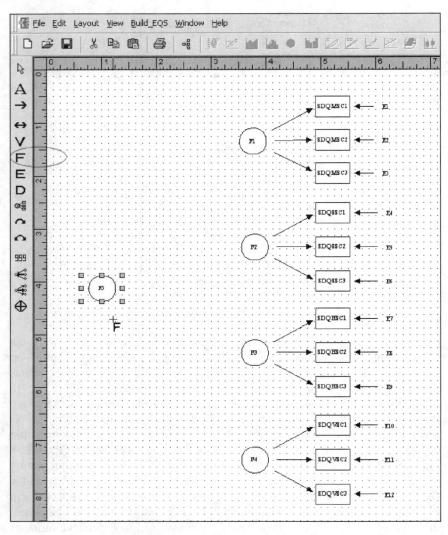

FIG. 2.37.   Toolbar icon and activation of the F (Factor) tool.

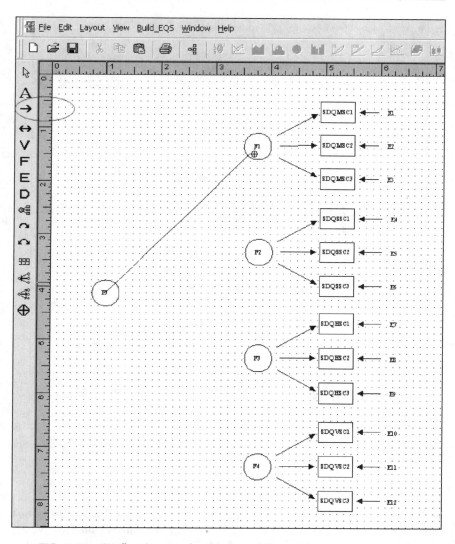

FIG. 2.38.   Toolbar icon and activation of the → (one-way arrow) tool.

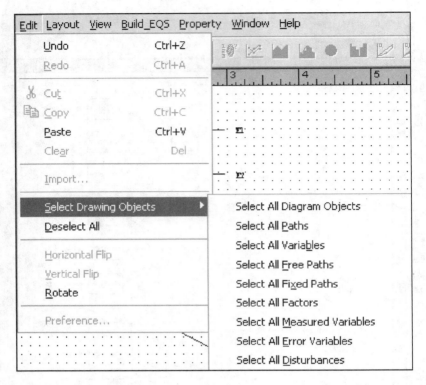

FIG. 2.39.   Edit drop-down menu showing the select Drawing Objects option.

snaps the arrow into correct position. So, that's it. Except for the asterisks, fixed 1's, and variable labeling, the completed model resembles the one shown in Fig. 2.2.

Full Structural Equation Model (see Fig. 2.3)

Because the building of this model encompasses most of the operations that have already been demonstrated, this material is not presented again. However, at least two other features of the DIAGRAMMER are helpful in building the models illustrated in this chapter; therefore, the discussion is limited to these features. The first addresses the issue of relocating various portions of the model during the construction process. This information is critical in the building of complex CFA (e.g., higher order, multitrait–multimethod) and full structural models. For example, the user may wish to move a section of the model to the center of the page but not piece by piece! To join these model components together so they operate as a single unit, click on the Edit menu, then Select Drawing Objects, and then Select All Diagram Objects (Fig. 2.39). Although a wide selection of choices is presented,

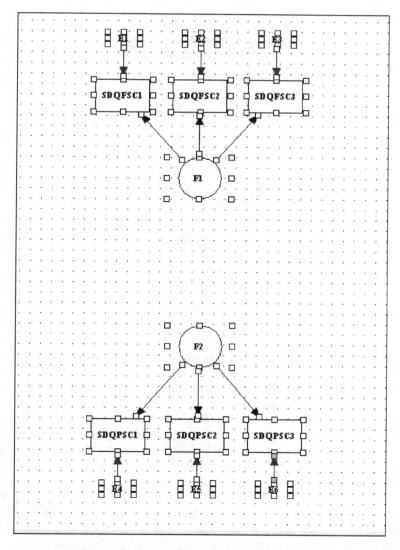

FIG. 2.40. Graphic handles associated with all model components.

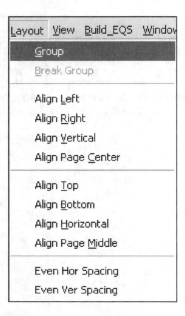

FIG. 2.41.   Layout drop-down menu showing the Group option.

only the first is relevant here. This action makes visible all the handles associated with every component in the partial model shown in Fig. 2.40. To amalgamate these component parts into a single object, click on the Layout tab and select Group from its drop-down menu (Fig. 2.41). Of course, the reverse situation is when the user wants to break up a single group to modify a specific component of the grouping. One example might be a situation where you wish to reassign the fixed factor loading of 1.00 to a different indicator variable. In this case, simply click on the grouped set of objects and then Break Group from the Layout menu, listed below Group but grayed out.

The second illustration addresses the correlation between Factors 1 and 2. This tool has to be the *crème de la crème* of EQS, and so it seems fitting to save the best until last. Of course, I am referring to the double-headed curved-arrow icon on the toolbar, as shown circled in Fig. 2.42. To construct the correlation symbol, click on this icon, move the mouse and click inside the F1 circle, draw a line joining the two factors by depressing the left button and dragging the cursor to inside the F2 circle; finally, click the left mouse button and then right-click to stop any further drawing action. The great thing about this tool, is that you no longer need to possess innate artistic skills to draw an arc (the bane of my SEM existence for so many years!). As soon as the mouse button is released, the DIAGRAMMER automatically draws the curved arrow and snaps it into place, as illustrated in Fig. 2.43.

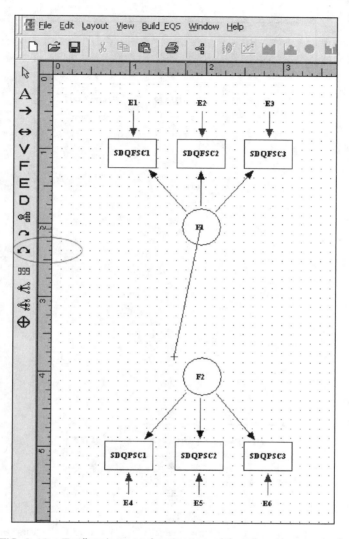

FIG. 2.42. Toolbar icon and activation of the curved arrow tool.

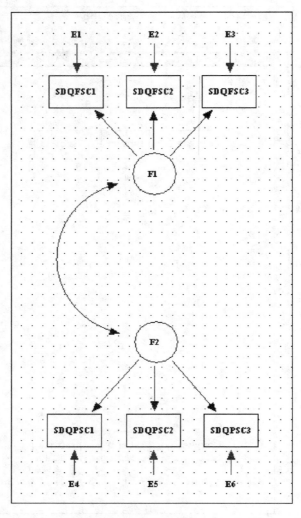

FIG. 2.43.   DIAGRAMMER-completed drawing of a double-headed arrow.

THE EQS OUTPUT FILE IN GENERAL

As discussed previously, to execute any EQS input file—whether created as a text file or as a model file built using the DIAGRAMMER—the user must select Run EQS from the BUILD_EQS drop-down menu. As soon as the program has finished running, the test results are placed in an output file that is given the default extension of *.out, in which the asterisk represents the name of the EQS input file. This file can be edited within EQS and with any text editor (Bentler & Wu, 2002).

Regardless of whether a text input file or a DIAGRAMMER model file was executed, as soon as the run has been completed, the output file is automatically fetched to the front window of the user's working space. The first part of the output file echoes the input file, which can be very helpful in identifying particular job runs. Details related to the output file are the topic of discussion throughout this book so are not addressed here.

If you created a model file using the DIAGRAMMER, you will have the added benefit of viewing the estimates directly from the model. When a model

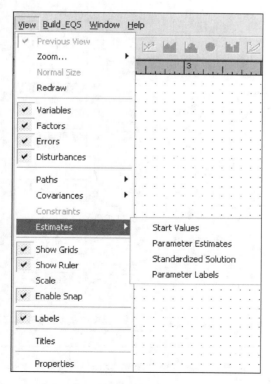

FIG. 2.44. View drop-down menu showing estimates → standardization solution.

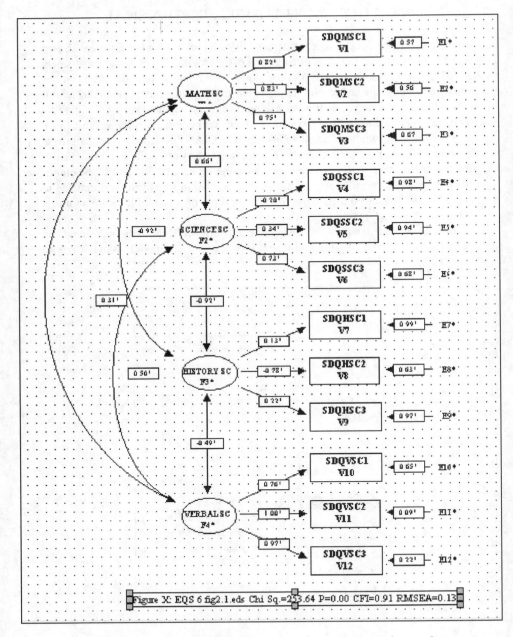

FIG. 2.45.　Standardization estimates and summary goodness-of-fit statistics related to Fig. 2.1.

file is executed, EQS automatically creates an /OUTPUT section. This command writes all estimates to an external file called eqsout.ets, which enables the DIAGRAMMER to read those estimates after the job is completed. To review the parameter estimates from the model, click the View tab on the Windows™ toolbar, then scroll down the menu and click on Estimates. As shown in Fig. 2.44, there are four options from which to choose. Clicking on either the Parameter estimates (unstandardized solution) or the Standardized solution causes the model to be redrawn with the estimates embedded in the paths. Figure 2.45 presents the standardized solution for the first-order CFA model shown in Fig. 2.1 and summarizes the χ^2 and probability values, along with two goodness-of-fit statistics (to be detailed in Chapter 3). Unfortunately, to capture this estimated model for viewing purposes, it was necessary to reduce its size to 75%, which resulted in a much reduced goodness-of-fit summary that could be viewed in total only by leaving the DIAGRAMMER handles in place.

EQS ERROR MESSAGES

Errors are inevitable, regardless of how familiar a user is with various computer environments and software packages.[10] Typically, error messages produced by a particular program provide some clue as to the location and correction of the error. This task for SEM software packages is substantially more difficult, given the combined complexities associated with both the data and the specified model. Nonetheless, compared with other SEM packages, EQS is exceptionally helpful in this regard.

Error messages in EQS fall into two categories: those considered minor and those considered more serious. Following are a few examples.

Minor Errors

These errors are typically of a syntactical nature. EQS automatically checks for such errors and prints a message, immediately following the Bentler–Weeks representation of the model in the output file, advising that a syntax error has occurred. If such an error is identified, the program automatically terminates. A few of the most common syntax errors are as follows:

- using key words that do not conform to the EQS naming convention
- forgetting to put a slash before the key word
- forgetting to put a semicolon after each statement
- forgetting to specify a name of the external file to be created by the RETEST option and to enclose this filename in single quotes
- forgetting to include the equals sign (=) and yes (no) following specification of the LMTEST, WTEST, and EFFECTS options

---

[10]If the model is created through the DIAGRAMMER or BUILD_EQS, syntactic errors will not be encountered in the input file.

Another minor error that can occur relates to the number of cases specified. If the actual number of cases differs from the number specified in the input file, EQS warns the user that this has occurred, and analyses are based on the number of cases in the data file. Unlike the previously described problems, the program continues with all computations.

Serious Errors

In the event that the program cannot logically correct the input errors, such errors are considered fatal with the result that the program terminates without completing the computations. These error messages generally relate to problems such as a matrix that may not be positive definite, start values that are bad, and a particular variable is linearly dependent on other parameters. (For excellent reviews of these types of problems, see Bentler & Chou, 1987; and Rindskopf, 1984.) Given these types of messages, users need to carefully review their content to resolve the problem.

In general, most EQS problems result from typographical or syntactical errors. I strongly urge you to re-examine your input file with a critical eye for syntax error before running the job. In the long run, it can save you many hours of distress!

OVERVIEW OF REMAINING CHAPTERS

Thus far, only the bricks and mortar of SEM applications using the EQS program have been introduced. As such, you have learned the basics regarding (a) concepts underlying SEM procedures, (b) components of the CFA and full models, (c) elements and structure of the EQS program, (d) creation of EQS input files, and (e) execution of EQS jobs. Now it's time to combine these bricks and mortar to build a variety of structures. The remainder of the book is devoted to an in-depth examination of basic EQS applications involving both the CFA and full models.

In presenting these examples from the literature, I have tried to address the diverse needs of my readers by including a potpourri of EQS setups. Some applications have the data matrix embedded in the input file, others draw from an external file; some include data in the form of a correlation matrix, others involve the input of raw data; some include start values, others do not. All data related to these applications are included in the CD located in a pocket at the back of the book. Given that personal experience is always the best teacher; I encourage you to work through these examples on your own computer. Taken together, the applications presented in the remaining 11 chapters should provide you with a comprehensive understanding of how EQS can be used to analyze various structural equation models based on an array of input data. Let's move on, then, to our first example.

II

Single Group Analyses

Confirmatory Factor Analytic Models

The Full Latent Variable Model

3

Application 1:
Testing for the Factorial
Validity of a Theoretical
Construct (First-Order
CFA Model)

Our first application examines a First-order CFA model designed to test the multidimensionality of a theoretical construct. Specifically, this application tests the hypothesis that self-concept (SC) for early adolescents (Grade 7) is a multidimensional construct composed of four factors: general SC (GSC), academic SC (ASC), English SC (ESC), and mathematics SC (MSC). The theoretical underpinning of this hypothesis derives from the hierarchical model of SC proposed by Shavelson, Hubner, and Stanton (1976). The example is taken from a study by Byrne and Worth Gavin (1996) in which four hypotheses related to the Shavelson et al. model were tested for three groups of children: preadolescents (Grade 3), early adolescents (Grade 7), and late adolescents (Grade 11). Only tests bearing on the multidimensional structure of SC, as it relates to Grade 7 children, are relevant to the present chapter. This study followed from earlier work in which the same four-factor structure of SC was tested for adolescents (see Byrne & Shavelson, 1986) and was part of a larger study that focused on the structure of social SC (Byrne & Shavelson, 1996). For a more extensive discussion of the substantive issues and the related findings, see the original Byrne and Worth Gavin (1996) article.

THE HYPOTHESIZED MODEL

At issue in this first application is the plausibility of a multidimensional SC structure for early adolescents. Although numerous studies have supported the multidimensionality of the construct for Grade 7 children, others have counter-argued that SC is less differentiated for children in their pre- and early-adolescent years (e.g., Harter, 1990). Thus, the argument could be made for a two-factor structure comprising only GSC and ASC. Still others postulate that SC is a uni-dimensional structure so that all facets of SC are embodied within a single SC construct (GSC). (For a review of the related literature, see Byrne, 1996.) The task presented here is to test the original hypothesis that SC is a four-factor structure comprising a general component (GSC), an academic component (ASC), and two subject-specific components (ESC and MSC) against two alternative hypotheses: (a) that SC is a two-factor structure comprising GSC and ASC, and (b) that SC is a one-factor structure in which there is no distinction between GSC and ASC. We now examine and test each of these hypotheses.

HYPOTHESIS 1:
Self-Concept Is a Four-Factor Structure

The model to be tested in Hypothesis 1 postulates a priori that SC is a four-factor structure composed of GSC, ASC, ESC, and MSC; it is presented schematically in Fig. 3.1, with asterisks representing parameters to the fully estimated.

Before discussing how to go about testing this model, let's first dissect the model and list its component parts, as follows:

1. There are four SC factors, as indicated by the four circles labeled GENERAL SC, ACADEMIC SC, ENGLISH SC, and MATH SC.
2. The four factors are intercorrelated, as indicated by the two-headed arrows.
3. There are 16 observed variables, as indicated by the 16 rectangles (SDQ2N01-SDQ2N43); they represent item-pairs from the General, Aca-demic, Verbal, and Math SC subscales of the *Self-Description Questionnaire II* (Marsh, 1992), respectively.
4. The observed variables load on the factors in the following pattern: SDQ2N01–SDQ2N37) load on Factor 1, SDQ3N04–SDQ2N40 load on Fac-tor 2, SDQ2N10–SDQ2N46 load on Factor 3, and SDQ2N07–SDQ2N43 load on Factor 4.
5. Each observed variable loads on one and only one factor.
6. Errors of measurement associated with each observed variable (E25–E40) are uncorrelated.

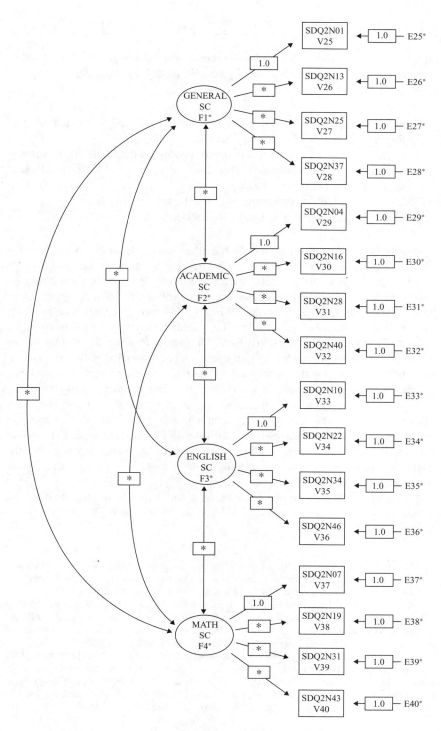

FIG. 3.1. Hypothesized four-factor model of self-concept.

After summarizing these observations, a more formal description of the hypothe-sized model is now presented. As such, the CFA model shown in Fig. 3.1 hypoth-esizes a priori that:

1. SC responses can be explained by four factors: General SC, Academic SC, English SC, and Math SC, respectively.
2. Each item-pair measure has a nonzero loading on the SC factor that it was designed to measure (termed a *target loading*) and a zero loading on all other factors (termed *nontarget loadings*).
3. The four SC factors, consistent with the theory, are correlated.
4. Error–uniquenesses[1] associated with each measure are uncorrelated.

Another way of conceptualizing the hypothesized model in Fig. 3.1 is within a matrix framework as shown in Table 3.1. Thinking about the model components in this format can be very helpful because it is consistent with the manner by which the results from SEM analyses are commonly reported in program output files. Although EQS, as well as other Windows™-based programs, also provides users with a graphical output, the labeled information is typically limited to the estimated values and their standard errors. The tabular representation of the model in Table 3.1 shows the pattern of parameters to be estimated within the frame-work of three matrices: the factor-loading matrix, the factor variance–covariance matrix, and the error variance–covariance matrix. For purposes of model identi-fication and latent variable scaling (see chap. 2), the first of each congeneric set of SC measures in the factor-loading matrix is set to 1.0,[2] all other parameters are freely estimated (as represented by the asterisk [*]). Likewise, as indicated in the variance–covariance matrix, all parameters are to be freely estimated. Finally, in the error–uniqueness matrix, only the error variances are estimated; all error covariances are presumed to be zero.[3]

Provided with these two perspectives, let's now move on to the actual testing of this four-factor hypothesized model. First, we review the EQS input file.

---

[1]The term *uniqueness* is used here in the factor-analytic sense to mean a composite of random measurement error and specific measurement error associated with a particular measuring instrument; in cross-sectional studies, the two cannot be separated (Gerbing & Anderson, 1984).

[2]A set of measures is said to be *congeneric* if each measure in the set purports to assess the same construct, except for errors of measurement (Jöreskog, 1971a). For example, as indicated in Table 3.1 and Fig. 3.1, SDQ2N01, SDQ2N13, SDQ2N25, and SDQ2N37 all serve as measures of general self-concept (GSC); therefore, they represent a congeneric set of indicator variables.

[3]For readers interested in comparing input and output files from both the EQS (2005) and LISREL (Jöreskog & Sörbom, 1996) programs, the present application provides a unique opportunity to do so. Although such details are by necessity limited and briefly described in the Byrne and Worth Gavin (1996) paper, they are dealt with more comprehensively in Byrne (1998), in which the same analyses presented here were conducted on the same data matrix using the LISREL 8 program.

TABLE 3.1

Pattern of Estimated Parameters for Hypothesized Four-Factor Model

Factor Loading Matrix

	Factors			
	GSC	ASC	ESC	MSC
Observed Measure	F_1	F_2	F_3	F_4
SDQ2N01 (V25)	1.0^a	0.0	0.0	0.0
SDQ2N13 (V26)	$*^b$	0.0	0.0	0.0
SDQ2N25 (V27)	*	0.0	0.0	0.0
SDQ2N37 (V28)	*	0.0	0.0	0.0
SDQ2N04 (V29)	0.0^c	1.0	0.0	0.0
SDQ2N16 (V30)	0.0	*	0.0	0.0
SDQ2N28 (V31)	0.0	*	0.0	0.0
SDQ2N40 (V32)	0.0	*	0.0	0.0
SDQ2N10 (V33)	0.0	0.0	1.0	0.0
SDQ2N22 (V34)	0.0	0.0	*	0.0
SDQ2N34 (V35)	0.0	0.0	*	0.0
SDQ2N46 (V36)	0.0	0.0	*	0.0
SDQ2N07 (V37)	0.0	0.0	0.0	1.0
SDQ2N19 (V38)	0.0	0.0	0.0	*
SDQ2N31 (V39)	0.0	0.0	0.0	*
SDQ2N43 (V40)	0.0	0.0	0.0	*

Factor Variance/Covariance Matrix

GSC	*			
ASC	*	*		
ESC	*	*	*	
MSC	*	*	*	*

Error Variance/Covariance Matrix

	V25	V26	V27	V28	V29	V30	V31	V32	V33	V34	V35	V36	V37	V38	V39	V40
SDQ2N01 (V25)	*															
SDQ2N13 (V26)	0.0	*														
SDQ2N25 (V27)	0.0	0.0	*													
SDQ2N37 (V28)	0.0	0.0	0.0	*												
SDQ2N04 (V29)	0.0	0.0	0.0	0.0	*											
SDQ2N16 (V30)	0.0	0.0	0.0	0.0	0.0	*										
SDQ2N28 (V31)	0.0	0.0	0.0	0.0	0.0	0.0	*									
SDQ2N40 (V32)	0.0	0.0	0.0	0.0	0.0	0.0	0.0	*								
SDQ2N10 (V33)	0.0	0.0	0.0	0.0	0.0	0.0	0.0	0.0	*							
SDQ2N22 (V34)	0.0	0.0	0.0	0.0	0.0	0.0	0.0	0.0	0.0	*						
SDQ2N34 (V35)	0.0	0.0	0.0	0.0	0.0	0.0	0.0	0.0	0.0	0.0	*					
SDQ2N46 (V36)	0.0	0.0	0.0	0.0	0.0	0.0	0.0	0.0	0.0	0.0	0.0	*				
SDQ2N07 (V37)	0.0	0.0	0.0	0.0	0.0	0.0	0.0	0.0	0.0	0.0	0.0	0.0	*			
SDQ2N19 (V38)	0.0	0.0	0.0	0.0	0.0	0.0	0.0	0.0	0.0	0.0	0.0	0.0	0.0	*		
SDQ2N31 (V39)	0.0	0.0	0.0	0.0	0.0	0.0	0.0	0.0	0.0	0.0	0.0	0.0	0.0	0.0	*	
SDQ2N43 (V40)	0.0	0.0	0.0	0.0	0.0	0.0	0.0	0.0	0.0	0.0	0.0	0.0	0.0	0.0	0.0	*

[a] parameter fixed to 1.0

[b] parameter to be estimated

[c] parameter fixed to 0.0

The EQS Input File

We proceed by examining the link between the CFA model presented in Fig. 3.1 and the translation of its specifications into a file interpretable to EQS. This input file is shown in Table 3.2.

As described by the /TITLE paragraph, this file represents the initially hypothesized model representing a four-factor structure. The /SPECIFICATIONS paragraph indicates that (a) the sample size is 265, (b) there are 46 observed variables, (c) the method of estimation is maximum likelihood, (d) the data are in raw matrix form, and (e) the data are in fixed format, as described by the Fortran statement (40F1.0,X,6F2.0). This expression tells the program to read 40 single-digit numbers, to skip one column, and then to read six double-digit numbers. The first 40 columns represent item scores on the SPPC (not used in the present study) and the SDQ2; the remaining six scores represent scores for the MASTENG1 through SMAT1 variables (not used in the present study). Finally, note that the data reside as an external file called "ASC7INDM.ess." However, a brief explanation of this specification is in order. Installation instructions accompanying EQS6.1 recommend that all files be kept in the program folder, in which case DATA specification in the input file would read as DATA='ASC7INDM.ess'. The reason for the modified input in Table 3.2 is because I prefer to keep my working files separate from the program files. Therefore, I need to specify to the program exactly where these files can be found. Likewise, if users wish to operate in the same manner, they would simply specify the location of their data in accordance with their own computer.

By now, you will no doubt find the information specified in the next four paragraphs (/LABELS; /EQUATIONS; /VARIANCES; /COVARIANCES) to be fairly straightforward; thus, further explanation is unnecessary. However, the final two paragraphs introduced by the keywords /PRINT and /LMTEST are new and require elaboration. The /PRINT paragraph provides for printing of additional information that the manual states "make sense of a model and the quality of the estimates" (Bentler, 2005, p. 91). Some examples include the printing of a specified number of digits (DI=n; default=3), effect decomposition (EF=YES; Default=No), and additional goodness-of-fit indexes (FIT=ALL), which is the case with this input file.[4] The /PRINT paragraph also allows for the generation of a RETEST file in which start values are automatically assigned to all estimated parameters by the program, a function that is illustrated in chap. 6.

The /LMTEST keyword requests that the Lagrange Multiplier Test (LM Test) be implemented to test hypotheses bearing on the statistical viability of specified

---

[4]EQS automatically includes this /PRINT ↳ FIT=ALL paragraph when the input file is formulated using BUILD_EQS.

TABLE 3.2
EQS Input for Initially Hypothesized Four-Factor Model

/TITLE
CFA OF ASC Structure - GRADE 7 "ASC7F4I"
Initial 4-factor Model
/SPECIFICATIONS
CASE=265; VAR=46; ME=ML; MA=RAW; FO='(40F1.0,X,6F2.0)';
DATA='C:\EQS61\Files\Books\Data\ASC7INDM.ess';
/LABELS

V1=SPPCN08;	V2=SPPCN18;	V3=SPPCN28;	V4=SPPCN38;	V5=SPPCN48;
V6=SPPCN58;	V7=SPPCN01;	V8=SPPCN11;	V9=SPPCN21;	V10=SPPCN31;
V11=SPPCN41;	V12=SPPCN51;	V13=SPPCN06;	V14=SPPCN16;	V15=SPPCN26;
V16=SPPCN36;	V17=SPPCN46;	V18=SPPCN56;	V19=SPPCN03;	V20=SPPCN13;
V21=SPPCN23;	V22=SPPCN33;	V23=SPPCN43;	V24=SPPCN53;	V25=SDQ2N01;
V26=SDQ2N13;	V27=SDQ2N25;	V28=SDQ2N37;	V29=SDQ2N04;	V30=SDQ2N16;
V31=SDQ2N28;	V32=SDQ2N40;	V33=SDQ2N10;	V34=SDQ2N22;	V35=SDQ2N34;
V36=SDQ2N46;	V37=SDQ2N07;	V38=SDQ2N19;	V39=SDQ2N31;	V40=SDQ2N43;

V41=MASTENG1; V42=MASTMAT1; V43=TENG1; V44=TMAT1; V45=SENG1; V46=SMAT1;
/EQUATIONS
V25= F1+E25;
V26= *F1+E26;
V27= *F1+E27;
V28= *F1+E28;
  V29= F2+E29;
  V30= *F2+E30;
  V31= *F2+E31;
  V32= *F2+E32;
    V33= F3+E33;
    V34= *F3+E34;
    V35= *F3+E35;
    V36= *F3+E36;
      V37= F4+E37;
      V38= *F4+E38;
      V39= *F4+E39;
      V40= *F4+E40;
/VARIANCES
F1 TO F4= *;
E25 TO E40= *;
/COVARIANCES
F1 TO F4= *;
/PRINT
FIT=ALL;
/LMTEST
SET=GVF, PEE;
/END

restrictions in the model;[5] in a CFA model, for example, that selected indicator variables load on specific factors. The basic idea underlying this test is to determine if, in a subsequent EQS run, certain parameters were specified as free rather than fixed, would it lead to a model that better represents the data? Although we are using the LM Test only to identify which fixed parameters, if freely estimated, would lead to a significantly better-fitting model, it is also used to assess the viability of equality constraints (an issue explored in chaps. 7–10). EQS produces univariate and multivariate χ^2 statistics that permit evaluation of the appropriateness of the specified restrictions; it also yields a "parameter change statistic" that represents the value that would be obtained if a particular fixed parameter were freely estimated in a future run.

The LM Test procedure provides for several options, all of which are fully described in the manual (Bentler, 2005). One of these options, the SET command, is included in the present input. This command allows the user to limit the LM Test to a subset of only fixed parameters in the model; otherwise, the program produces numerous and often irrelevant modification indexes. In this CFA model, for example, misspecification can arise from two possible sources: (a) one or more of the item-pairs is loading on a nontarget factor, and (b) error terms associated with two or more of the indicator variables may be correlated. As such, the factor loadings and error terms that are fixed to a value of 0.0 are of substantial interest. Statistically significant LM χ^2 values would argue for the presence of factor cross-loadings (i.e., a loading on more than one factor) and error covariances (correlated errors), respectively.

EQS follows SEM convention in its coding for the SET command: a Greek letter designates the matrix of which a particular parameter is an element. However, unlike the LISREL program in which there are eight such matrices, EQS functions with only three: a variance–covariance matrix of independent factors (PHI), a regression (or coefficient) matrix involving both independent and dependent variables (GAMMA), and a regression matrix involving only dependent variables (BETA). This minimal set of matrices arises from the EQS requirement that all variables be designated as either independent or dependent variables; only dependent variables can have equations, and only independent variables can have variances and covariances. Coding for the SET command comprises three letters: the first represents the matrix (P, G, or B) and the remaining two represent a sub-matrix of one of those matrices. For example, the input file in Table 3.2 shows SET=GVF, PEE. The letter G represents the GAMMA matrix, and the double letters VF indicate the regression of the dependent V's on the independent F's (i.e., the factor loadings). Likewise, the letter P stands for the PHI matrix and the

<hr>

[5]The LM Test is analagous to the so-called Modification Indices in LISREL. However, there is at least one very important difference between the two: whereas the LM Test operates multivariately in determining misspecifed parameters in a model, the LISREL Modification Indices operate univariately.

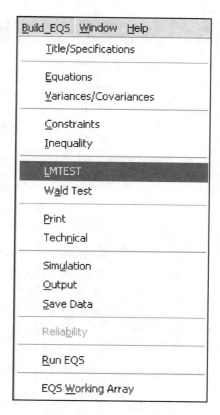

FIG. 3.2. Build EQS drop-down menu showing selection of LMTest.

double letters EE for the covariance between two error terms (i.e., correlations among the independent error terms).

In building an EQS input file, using the BUILD_EQS, specification of the LM Test is implemented following completion of the /VAR and /COV paragraphs. To begin the process, drop down the BUILD_EQS menu and select LMTEST, as highlighted in Fig. 3.2. Clicking on LMTEST subsequently yields the Build LMtest dialog box presented in Fig. 3.3. As shown here, only the boxes related to factor loadings (GVF) and error covariances (PEE) are checked. However, note that when the dialog box is first opened, you will find several other options are checked albeit not the ones that we have selected here. Simply Click on these other boxes to delete the checkmark. Once this dialog box has been completed, click OK and the /LMTEST paragraph will be added to the input file.[6]

---

[6]Alternatively, this choice could have been programmed via the Preference dialog box (see Fig. 2.5).

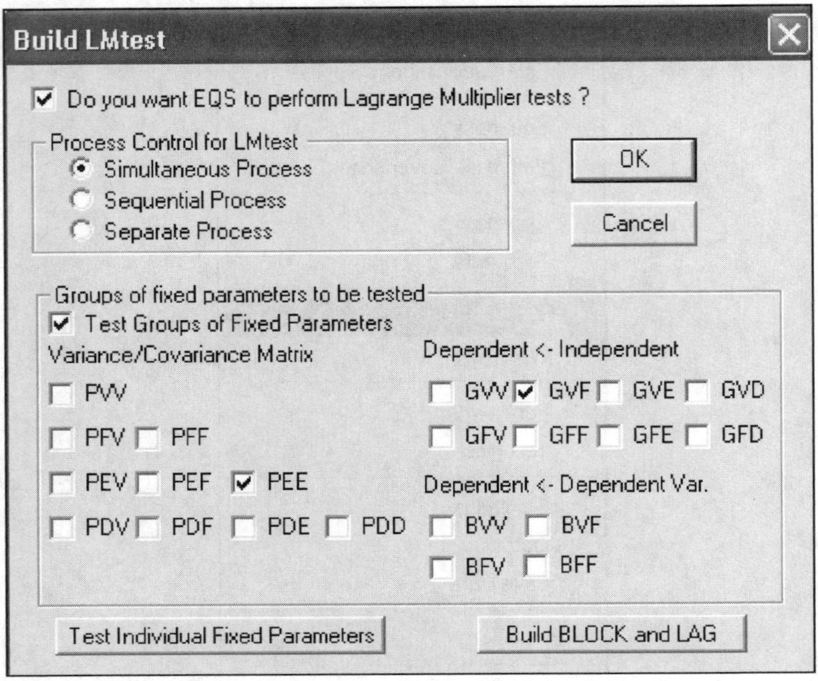

FIG. 3.3. Build LMTest dialog box showing fixed parameters under test.

Before leaving this topic of the LM Test, one vitally important caveat needs to be stressed. It bears on two factors: (a) the LM Test is based solely on statistical criteria, and (b) virtually any fixed parameter (constrained either to zero or some nonzero value) is eligible for testing. Thus, it is critical that the researcher heed the substantive theory before relaxing constraints as may be suggested by the LM statistics. Model respecification in which certain parameters have been set free must be substantiated by sound theoretical rationale; it also demands that heed be paid to the issue of identification.

The EQS Output File

We turn now to the EQS output resulting from the input file shown in Table 3.2. For didactic purposes, the entire output (except for the descriptive statistics section, which is addressed in chap. 4) is provided for the initially hypothesized model in Application 1 only; hereafter, selected portions of the output are displayed. To facilitate the presentation and discussion of results, this material is divided into three subsections: (a) model specification and analysis summary, (b) model assessment, and (c) model misspecification.

Model Specification and Analysis Summary. Given the known problems that can occur with analyses based on the correlation matrix (see, e.g., Bollen, 1989a; Boomsma, 1985; Cudeck, 1989; and Jöreskog & Sörbom, 1988), EQS automatically analyzes the covariance matrix when data are in raw matrix form. If, however, you wish to use data that are in the form of a correlation matrix, simply include the standard deviations (as shown in chap. 2) and EQS will again base the analyses on the covariance matrix. Conversely, should you wish (for any reason) to have the program base analyses on the correlation matrix, the program automatically presents a warning message advising that "statistics may not be meaningful due to analyzing a correlation matrix" (Byrne, 1994a, p. 49). Nonetheless, the program can still analyze the correlation matrix, but the ANAL=CORR command must be included, as noted in chap. 2. Shown in Table 3.3 is the covariance matrix to be analyzed in the present example.

EQS automatically decodes the input file to generate a model specification based on the Bentler–Weeks designation of dependent and independent variables. As shown in Table 3.3, there are 16 dependent variables (i.e., 16 observed variables) and 20 independent variables (i.e., four factors and 16 error terms). There are also 38 free parameters (i.e., 12 factor loadings, four factor variances, six factor covariances, 16 error variances) and 20 fixed nonzero parameters (four factor loadings, 16 error regression paths). This summary of the model is helpful in at least two ways. First, it enables you to verify that the labeled figure is consistent with the input file. In other words, is the specified model the one that you were expecting to analyze? Second, it enables you to quickly calculate degrees of freedom. In the present case, given 38 freely estimated parameters and 136 (16 [17]/2) pieces of information (see chap. 2), we know we are working with 98 (136 minus 38) degrees of freedom.

Following the Bentler–Weeks representation are two summary pieces of information: the first represents the numerical value of the matrix determinant value and the second represents a summary statement regarding the technical acceptability of the model parameters—basically, the program checks on the identification status of all parameters. Ideally, the message "PARAMETER ESTIMATES APPEAR IN ORDER, NO SPECIAL PROBLEMS WERE ENCOUNTERED DURING OPTIMIZATION" appears, as shown. It is important to locate this message prior to any interpretation of results; accordingly, we can be confident that the estimates in the present application are appropriate.

On the other hand, if the program encounters difficulties in the estimation process, the message locates the problematic parameter and prints out a Condition Code that pinpoints the obstacle contributing to its lack of identification. Basically, such problems relate to two situations. First, a parameter is linearly dependent on other parameters in the model, thereby causing the covariance matrix to be singular; the message appears as "LINEARLY DEPENDENT ON OTHER PARAMETERS." This situation occurs because either the parameter is underidentified in the model or it is empirically underidentified as a consequence of the data.

TABLE 3.3
EQS Output for Initially Hypothesized Four-Factor Model: Specification and Analysis Summary

---

COVARIANCE MATRIX TO BE ANALYZED: 16 VARIABLES (SELECTED FROM 46 VARIABLES)
BASED ON   265 CASES.

		SDQ2N01 V 25	SDQ2N13 V 26	SDQ2N25 V 27	SDQ2N37 V 28	SDQ2N04 V 29
SDQ2N01	V 25	1.818				
SDQ2N13	V 26	.684	1.845			
SDQ2N25	V 27	.752	.503	1.505		
SDQ2N37	V 28	.476	.656	.430	1.311	
SDQ2N04	V 29	.420	.665	.301	.470	1.963
SDQ2N16	V 30	.466	.554	.394	.579	.752
SDQ2N28	V 31	.377	.478	.349	.541	.692
SDQ2N40	V 32	.452	.542	.434	.663	.516
SDQ2N10	V 33	.351	.411	.253	.324	.595
SDQ2N22	V 34	.266	.343	.258	.301	.371
SDQ2N34	V 35	.363	.463	.284	.314	.231
SDQ2N46	V 36	.379	.374	.174	.225	.349
SDQ2N07	V 37	.562	.514	.544	.582	.885
SDQ2N19	V 38	.497	.566	.348	.477	.727
SDQ2N31	V 39	.576	.653	.579	.716	.882
SDQ2N43	V 40	.274	.474	.332	.345	.493

		SDQ2N16 V 30	SDQ2N28 V 31	SDQ2N40 V 32	SDQ2N10 V 33	SDQ2N22 V 34
SDQ2N16	V 30	1.539				
SDQ2N28	V 31	.948	1.775			
SDQ2N40	V 32	.878	.929	1.848		
SDQ2N10	V 33	.583	.519	.639	1.327	
SDQ2N22	V 34	.580	.507	.577	.586	1.190
SDQ2N34	V 35	.189	.080	.327	.512	.348
SDQ2N46	V 36	.473	.451	.605	.545	.527
SDQ2N07	V 37	1.022	.978	.890	.246	.246
SDQ2N19	V 38	1.002	1.063	1.039	.350	.366
SDQ2N31	V 39	1.075	1.124	1.017	.341	.371
SDQ2N43	V 40	.746	.747	.837	.226	.187

		SDQ2N34 V 35	SDQ2N46 V 36	SDQ2N07 V 37	SDQ2N19 V 38	SDQ2N31 V 39
SDQ2N34	V 35	2.901				
SDQ2N46	V 36	.454	1.682			
SDQ2N07	V 37	-.328	.213	3.173		
SDQ2N19	V 38	-.080	.161	2.003	2.870	
SDQ2N31	V 39	-.123	.331	2.247	1.763	2.466
SDQ2N43	V 40	-.067	.347	1.435	1.444	1.433

		SDQ2N43 V 40
SDQ2N43	V 40	1.962

BENTLER—WEEKS STRUCTURAL REPRESENTATION:

NUMBER OF DEPENDENT VARIABLES = 16
    DEPENDENT V'S :   25   26   27   28   29   30   31   32   33   34
    DEPENDENT V'S :   35   36   37   38   39   40

NUMBER OF INDEPENDENT VARIABLES = 20
    INDEPENDENT F'S :   1   2   3   4
    INDEPENDENT E'S :   25   26   27   28   29   30   31   32   33   34
    INDEPENDENT E'S :   35   36   37   38   39   40

NUMBER OF FREE PARAMETERS = 38
NUMBER OF FIXED NONZERO PARAMETERS = 20

PARAMETER ESTIMATES APPEAR IN ORDER,
NO SPECIAL PROBLEMS WERE ENCOUNTERED DURING OPTIMIZATION.

(For an extensive explanation of empirical identification [and underidentification], see Bollen, 1989a; Kenny, 1979; Kline, 1998; Maruyama, 1998; Rindskopf, 1984; and Wothke, 1993.) The second situation results from the presence of boundary parameters—those with values close to the boundary of admissible values; typical examples are correlation estimates greater than 1.00 and variance estimates that are zero or some negative value. In contrast to LISREL, which places no constraints on these parameters, EQS forces them to be held to a boundary value (i.e., 1.00 or zero). As such, the presence of boundary parameters in EQS generates one of two Condition Code messages: (a) "CONSTRAINED AT UPPER BOUND" or (b) "CONSTRAINED AT LOWER BOUND." (For greater elaboration on the cause and alternative approaches to addressing these difficulties, see Bentler, 2005; Bentler & Chou, 1987; Bollen, 1989a; and Rindskopf, 1984.)

Model Assessment. Of primary interest in SEM is the extent to which a hypothesized model "fits" or, in other words, adequately describes the sample data. Given findings of an inadequate goodness-of-fit, the next logical step is to detect the source of misfit in the model. Ideally, evaluation of model fit should derive from a variety of perspectives based on several criteria that can assess model fit. In particular, these criteria focus on the adequacy of (a) the model as a whole, and (b) the individual parameter estimates.

Model as a Whole

Before turning to this section of the EQS output, it is worthwhile to review five important aspects of fitting hypothesized models: (a) the rationale on which the model-fitting process is based, (b) the issue of statistical significance, (c) the estimation process, (d) the residual covariance matrices and (e) the goodness-of-fit statistics.

The Model-Fitting Process. In chap. 1, I presented a general description of this process and noted that the primary task is to determine the goodness-of-fit between the hypothesized model and the sample data. In other words, the researcher specifies a model and then uses the sample data to test the model.

With a view to helping you gain a better understanding of the material to be presented next in the output file, let's take a few moments to recast this model-fitting process within a more formalized framework. As such, let S represent the sample covariance matrix (of observed variable scores), Σ (sigma) the population covariance matrix, and θ (theta) a vector that comprises the model parameters. As such, $\Sigma(\theta)$ represents the restricted covariance matrix implied by the model (i.e., the specified structure of the hypothesized model). In SEM, the null hypothesis (H_0) being tested is that the postulated model holds in the population [i.e., $\Sigma = \Sigma(\theta)$]. In contrast to traditional statistical procedures, however, the researcher hopes *not* to reject H_0 (but see MacCallum, Browne, & Sugarawa, 1996, for proposed changes to this hypothesis-testing strategy).

The issue of statistical significance. The rationale underlying the practice of statistical significance testing has generated a plethora of criticism over at least the past four decades. Indeed, Cohen (1994) noted that, despite Rozeboom's (1960) admonition 45 years ago that "the statistical folkways of a more primitive past continue to dominate the local scene" (p. 417), this dubious practice still persists. (For an array of supportive as well as opposing views with respect to this article by a number of researchers, see the *American Psychologist* [1995], *50*, 1098–1103.) In light of this historical bank of criticism, together with the current pressure by methodologists to cease this traditional ritual (see, e.g., Cohen, 1994; Kirk, 1996; Schmidt, 1996; and Thompson, 1996), the Board of Scientific Affairs for the American Psychological Association appointed a task force to study the feasibility of phasing out the use of null hypothesis testing procedures, as described in course texts and reported in journal articles. Consequently, the end of statistical significance testing relative to traditional statistical methods may soon be a reality.

Statistical significance testing with respect to the analysis of covariance structures, however, is somewhat different in that it is driven by degrees of freedom involving the number of elements in the sample covariance matrix and the number of parameters to be estimated. Nonetheless, it is interesting that many of the issues raised with respect to the traditional statistical methods (e.g., practical significance, importance of confidence intervals, and importance of replication) have long been addressed in SEM applications. Indeed, it was this very issue of practical "nonsignificance" in model testing that led Bentler and Bonett (1980) to develop one of the first subjective indexes of fit (i.e., the NFI). Their work subsequently spawned the development of numerous additional practical indexes of fit, many of which are included in the EQS output shown in Table 3.5. Likewise, the early work of Steiger (1990; and Steiger & Lind, 1980) precipitated the call for use of confidence intervals in the reporting of SEM findings (see, e.g., MacCallum et al., 1996). Finally, the classic paper by Cliff (1983) denouncing the proliferation of post hoc model-fitting and criticizing the apparent lack of concern for the dangers of overfitting models to trivial effects arising from capitalization on chance factors, spirited the development of evaluation indexes (Browne & Cudeck, 1989; and Cudeck & Browne, 1983), as well as a general call for the increased use of cross-validation procedures (see, e.g., MacCallum et al., 1992, 1994).

The estimation process.   The primary focus of the estimation process in SEM is to yield parameter values such that the discrepancy (i.e., residual) between the sample covariance matrix S and the population covariance matrix implied by the model $[\Sigma(\theta)]$ is minimal. This objective is achieved by minimizing a discrepancy function, $F[S, \Sigma(\theta)]$, such that its minimal value (F_{min}) reflects the point in the estimation process where the discrepancy between S and $\Sigma(\theta)$ is least $[S - \Sigma(\theta) =$ minimum]. Taken together, then, F_{min} serves as a measure of the extent to which S differs from $\Sigma(\theta)$; any discrepancy between the two is captured by the residual covariance matrix. In EQS, information related to these residuals is presented first, followed by the global goodness-of-fit indexes. Table 3.4 summarizes the residual covariance matrices related to the hypothesized model.

TABLE 3.4
EQS Output for Initially Hypothesized Four-Factor Model: Residuals

RESIDUAL COVARIANCE MATRIX (S-SIGMA):

		SDQ2N01 V 25	SDQ2N13 V 26	SDQ2N25 V 27	SDQ2N37 V 28	SDQ2N04 V 29
SDQ2N01	V 25	.000				
SDQ2N13	V 26	.018	.000			
SDQ2N25	V 27	.229	-.063	.000		
SDQ2N37	V 28	-.098	.033	-.059	.000	
SDQ2N04	V 29	.003	.214	-.053	.080	.000
SDQ2N16	V 30	-.067	-.022	-.058	.081	.031
SDQ2N28	V 31	-.142	-.084	-.093	.056	-.010
SDQ2N40	V 32	-.072	-.026	-.012	.173	-.194
SDQ2N10	V 33	-.005	.025	-.050	-.009	.129
SDQ2N22	V 34	-.051	.000	-.011	.004	-.043
SDQ2N34	V 35	.124	.204	.081	.091	-.080
SDQ2N46	V 36	.079	.049	-.081	-.056	-.044
SDQ2N07	V 37	-.075	-.177	.002	-.013	.009
SDQ2N19	V 38	-.039	-.015	-.108	-.024	-.010
SDQ2N31	V 39	-.031	-.005	.062	.149	.048
SDQ2N43	V 40	-.143	.021	-.024	-.046	-.081

		SDQ2N16 V 30	SDQ2N28 V 31	SDQ2N40 V 32	SDQ2N10 V 33	SDQ2N22 V 34
SDQ2N16	V 30	.000				
SDQ2N28	V 31	.050	.000			
SDQ2N40	V 32	-.028	.044	.000		
SDQ2N10	V 33	-.012	-.061	.053	.000	
SDQ2N22	V 34	.050	-.009	.055	-.010	.000
SDQ2N34	V 35	-.210	-.309	-.066	.062	-.051
SDQ2N46	V 36	-.029	-.039	.111	-.021	.025
SDQ2N07	V 37	-.098	-.114	-.213	-.085	-.049
SDQ2N19	V 38	.060	.144	.111	.071	.118
SDQ2N31	V 39	.008	.084	-.034	.025	.090
SDQ2N43	V 40	.012	.031	.114	.009	-.007

		SDQ2N34 V 35	SDQ2N46 V 36	SDQ2N07 V 37	SDQ2N19 V 38	SDQ2N31 V 39
SDQ2N34	V 35	.000				
SDQ2N46	V 36	.075	.000			
SDQ2N07	V 37	-.551	-.067	.000		
SDQ2N19	V 38	-.267	-.075	.055	.000	
SDQ2N31	V 39	-.335	.065	.042	-.092	.000
SDQ2N43	V 40	-.213	.164	-.082	.168	-.012

		SDQ2N43 V 40
SDQ2N43	V 40	.000

AVERAGE ABSOLUTE COVARIANCE RESIDUALS =	.0684
AVERAGE OFF-DIAGONAL ABSOLUTE COVARIANCE RESIDUALS =	.0775

(Continued)

TABLE 3.4
(Continued)

STANDARDIZED RESIDUAL MATRIX:

		SDQ2N01 V 25	SDQ2N13 V 26	SDQ2N25 V 27	SDQ2N37 V 28	SDQ2N04 V 29
SDQ2N01	V 25	.000				
SDQ2N13	V 26	.010	.000			
SDQ2N25	V 27	.138	-.038	.000		
SDQ2N37	V 28	-.064	.021	-.042	.000	
SDQ2N04	V 29	.002	.112	-.031	.050	.000
SDQ2N16	V 30	-.040	-.013	-.038	.057	.018
SDQ2N28	V 31	-.079	-.046	-.057	.036	-.006
SDQ2N40	V 32	-.039	-.014	-.007	.111	-.102
SDQ2N10	V 33	-.003	.016	-.035	-.007	.080
SDQ2N22	V 34	-.034	.000	-.008	.004	-.028
SDQ2N34	V 35	.054	.088	.039	.047	-.034
SDQ2N46	V 36	.045	.028	-.051	-.038	-.024
SDQ2N07	V 37	-.031	-.073	.001	-.007	.004
SDQ2N19	V 38	-.017	-.006	-.052	-.012	-.004
SDQ2N31	V 39	-.014	-.002	.032	.083	.022
SDQ2N43	V 40	-.076	.011	-.014	-.029	-.041

		SDQ2N16 V 30	SDQ2N28 V 31	SDQ2N40 V 32	SDQ2N10 V 33	SDQ2N22 V 34
SDQ2N16	V 30	.000				
SDQ2N28	V 31	.030	.000			
SDQ2N40	V 32	-.017	.025	.000		
SDQ2N10	V 33	-.009	-.040	.034	.000	
SDQ2N22	V 34	.037	-.006	.037	-.008	.000
SDQ2N34	V 35	-.099	-.136	-.028	.032	-.028
SDQ2N46	V 36	-.018	-.022	.063	-.014	.017
SDQ2N07	V 37	-.044	-.048	-.088	-.042	-.025
SDQ2N19	V 38	.028	.064	.048	.036	.064
SDQ2N31	V 39	.004	.040	-.016	.014	.053
SDQ2N43	V 40	.007	.017	.060	.005	-.004

		SDQ2N34 V 35	SDQ2N46 V 36	SDQ2N07 V 37	SDQ2N19 V 38	SDQ2N31 V 39
SDQ2N34	V 35	.000				
SDQ2N46	V 36	.034	.000			
SDQ2N07	V 37	-.181	-.029	.000		
SDQ2N19	V 38	-.093	-.034	.018	.000	
SDQ2N31	V 39	-.125	.032	.015	-.034	.000
SDQ2N43	V 40	-.089	.090	-.033	.071	-.005

		SDQ2N43 V 40
SDQ2N43	V 40	.000

AVERAGE ABSOLUTE STANDARDIZED RESIDUALS = .0342
AVERAGE OFF-DIAGONAL ABSOLUTE STANDARDIZED RESIDUALS = .0388

TABLE 3.4
(Continued)

```
LARGEST STANDARDIZED RESIDUALS:
NO.   PARAMETER    ESTIMATE    NO.   PARAMETER    ESTIMATE
---   ---------    --------    ---   ---------    --------
 1    V37, V35      -.181      11    V40, V35      -.089
 2    V27, V25       .138      12    V35, V26       .088
 3    V35, V31      -.136      13    V37, V32      -.088
 4    V39, V35      -.125      14    V39, V28       .083
 5    V29, V26       .112      15    V33, V29       .080
 6    V32, V28       .111      16    V31, V25      -.079
 7    V32, V29      -.102      17    V40, V25      -.076
 8    V35, V30      -.099      18    V37, V26      -.073
 9    V38, V35      -.093      19    V40, V38       .071
10    V40, V36       .090      20    V38, V34       .064
```

```
DISTRIBUTION OF STANDARDIZED RESIDUALS
    ---------------------------------
   !                              !
80-!                              -
   !                              !
   !            *                 !          RANGE      FREQ   PERCENT
   !            *                 !
   !            *  *              !      1  -0.5  -  --      0    .00%
60-!            *  *              -      2  -0.4  -  -0.5    0    .00%
   !            *  *              !      3  -0.3  -  -0.4    0    .00%
   !            *  *              !      4  -0.2  -  -0.3    0    .00%
   !            *  *              !      5  -0.1  -  -0.2    4   2.94%
40-!            *  *              -      6   0.0  -  -0.1   68  50.00%
   !            *  *              !      7   0.1  -   0.0   61  44.85%
   !            *  *              !      8   0.2  -   0.1    3   2.21%
   !            *  *              !      9   0.3  -   0.2    0    .00%
20-!            *  *              -      A   0.4  -   0.3    0    .00%
   !            *  *              !      B   0.5  -   0.4    0    .00%
   !            *  *              !      C   ++   -   0.5    0    .00%
   !         *  *  *  *           !      ---------------------------------
    ---------------------------------    TOTAL          136 100.00%
    1  2  3  4  5  6  7  8  9  A  B  C   EACH "*" REPRESENTS 4 RESIDUALS
```

Residual covariance matrices. Each element in the residual matrix represents the discrepancy between the covariances in $\Sigma(\theta)$ and those in S [i.e., $\Sigma(\theta) - $ S]; that is, there is one residual for each pair of observed variables (Jöreskog, 1993). In the case of this hypothesized model, for example, the residual matrix would contain $[(16 \times 17)/2] = 136$ elements. It is worth noting that, as in conventional regression analysis, the residuals are not independent of one another. Thus, any attempts to test them (in the strict statistical sense) would be inappropriate. In essence, only their magnitude is of interest in alerting the researcher to possible areas of model misfit.

EQS provides both unstandardized and standardized residual covariance matrices. Given that a model describes the data well, these residual values should be small and evenly distributed. Large residuals associated with particular parameters indicate their misspecification in the model, thereby affecting the overall model misfit. For both the unstandardized and standardized residual matrices, EQS computes two averages: one based on all elements of the lower triangular matrix, the other ignoring the diagonal elements. Typically, the off-diagonal elements play a more major role in the effect of goodness-of-fit χ^2 statistics (Bentler, 2005). Based on an ordering from large to small, the program then lists the 20 largest standardized residuals and designates which pairs of variables are involved. Finally, a frequency distribution of the standardized residuals is presented. Ideally, this distribution should be symmetric and centered around zero.

Because the fitted residuals are dependent on the unit of measurement of the observed variables, they can be difficult to interpret; thus, their standardized values are typically examined. Standardized residuals are fitted residuals divided by their asymptotically (large sample) standard errors (Jöreskog & Sörbom, 1988). As such, they are analogous to Z-scores and are therefore the easier of the two sets of residual values to interpret. In essence, they represent estimates of the number of standard deviations the observed residuals are from the zero residuals that would exist if model fit were perfect [i.e., $\Sigma(\theta) - S = .0$]. Values >2.58 are considered large (Jöreskog & Sörbom, 1988). In examining the standardized residual information in Table 3.4, we see that the average off-diagonal value is .0342, whereas the largest off-diagonal value is .0388, both of which reflect a very good fit to the data. Finally, a review of the frequency distribution reveals most residual values (94.85%) to fall between −.1 and .1. Of the remaining residuals, 2.94% fall between −0.1 and −0.2 (see values −1.81, .136, .125, .102) and 2.21% fall between 0.1 and 0.2 (see values .138, .112, .111). From this information, we can conclude that although there may be some minimal discrepancy in fit between the hypothesized model and the sample data, overall, the model as a whole appears to be quite well fitting.

The goodness-of-fit statistics.   Let's turn now to the goodness-of-fit statistics presented in Table 3.5. Here we find statistics reported for several goodness-of-fit values, all of which relate to the model as a whole.[7] The first of these values represents the INDEPENDENCE CHI-SQUARE statistic ($\chi^2_{(120)} = 1696.728$), as it relates to the Independence model. This model (also termed the *null* model) is so named because it represents complete independence from all variables in the model (i.e., all variables in the model are mutually uncorrelated). Although other baseline models have been proposed (see, e.g., Sobel & Bohrnstedt, 1985), Rigdon (1996) noted that beginning with the work of Tucker and Lewis (1973), the independence baseline model is the one most widely used. Indeed, Bentler and Bonett (1980) argued that in large samples, the independence model serves as a good baseline against which to compare alternative models to evaluate the gain in improved fit. That is, given a sound hypothesized model, one would expect the χ^2 value for the independence model to be extremely high, thereby indicating excessive misfit; such is the case with the present example.

---

[7]Had the /PRINT paragraph not been included in the input file, only the default goodness-of-fit indexes would have been reported; these include all statistics down to and including the CFI.

TABLE 3.5

EQS Output for Initially Hypothesized Four-Factor Model: Goodness-of-Fit Statistics

```
GOODNESS OF FIT SUMMARY FOR METHOD = ML

INDEPENDENCE MODEL CHI-SQUARE     =    1696.728 ON    120 DEGREES OF FREEDOM

INDEPENDENCE AIC =  1456.72826    INDEPENDENCE CAIC =    907.16068
      MODEL AIC =   -37.48818          MODEL CAIC =  -486.30170

CHI-SQUARE =       158.512 BASED ON        98 DEGREES OF FREEDOM
PROBABILITY VALUE FOR THE CHI-SQUARE STATISTIC IS          .00011

THE NORMAL THEORY RLS CHI-SQUARE FOR THIS ML SOLUTION IS          152.727.


FIT INDICES
-----------

BENTLER-BONETT       NORMED FIT INDEX =      .907
BENTLER-BONETT NON-NORMED FIT INDEX =      .953
COMPARATIVE FIT INDEX (CFI)          =      .962
BOLLEN    (IFI) FIT INDEX            =      .962
MCDONALD (MFI) FIT INDEX             =      .892
LISREL     GFI  FIT INDEX            =      .933
LISREL    AGFI  FIT INDEX            =      .906
ROOT MEAN-SQUARE RESIDUAL (RMR)      =      .104
STANDARDIZED RMR                     =      .048
ROOT MEAN-SQUARE ERROR OF APPROXIMATION (RMSEA)      =      .048
90% CONFIDENCE INTERVAL OF RMSEA  (       .034,       .062)

                       ITERATIVE SUMMARY
                    PARAMETER
ITERATION           ABS CHANGE        ALPHA              FUNCTION
    1                .584046          .50000              3.03565
    2                .313485         1.00000              1.36061
    3                .076048         1.00000               .62068
    4                .038441         1.00000               .60229
    5                .004573         1.00000               .60056
    6                .003231         1.00000               .60044
    7                .000542         1.00000               .60042
```

Now skip down three lines to the chi-square value reported for the hypothesized four-factor model. The value of 158.512 represents the discrepancy between the unrestricted sample covariance matrix S and the restricted covariance matrix $\Sigma(\theta)$ and, in essence, represents the Likelihood Ratio Test statistic, most commonly expressed as a chi-square (χ^2) statistic. This statistic is equal to $(N - 1)F_{min}$ (i.e., sample size minus 1 multiplied by the minimum fit function) and in large samples is distributed as a central χ^2 with degrees of freedom equal to $1/2(p)(p + 1) - t$, where p is the number of observed variables and t is the number of parameters to be estimated (Bollen, 1989a). In general, $H_0 : \Sigma = \Sigma(\theta)$ is equivalent to the hypothesis that $\Sigma - \Sigma(\theta) = 0$; the χ^2 test, then, simultaneously tests the extent to which all residuals in $\Sigma - \Sigma(\theta)$ are zero (Bollen, 1989a). Framed somewhat differently, the null hypothesis (H_0) postulates that specification of the factor loadings, factor variances–covariances, and error variances for the model under study are valid; the χ^2 test simultaneously tests the extent to which this specification is true. The probability value associated with χ^2 represents the likelihood of obtaining a χ^2 value that exceeds the χ^2 value when H_0 is true. Thus, the higher the probability associated with χ^2, the closer the fit between the hypothesized model (under H_0) and the perfect fit (Bollen, 1989a).

The test of H_0—that SC is a four-factor structure as depicted in Fig. 3.1— yielded a χ^2 value of 158.512, with 98 degrees of freedom and a probability of less than .0001 (p < .0001), thereby suggesting that the fit of the data to the hypothesized model is not entirely adequate. Interpreted literally, this test statistic indicates that given the present data, the hypothesis bearing on SC relations, as summarized in the model, represents an unlikely event (i.e., occurring less than one time in a thousand under the null hypothesis) and should be rejected. The sensitivity of the χ^2 likelihood ratio test to sample size, however, is well known and is addressed shortly.

In addition to furnishing χ^2 statistics for the independence and hypothesized models, EQS provides for the evaluation of both models based on Akaike's (1987) Information Criterion (AIC) and Bozdogan's (1987) consistent version of the AIC (CAIC). Both criteria address the issue of parsimony in the assessment of model fit; that is, statistical goodness-of-fit as well as the number of estimated parameters are taken into account. However, Bozdogan (1987) noted that the AIC carried a penalty only as it related to degrees of freedom (thereby reflecting the number of estimated parameters in the model) and not to sample size; he subsequently proposed the CAIC, which takes sample size into account (Bandalos, 1993). Although both criteria were developed for maximum likelihood (ML) estimation, they are applied to all estimation methods in EQS.

The AIC and CAIC are used in the comparison of two or more models with smaller values representing a better fit of the hypothesized model (Hu & Bentler, 1995). The AIC and CAIC indexes also share the same conceptual framework; as such, they reflect the extent to which parameter estimates from the original sample will cross-validate in future samples (Bandalos, 1993). Returning to the output, we see that the AIC statistic for both the independence and hypothesized models is substantially smaller than the χ^2 statistic.[8]

Before reviewing the remaining goodness-of-fit statistics, let's first return to the issue of χ^2 sensitivity. In particular, both the sensitivity of the Likelihood Ratio Test to sample size and its basis on the central χ^2 distribution, which assumes that the model fits perfectly in the population (i.e., that H_0 is correct), have led to problems of fit that are now widely known. Because the χ^2 statistic equals $(N - 1)F_{min}$, this value tends to be substantial when the model does not hold and sample size is large (Jöreskog & Sörbom, 1993). Yet, the analysis of covariance structures is grounded in large sample theory. As such, large samples are critical to obtaining precise parameter estimates, as well as to the tenability of asymptotic

---

[8]Readers are referred to the EQS manual (Bentler, 2005) for an explanation of the CAIC.

distributional approximations (MacCallum et al., 1996). Thus, findings of well-fitting hypothesized models, where the χ^2 value approximates the degrees of freedom, have proven to be unrealistic in most SEM empirical research. More common are findings of a large χ^2 relative to degrees of freedom, thereby indicating a need to modify the model to better fit the data (Jöreskog & Sörbom, 1993). Thus, results related to the test of the hypothesized model are not unexpected. Indeed, given this problematic aspect of the Likelihood Ratio Test and the fact that postulated models (no matter how good) can only ever fit real-world data approximately and never exactly, MacCallum et al. (1996) proposed changes to the traditional hypothesis-testing approach in covariance structure modeling. (For an extended discussion of these changes, see MacCallum et al., 1996.)

Researchers addressed the χ^2 limitations by developing goodness-of-fit indexes that take a more pragmatic approach to the evaluation process. To this end, the past two decades have witnessed a plethora of newly developed fit indexes as well as unique approaches to the model-fitting process (for reviews, see, e.g., Gerbing & Anderson, 1993; Hu & Bentler, 1995; Marsh, Balla, & McDonald, 1988; and Tanaka, 1993). These criteria, referred to as "subjective," "practical," or "ad hoc" indexes of fit, are now commonly used as adjuncts to the χ^2 statistic. At the time of writing this book, EQS users are able to select from 10 of these indexes, as reproduced in Table 3.5 (but only if the /PRINT $\hookrightarrow$ Fit = All is specified in the input file).

The first four fit indexes listed in the output (see Table 3.5) fall into the category of comparative (Browne, MacCallum, Kim, Andersen, & Glaser, 2002) or incremental (Hu & Bentler, 1995, 1999) fit indexes. These indexes measure the proportionate improvement in fit by comparing a hypothesized model with a more restricted, nested baseline model.[9] As discussed previously, the independence (or *null*) model is typically the most commonly used baseline model (Hu & Bentler, 1999; and Rigdon, 1996).

For more than two decades, Bentler and Bonett's (1980) Normed Fit Index (NFI) has been the practical criterion of choice, as evidenced in large part by the current "classic" status of its original paper (Bentler, 1992; and Bentler & Bonett, 1987). However, addressing evidence that the NFI has shown a tendency to underestimate fit in small samples, Bentler (1990) revised the NFI to consider sample size and proposed the Comparative Fit Index (CFI). Values for both the NFI and CFI range from zero to 1.00 and are derived from comparison between the hypothesized and independence models, as described previously. As such, each provides a measure of complete covariation in the data. Although a value $> .90$ was originally considered representative of a well-fitting model (see Bentler, 1992), a revised cutoff value close to 0.95 has been advised (Hu & Bentler, 1999). Although both indexes of fit

---

[9]Nested models are hierarchically related to one another in the sense that their parameter sets are subsets of one another (i.e., particular parameters are freely estimated in one model but fixed to zero in a second model) (Bentler & Chou, 1987; and Bollen, 1989a).

are reported in the EQS output, Bentler (1990) suggested that the CFI should be the index of choice. The program also reports the Non-Normed Fit Index (NNFI), a variant of the NFI that takes model complexity into account. Values for the NNFI can exceed those reported for the NFI and can also fall outside the zero to 1.00 range.

As shown in Table 3.5, all three indexes (NFI = .907, NNFI = .953, CFI = .962) were consistent in suggesting that the hypothesized model represented an adequate fit to the data, albeit the value reported for the NFI reflected only a marginally well-fitting model. However, considering the CFI to be the most appropriate index of the three, we consider the fit of this model to be satisfactory.

The Incremental Fit Index (IFI; Bollen, 1989b) represents a derivative of the NFI; as with both the NFI and CFI, the IFI coefficient values range from zero to 1.00, with values close to 0.95 indicating superior fit (see Hu & Bentler, 1999). More specifically, the IFI was developed to address the issues of parsimony and sample size, which were known to be associated with the NFI. As such, its computation is basically the same as the NFI, except that degrees of freedom are considered. Thus, it is not surprising that the finding of IFI = .962 is consistent with that of the CFI in reflecting a well-fitting model.

The next three fit indexes reported in the output file in Table 3.5 (i.e., MFI, GFI, and AGFI) belong to the category of "absolute" fit indexes. In contrast to the previous incremental fit indexes, the absolute fit indexes do not rely on comparison with a reference model to determine the amount of improvement in model fit; rather, they depend only on how well the hypothesized model fits the sample data (Browne et al., 2002; and Hu & Bentler, 1999). Nonetheless, Hu and Bentler (1999, p. 2) noted that "an implicit or explicit comparison may be made to a saturated model that exactly reproduces the sample covariance matrix."[10] The McDonald Fit Index (MFI; McDonald, 1989) represents a normed measure of the centrality parameter that transforms the rescaled noncentrality parameter,[11] which assesses model misfit (Hu & Bentler, 1995). Although the MFI is similar to the RMSEA (described shortly), it does not provide for a fit-per-degree-of-freedom interpretation. The Goodness-of-Fit Index (GFI; Jöreskog & Sörbom, 1984) is

---

[10] A saturated model is one in which the number of estimated parameters equals the number of data points (i.e., variances and covariances of the observed variables as in the case of the just-identified model). Conceptualized within the framework of a continuum, the saturated (i.e., least restricted) model would represent one extreme endpoint, whereas the independence (the most restricted) model would represent the other; a hypothesized model always represents a point somewhere between the two.

[11] The noncentrality parameter is a fixed parameter with associated degrees of freedom and can be denoted as $\chi^2_{(df,\lambda)}$. Essentially, it functions as a measure of the discrepancy between Σ and $\Sigma(\theta)$ and thus can be regarded as a "population badness-of-fit" (Steiger, 1990). As such, the greater the discrepancy between Σ and $\Sigma(\theta)$, the larger the λ value. It is now easy to see that the central χ^2 statistic is a special case of the noncentral χ^2 distribution when $\lambda = 0.0$. (For an excellent discussion and graphic portrayal of differences between the central and noncentral χ^2 statistics, see MacCallum et al., 1996.)

a measure of the relative amount of variance and covariance in S that is jointly explained by Σ. The AGFI differs from the GFI only in the fact that it adjusts for the number of degrees of freedom in the specified model. As such, it addresses the issue of parsimony by incorporating a penalty for the inclusion of additional parameters. Although the GFI and AGFI are commonly reported in the SEM literature, Hu and Bentler (1998) recommended against their use as indexes of fit. In addition to being insufficiently and inconsistently sensitive to model misspecification, Marsh et al. (1988) have shown both indexes to be strongly influenced by sample size.

Although values reported for these three absolute fit indexes range from zero to 1.0, the MFI can exceed 1.0 due to sampling error (Browne et al., 2002; and Hu & Bentler, 1995, 1999), and it is possible for both the GFI and AGFI to be negative (Jöreskog and Sörbom, 1993). The latter, of course, should not occur because it would reflect the fact that the model fits worse than no model at all. Although values greater than 0.90 for the GFI and AGFI are considered to represent a well-fitting model, Hu and Bentler (1999) suggested a cutoff score of .89 for the MFI. Based on the MFI, GFI, and AGFI values reported in Table 3.5 (.892, .933, and .906, respectively), albeit cognitive of their deficiencies noted earlier, we can again conclude that the hypothesized model fits the sample data fairly well.

Finally, although the last three indexes listed in Table 3.5 (i.e., RMR, SRMR, and RMSEA) are also categorized as absolute fit indexes, Browne et al. (2002, p. 405) termed them more specifically as "absolute *misfit* indices." Although both sets of indexes depend only on the fit of the hypothesized model, the absolute fit indexes (MFI, GFI, and AGFI in this instance) increase as goodness-of-fit improves, whereas the absolute misfit indexes decrease as goodness-of-fit improves and attain their lower-bound value of zero when the model fits perfectly (Browne et al., 2002).

The root mean square residual (RMR) represents the average residual value derived from the fitting of the variance–covariance matrix for the hypothesized model $\Sigma(\theta)$ to the variance–covariance matrix of the sample data (S). However, because these residuals are relative to the sizes of the observed variances and covariances, they are difficult to interpret. Thus, they are best interpreted in the metric of the correlation matrix (Hu & Bentler, 1995; and Jöreskog & Sörbom, 1989). Therefore, the standardized RMR (SRMR) represents the average value across all standardized residuals and ranges from zero to 1.00; in a well-fitting model, this value is small—say .05 or less. Review of the output in Table 3.5 shows that the unstandardized residual value reported for the hypothesized model is .104, whereas the SRMR value is .048. Given that the SRMR represents the average discrepancy between the observed sample and hypothesized correlation matrices, we can interpret this value as meaning that the model explains the correlations to within an average error of .043 (Hu & Bentler, 1995).

The Root Mean Square Error of Approximation (RMSEA) and the conceptual framework within which it is embedded were first proposed by Steiger and Lind in 1980, yet the RMSEA has only recently been recognized as one of the most informative criteria in covariance structure modeling. The RMSEA considers the error of approximation in the population and asks the question, "How well would the model, with unknown but optimally chosen parameter values, fit the population covariance matrix if it were available?" (Browne & Cudeck, 1993, pp. 137–8). This discrepancy, as measured by the RMSEA, is expressed per degree of freedom, thus making it sensitive to the number of estimated parameters in the model (i.e., the complexity of the model). Values less than .05 indicate good fit, and values as high as .08 represent reasonable errors of approximation in the population (Browne & Cudeck, 1993). MacCallum et al. (1996) elaborated on those cutpoints and noted that RMSEA values ranging from .08 to .10 indicate mediocre fit and those greater than .10 indicate poor fit. Although Hu and Bentler (1999) suggested a value of .06 to indicate good fit between the hypothesized model and the observed data, they cautioned that when sample size is small, the RMSEA tends to over-reject true population models. Noting that these criteria are based solely on subjective judgment and therefore cannot be regarded as infallible or correct, Browne and Cudeck (1993) and MacCallum et al. (1996) nonetheless argued, that they would appear to be more realistic than a requirement of exact fit, where RMSEA = 0.0. (For a generalization of the RMSEA to multiple independent samples, see Steiger, 1998.)

Overall, MacCallum and Austin (2000) strongly recommended routine use of the RMSEA for at least three reasons: (a) it would appear to be adequately sensitive to model misspecification (Hu & Bentler, 1998); (b) commonly used interpretative guidelines would appear to yield appropriate conclusions regarding model quality (Hu & Bentler, 1998, 1999); and (c) it is possible to build confidence intervals around RMSEA values.

Addressing Steiger's (1990) call for the use of confidence intervals to assess the precision of RMSEA estimates, EQS reports a 90% interval around the RMSEA value. In contrast to point estimates of model fit (which do not reflect the imprecision of the estimate), confidence intervals can yield this information, thereby providing the researcher with more assistance in the evaluation of model fit. Thus, MacCallum et al. (1996) strongly urged the use of confidence intervals in practice. Presented with a small RMSEA, albeit a wide confidence interval, a researcher would conclude that the estimated discrepancy value is quite imprecise, thereby negating any possibility of accurately determining the degree of fit in the population. In contrast, a narrow confidence interval would argue for good precision of the RMSEA value in reflecting model fit in the population (MacCallum et al., 1996).

Table 3.5 shows that the RMSEA value for the hypothesized model is .048, with the 90% confidence interval ranging from .034 to .062. Interpretation of the confidence interval indicates that we can be 90% confident that the true RMSEA value in the population will fall within the bounds of .034 and .062, which represents a good degree of precision. Given that (a) the RMSEA point estimate is <.05 (.048), and (b) the upper bound of the 90% interval is .062, which is less than the value suggested by Browne and Cudeck (1993)—albeit equal to the cut-off value proposed by Hu and Bentler (1999)—we can conclude that the initially hypothesized model fits the data well.

Before leaving this discussion of the RMSEA, it is important to note that confidence intervals can be influenced seriously by sample size as well as model complexity (MacCallum et al., 1996). For example, if sample size is small and the number of estimated parameters is large, the confidence interval will be wide. Given a complex model (i.e., a large number of estimated parameters), a large sample size would be required to obtain a reasonably narrow confidence interval. Conversely if the number of parameters is small, then the probability of obtaining a narrow confidence interval is high, even for samples of rather moderate size (MacCallum et al., 1996).

Having worked your way through these goodness-of-fit measures, you no doubt are feeling totally overwhelmed and wondering what to do with all this information! Although the entire set of fit indexes does not need to be reported, such an array can provide a good sense of how well a model fits the sample data. But how does one choose which indexes are appropriate in the assessment of model fit? Unfortunately, this choice is not a simple one, primarily because particular indexes have been shown to operate somewhat differently given the sample size, estimation procedure, model complexity, and/or violation of the underlying assumptions of multivariate normality and variable independence. Thus, Hu and Bentler (1995) cautioned, that in choosing which goodness-of-fit indexes to use in the assessment of model fit, careful consideration of these critical factors is essential. In reporting results for the remaining applications in this book, goodness-of-fit indexes are limited to the CFI, SRMR, and RMSEA, along with the related χ^2 value and RMSEA 90% confidence interval. Readers who want further elaboration on these goodness-of-fit statistics with respect to their formulae and functions—and/or the extent to which they are affected by sample size, estimation procedures, misspecification, and/or violations of assumptions—are referred to Bandalos, 1993; Bentler & Yuan, 1999; Bollen, 1989a; Browne & Cudeck, 1993; Curran, West, & Finch, 1996; Fan, Thompson, & Wang, 1999; Finch, West, & MacKinnon, 1997; Gerbing & Anderson, 1993; Hu & Bentler, 1995, 1998, 1999; Hu, Bentler, & Kano, 1992; Jöreskog & Sörbom, 1993; La Du & Tanaka, 1989; Marsh et al., 1988; Mulaik, James, van Altine, Bennett, Lind, & Stilwell, 1989; Raykov & Widaman, 1995; Sugawara & MacCallum, 1993; Tomarken & Waller, 2005; Weng & Cheng, 1997; West, Finch, & Curran, 1995; Wheaton, 1987; and Williams & Holahan, 1994. For an annotated bibliography, see Austin & Calderón, 1996.

To finalize this subsection on model assessment, I wish to leave you with this important reminder: global fit indexes alone cannot possibly envelop all that needs to be known about a model to judge the adequacy of its fit to the sample data. As Sobel and Bohrnstedt (1985, p. 158) so cogently stated two decades ago, "Scientific progress could be impeded if fit coefficients (even appropriate ones) are used as the primary criterion for judging the adequacy of a model." They further posited that despite the problematic nature of the χ^2 statistic, exclusive reliance on goodness-of-fit indexes is unacceptable. Indeed, fit indexes provide no guarantee that a model is useful. In fact, it is entirely possible for a model to fit well and still be incorrectly specified (Wheaton, 1987). (For an excellent review of ways by which such a seemingly dichotomous event can happen, see Bentler and Chou, 1987.) Fit indexes yield information bearing only on the model's *lack of fit*. More important, they can in no way reflect the extent to which the model is plausible; *this judgment rests squarely on the shoulders of the researcher*. Thus, assessment of model adequacy must be based on multiple criteria that take into account theoretical, statistical, and practical considerations.

The last piece of information related to overall model fit appearing on the output in Table 3.5 is the ITERATIVE SUMMARY. Here we see a synopsis of the number of iterations required for a convergent solution and the mean absolute change in parameter estimates (PARAMETER ABS CHANGE) associated with each iteration. The best scenario is a situation in which only a few iterations are needed to reach convergence; after the first two or three iterations, the change in parameter estimates stabilizes and remains minimal. As indicated in Table 3.5, this is the case with our CFA model, in which only seven iterations were needed to reach convergence. After the first three iterations, the parameter values remained relatively stable.

At the very worst, the number of iterations exceeds the default value of 30, resulting in nonconvergence; as such, the iterative process terminates and a message warning the user not to trust the output is issued. If this problem is presented, it is unlikely that a simple resubmission of the job with a requested extension in the number of iterations (e.g., /TECHNICAL $\hookrightarrow$ Iter = 500;) will resolve the dilemma. Rather, the user should look for other means of resolution. In my experience, I have found this situation to be easily solved just by attending to the start values. If start values were not included in the input file, then add them; if they were included, make a few modifications. Given that start values were included, lack of convergence occurs most often due to a wide discrepancy between the start values and actual estimated values related to only a few parameters. A typical example is one in which the start value is positive but the actual estimate is negative. A quick way to determine more appropriate start values is to review the estimates provided with the failed output; despite the fact that many of these estimates may be inaccurate, they can often guide the user to a start value that better approximates the actual estimated value. The most efficient approach to achieving more appropriate start values is to use the RETEST option provided by EQS. This option is introduced and discussed in Chap. 6.

A final point about Table 3.5 is the FUNCTION column. In general, EQS minimizes a fit function and when iterations stop, this value should be at the minimum value, with $\chi^2 = (N - 1) \times$ Function. Within the context of the current model, this formulation gives a χ^2 value of $264 \times 0.60042 = 158.51$.

Assessment of Individual Parameter Estimates

This discussion of model fit assessment has thus far concentrated on the model as a whole. Now, we turn our attention to the fit of individual parameters in the model. There are two aspects of concern: (a) the appropriateness of the estimates, and (b) their statistical significance. Parameter estimates and related information are presented in Table 3.6.

Feasibility of parameter estimates. The initial step in assessing the fit of individual parameters in a model is to determine the viability of their estimated values. Specifically, parameter estimates should exhibit the correct sign and size and be consistent with the underlying theory. Any estimates falling outside the admissable range signal a clear indication that either the model is wrong or the input matrix lacks sufficient information. Examples of parameters exhibiting unreasonable estimates are correlations >1.00, negative variances, and covariance or correlation matrices that are not positive definite.

Appropriateness of standard errors. Another indicator of poor model fit is the presence of standard errors that are excessively large or small. For example, if a standard error approaches zero, the test statistic for its related parameter cannot be defined (Bentler, 2005). Likewise, standard errors that are extremely large indicate parameters that cannot be determined (Jöreskog & Sörbom, 1989). Because standard errors are influenced by the units of measurement in observed and/or latent variables, as well as the magnitude of the parameter estimate itself, no definitive criterion of "small" and "large" has been established (Jöreskog & Sörbom, 1989).

Statistical significance of parameter estimates. The test statistic here represents the parameter estimate divided by its standard error; as such, it operates as a Z-statistic in testing that the estimate is statistically different from zero. Based on an α level of .05, the test statistic needs to be $> \pm1.96$ before the hypothesis (i.e., that the estimate $= 0.0$) can be rejected. Nonsignificant parameters, with the exception of error variances, can be considered unimportant to the model; in the interest of scientific parsimony, albeit given an adequate sample size, they should be deleted from the model. Conversely nonsignificant parameters can be indicative of a sample size that is too small (Jöreskog, pers. comm., January 1997). Finally, conclusions based on a series of univariate tests, as in this case, may differ from those based on a multivariate test in which a set of parameters is considered simultaneously. Although this multivariate option is available to EQS users via the Wald Test (WTest; Wald, 1943), it is not considered herein due to space constraints but is illustrated in subsequent chapters.

Scanning the output in the printout presented in Table 3.6, we see that the unstandardized estimates are presented first, followed by the standardized solution. Both sets of estimates are presented separately for the measurement equations, the variances, and the covariances. Looking more closely at the unstandardized estimates, we see that for variables SDQ2N01 (V25), SDQ2N04 (V29), SDQ2N10 (V33),

TABLE 3.6

EQS Output for Initially Hypothesized Four-Factor Model: Parameter Estimates

---

MEASUREMENT EQUATIONS WITH STANDARD ERRORS AND TEST STATISTICS
STATISTICS SIGNIFICANT AT THE 5% LEVEL ARE MARKED WITH @.

SDQ2N01 =V25 =   1.000 F1   + 1.000 E25

SDQ2N13 =V26 =   1.084*F1   + 1.000 E26
        .154
       7.027@

SDQ2N25 =V27 =   .851*F1   + 1.000 E27
        .132
       6.437@

SDQ2N37 =V28 =   .935*F1   + 1.000 E28
        .131
       7.117@

SDQ2N04 =V29 =   1.000 F2   + 1.000 E29

SDQ2N16 =V30 =   1.278*F2   + 1.000 E30
        .150
       8.507@

SDQ2N28 =V31 =   1.247*F2   + 1.000 E31
        .154
       8.083@

SDQ2N40 =V32 =   1.259*F2   + 1.000 E32
        .157
       8.037@

SDQ2N10 =V33 =   1.000 F3   + 1.000 E33

SDQ2N22 =V34 =   .889*F3   + 1.000 E34
        .103
       8.643@

SDQ2N34 =V35 =   .670*F3   + 1.000 E35
        .148
       4.528@

SDQ2N46 =V36 =   .843*F3   + 1.000 E36
        .117
       7.212@

SDQ2N07 =V37 =   1.000 F4   + 1.000 E37

SDQ2N19 =V38 =   .841*F4   + 1.000 E38
        .058
      14.471@

SDQ2N31 =V39 =   .952*F4   + 1.000 E39
        .049
      19.475@

SDQ2N43 =V40 =   .655*F4   + 1.000 E40
        .049
      13.273@

TABLE 3.6
(Continued)

VARIANCES OF INDEPENDENT VARIABLES

```
            V                      F
            ---                    ---
                    I F1 - F1      .615*
                    I              .138
                    I              4.452@
                    I
                    I F2 - F2      .563*
                    I              .127I
                    I              4.446@
                    I
                    I F3 - F3      .671*
                    I              .117
                    I              5.739@
                    I                I
                    I F4 - F4      2.316*
                    I              .274
                    I              8.443@
                    I
                    E                      D
                    ---                    ---
E25 -SDQ2N01        1.203*
                    .126
                    9.524@

E26 -SDQ2N13        1.123*
                    .125
                    9.003@

E27 -SDQ2N25        1.061*
                    .107
                    9.882@

E28 -SDQ2N37        .773*
                    .088
                    8.797@

E29 -SDQ2N04        1.399*
                    .129
                    10.879@

E30 -SDQ2N16        .618*
                    .069
                    9.005@

E31 -SDQ2N28        .900*
                    .090
                    9.943@

E32 -SDQ2N40        .955*
                    .095
                    10.009@

E33 -SDQ2N10        .656*
                    .083
                    7.926@
```

(Continued)

TABLE 3.6
(Continued)

E34 -SDQ2N22	.660*	
	.076	
	8.718@	
E35 -SDQ2N34	2.600*	
	.234	
	11.108@	
E36 -SDQ2N46	1.205*	
	.119	
	10.164@	
E37 -SDQ2N07	.858*	
	.100	
	8.537@	
E38 -SDQ2N19	1.232*	
	.122	
	10.132@	
E39 -SDQ2N31	.366*	
	.065	
	5.639@	
E40 -SDQ2N43	.967*	
	.093	
	10.453@	

COVARIANCES AMONG INDEPENDENT VARIABLES

```
 V                         F
 ---                       ---
 I F2 -  F2                .416*
 I F1 -  F1                .079
 I                         5.282@
 I
 I F3 -  F3                .356*
 I F1 -  F1                .072
 I          '             4.937@
 I
 I F4 -  F4                .637*
 I F1 -  F1                .119
 I                         5.375@
 I
 I F3 -  F3                .466*
 I F2 -  F2                .079
 I                         5.911@
 I
 I F4 -  F4                .876*
 I F2 -  F2                .135
 I                         6.508@
 I
 I F4 -  F4                .332*
 I F3 -  F3                .101
 I                         3.302@
```

TABLE 3.6
(Continued)

STANDARDIZED SOLUTION:			R-SQUARED
SDQ2N01 =V25 =	.581 F1	+ .814 E25	.338
SDQ2N13 =V26 =	.626*F1	+ .780 E26	.391
SDQ2N25 =V27 =	.544*F1	+ .839 E27	.296
SDQ2N37 =V28 =	.640*F1	+ .768 E28	.410
SDQ2N04 =V29 =	.536 F2	+ .844 E29	.287
SDQ2N16 =V30 =	.774*F2	+ .634 E30	.598
SDQ2N28 =V31 =	.702*F2	+ .712 E31	.493
SDQ2N40 =V32 =	.695*F2	+ .719 E32	.483
SDQ2N10 =V33 =	.711 F3	+ .703 E33	.506
SDQ2N22 =V34 =	.668*F3	+ .745 E34	.446
SDQ2N34 =V35 =	.322*F3	+ .947 E35	.104
SDQ2N46 =V36 =	.532*F3	+ .847 E36	.283
SDQ2N07 =V37 =	.854 F4	+ .520 E37	.730
SDQ2N19 =V38 =	.756*F4	+ .655 E38	.571
SDQ2N31 =V39 =	.923*F4	+ .385 E39	.851
SDQ2N43 =V40 =	.712*F4	+ .702 E40	.507

CORRELATIONS AMONG INDEPENDENT VARIABLES

```
       V                    F
      ---                  ---
            I F2 - F2      .707*
            I F1 - F1
            I
            I F3 - F3      .555*
            I F1 - F1
            I
            I F4 - F4      .534*
            I F1 - F1
            I
            I F3 - F3      .758*
            I F2 - F2
            I
            I F4 - F4      .767*
            I F2 - F2
            I
            I F4 - F4      .266*
            I F3 - F3
            I
```

and SDQ2N07 (V37), all information appears on one line only—these represent the fixed factor-loading parameters; therefore, no estimated values are presented. For each of the estimated (*) parameters, however, there are three lines of output: the estimated value is presented first, the standard error second, and the test statistic last, with statistically significant parameters assigned an @. Review of the unstandardized solution in Table 3.6 shows all estimates to be reasonable as well as statistically significant; all standard errors also appear to be in good order.

In the standardized solution, all variables are rescaled to have a variance of 1.0. In EQS, standardization is applied to all variables in the linear structural equation system, including errors and disturbances. As a result, all coefficients in the equations have a similar interpretation and the magnitude of their standardized values may be easier to interpret than that of coefficients obtained from the covariance or raw data metric (Bentler, 2005).[12] In contrast to the unstandardized solution, information related to the standardized solution is summarized on one line, along with a related R^2 value (i.e., the squared multiple correlation) appearing in the column to the right labeled R-SQUARED (see Aiken, West, & Pitts, 2003, p. 485). Each measured (or dependent, in the Bentler–Weeks sense) variable is accompanied by an R^2 value representing the proportion of variance accounted for by its related factor (or independent predictor variable). It is computed by subtracting the square of the error term from 1.0 (i.e., $1.0 - E^2$). Bentler (2005) notes that in the event that a particular R^2 cannot be computed or that it differs by more than 0.01 from the corresponding Bentler–Raykov corrected R^2 value (Bentler & Raykov, 2000), the corrected R^2 value will be printed below.

In reviewing the standardized estimates, the user should verify that particular parameter values are consistent with the literature. For example, within the context of the present application, it is of interest to inspect correlations among the SC factors for their consistency with previously reported values; in the present example, these estimates are as expected.

Three additional features of the standardized solution are note worthy. First, in the event that some variances are estimated as negative values, the standardized solution cannot be obtained because the computation requires the square roots of these values; if such is the case, no standardized solution will be printed. Second, in the standardized solution, parameters that were previously fixed to 1.0 take on new values. Finally, note the absence of output for the variances of the independent variables. This is because in standardizing the estimates, the variances automatically take on a value of 1.00.

Model Misspecification.   Determination of misfitting parameters is accomplished in EQS by means of the LM Test. As discussed previously, fixed parameters—as specified in the input file—are assessed both univariately and multivariately to identify parameters that would contribute to a significant drop in χ^2 if they were to be freely estimated in a subsequent EQS run. More specifically, information is presented first for univariate LM Tests of model parameters constrained either to 0.0 or to some nonzero value. If any of the univariate tests yield statistically significant results, the program then proceeds with a

---

[12]The standardized solution in EQS is not the same as the one in the LISREL output. In the latter, neither the measured variables, error terms, nor disturbances in equations (not present in first-order CFA models) are standardized (Bentler, 2005).

multivariate test of fixed parameters. As such, it proceeds with a forward stepwise procedure that selects as the next parameter to be added to the multivariate test, the single fixed parameter that provides the largest increase in the multivariate χ^2 statistic (Bentler, 2005). Results related to these LM Tests are presented in Table 3.7.

Univariate Test Statistics

Review of these results shows eight columns of information. Column 1 simply assigns a number to the parameter being tested. Column 2 assigns a dual numerical code to the parameter under test. In a simultaneous test of parameters, which is the case here, the first digit will always be 2, as shown in Table 3.7. The second digit refers to the submatrix number in which the parameter resides (1 to 22). However, if the parameter has been fixed to a nonzero value, the second digit will be zero. (There is no reason to remember this information; it is presented solely in the interest of completeness.) Column 3 lists the parameter under test.

Column 4 presents the univariate LM χ^2 test statistic, which has 1 degree of freedom; Column 5 presents its related statistical probability. These values result from testing the hypothesized constraint that the selected parameter is equal to zero. Interpreted literally, given a probability of less than .05, this hypothesis must be rejected, thereby indicating some evidence of misspecification in the model. However, Bentler (2005) cautions that because these LM univariate tests are correlated and can be applied repeatedly to test a variety of single restrictions, they should not be used to determine what the simultaneous effect of several restrictions may be. Such decisions should always be based on the multivariate LM Test results.

Column 6, labeled Hancock 98 df Prob presents LM Test probabilities based on Hancock's (1999) multiple comparison rationale. This criterion was developed for use in SEM as an analog to the Scheffé test (1953) used in ANOVA to control for family-wise Type I errors. These probabilities represent an evaluation of each LM χ^2 statistic based on degrees of freedom for the current model (98 in the present case) rather than the usual 1 degree of freedom. Hancock's criterion provides for an extremely conservative approach (too conservative, in my experience) to model testing that can help control Type I error in exploratory (i.e., post hoc) model modification.

Columns 7 and 8 present the unstandardized and standardized parameter change statistic, respectively.[13] For each parameter tested via the LM Test, the parameter change statistic represents its estimated value if this parameter is freely estimated in a subsequent test of the model. Such information can be helpful in determining whether a parameter identified by the LM Test is justified to stand as a candidate for respecification as a freely estimated parameter. In other words, is the estimated

---

[13]This is sometimes referred to as the expected parameter change statistic.

TABLE 3.7
EQS Output for Initially Hypothesized Four-Factor Model: Modification Indexes

LAGRANGE MULTIPLIER TEST (FOR ADDING PARAMETERS)
ORDERED UNIVARIATE TEST STATISTICS

NO	CODE	PARAMETER	CHI-SQUARE	PROBABILITY	HANCOCK 98 DF PROBABILITY	PARAMETER CHANGE	STANDARDIZED CHANGE
1	2 6	E39,E38	17.753	.000	1.000	-.333	-.495
2	2 6	E27,E25	16.986	.000	1.000	.360	.319
3	2 12	V37,F2	11.205	.001	1.000	-.563	-.421
4	2 6	E39,E37	10.660	.001	1.000	.306	.546
5	2 6	E32,E29	9.264	.002	1.000	-.243	-.210
6	2 12	V37,F3	9.200	.002	1.000	-.299	-.205
7	2 6	E40,E38	8.255	.004	1.000	.222	.203
8	2 12	V39,F1	7.404	.007	1.000	.293	.238
9	2 12	V35,F4	7.313	.007	1.000	-.200	-.077
10	2 12	V35,F2	7.307	.007	1.000	-.657	-.514
11	2 12	V28,F2	6.910	.009	1.000	.491	.571
12	2 6	E29,E26	6.514	.011	1.000	.221	.177
•	•	•	•	•	•	•	•
•	•	•	•	•	•	•	•
•	•	•	•	•	•	•	•
•	•	•	•	•	•	•	•
170	2 0	V33,F3	.000	1.000	1.000	.000	.000
171	2 0	V25,F1	.000	1.000	1.000	.000	.000
172	2 0	V29,F2	.000	1.000	1.000	.000	.000

MULTIVARIATE LAGRANGE MULTIPLIER TEST BY SIMULTANEOUS PROCESS IN STAGE 1
PARAMETER SETS (SUBMATRICES) ACTIVE AT THIS STAGE ARE: PEE GVF

		CUMULATIVE MULTIVARIATE STATISTICS			UNIVARIATE INCREMENT			
							HANCOCK'S SEQUENTIAL	
STEP	PARAMETER	CHI-SQUARE	D.F.	PROB.	CHI-SQUARE	PROB.	D.F.	PROB.
1	E39,E38	17.753	1	.000	17.753	.000	98	1.000
2	E27,E25	34.739	2	.000	16.986	.000	97	1.000
3	E32,E29	44.003	3	.000	9.264	.002	96	1.000
4	V35,F4	51.317	4	.000	7.313	.007	95	1.000
5	E40,E32	58.310	5	.000	6.993	.008	94	1.000
6	E29,E26	63.870	6	.000	5.560	.018	93	1.000
7	E33,E29	68.972	7	.000	5.102	.024	92	1.000
8	E40,E36	73.905	8	.000	4.933	.026	91	1.000
9	E32,E28	78.590	9	.000	4.685	.030	90	1.000
10	V39,F1	82.726	10	.000	4.136	.042	89	1.000
11	E39,E37	87.433	11	.000	4.707	.030	88	1.000

NOTES: LAGRANGIAN MULTIPLIER TEST REQUIRED   59325 WORDS OF MEMORY.
            PROGRAM ALLOCATES 2000000 WORDS.
        1
            Execution begins at 10:55:35
            Execution ends at 10:55:37

difference in the magnitude of the parameter estimate sufficient to justify inclusion of its specification in the model?[14]

Let's review two entries in the LM Test univariate results reported in Table 3.7. In Entry No. 1, the first parameter tested is E39, E38, an error covariance between V39 and V38. The test that this parameter equals zero produced a univariate LM $\chi^2_{(1)}$ of 17.753, ($p = .000$), thereby indicating that this hypothesized restriction is not tenable. In contrast, the Hancock's Criterion shows a probability value of 1.000, indicating that the parameter is tenable and need not be considered in any respecification of the model. (This criterion is elaborated on in chap. 4 in which adherence to its results runs counter to reasonable model respecification.[15] The unstandardized parameter change statistic indicates that if this parameter were freely estimated, its estimated value would be $-.333$; the standardized value would be $-.495$. In Entry No. 170 (most parameter values were deleted from the table due to space limitations), the parameter tested is V33,F3, a factor loading that was constrained to 1.0 for purposes of model identification. Relatedly, the second digit in the code is 0, and the LM χ^2 is 0 ($p=1.00$), as it should be.

Immediately following the univariate test statistics, the program identifies the parameter sets, or submatrices, to be included in the analyses; in this case, the parameters of interest are the error covariances (PEE) and factor loadings (GVF).

Multivariate Test Statistics

Here, information is summarized by means of nine columns. Column 1 represents the step in the forward stepwise procedure at which the selected parameter is included in the analysis. Column 2 identifies this parameter, and Columns 3, 4, and 5 cite the multivariate LMχ^2 statistic, degrees of freedom, and probability value, respectively. Based on the work of Bentler and Chou (1987), a unique feature of the EQS program is that it breaks down the multivariate LM Test into a series of incremental univariate tests; these results are presented in Columns 6 and 7. (For an elaboration of both the rationale and details of this procedure, see Bentler, 2005.) Decisions regarding possible misspecification followed by respecification of the model are based on these incremental univariate statistics. In targeting misfitting parameters, within the context of Columns 6 and 7, the user typically looks for parameters whose χ^2 values stand apart from the rest and probabilities $<.05$. For example, in Table 3.7, there is a substantial drop between the first two χ^2 values and the remaining χ^2 values. Thus, we focus on these two parameters (E39,E38; E27,E25), each of which represent error covariances. However, incremental univariate LMχ^2 values of 17.753 and 16.986, with standardized parameter

---

[14]Bentler (2005) cautioned, however, that because these parameter change statistics are sensitive to the way by which variables and factors are scaled or identified, their absolute value is sometimes difficult to interpret.

[15]The conditions for optimal use of this statistic remain to be determined.

change values of -.495 and .319, respectively—particularly as they relate to error covariances—can be considered of little concern and, therefore, not worthy of inclusion in an already well-fitting and adequately specified model. Finally, degrees of freedom and probability values related to the Hancock criterion are presented in Columns 8 and 9, respectively. The two columns are needed because in the sequential test of parameters, the model degrees of freedom will necessarily decrease by one with each univariate increment to the multivariate $LM\chi^2$. As expected, the probability values in Column 9 are consistently 1.000.

Post Hoc Analyses

In general, at this point in the analysis, a researcher can decide whether or not to respecify and reestimate the model. If he or she elects to follow this route, it is important to realize that analyses are now framed within an exploratory rather than a confirmatory mode. In other words, once a hypothesized CFA model, for example, has been rejected, it spells the end of the CFA approach in its truest sense. Although CFA procedures continue to be used in any respecification and reestimation of the model, these analyses are exploratory in the sense that they focus on the detection of misfitting parameters in the originally hypothesized model. Such post hoc analyses are conventionally termed *specification searches* (MacCallum, 1986). (The issue of post hoc model-fitting is addressed further in chap. 8 in the cross-validation subsection.)

The ultimate decision underscoring whether or not to proceed with a specification search is twofold. First and foremost, the researcher must determine whether the estimation of the targeted parameter is substantively meaningful. If, indeed, it makes no sound substantive sense to free up the parameter exhibiting the largest multivariate LM χ^2 value, the researcher may consider the parameter having the next largest value (Jöreskog, 1993). Second, whether the respecified model would lead to an overfitted model needs to be considered. The issue here is tied to the idea of knowing when to stop fitting the model or, as Wheaton (1987, p. 123) phrased the problem, "knowing . . . how much fit is enough without being too much fit." In general, overfitting a model involves the specification of additional parameters in the model after having determined a criterion that reflects a minimally adequate fit. For example, an overfitted model can result from the inclusion of additional parameters that (a) are "fragile" in the sense of representing weak effects that are not likely replicable, (b) lead to a significant inflation of standard errors, and (c) influence primary parameters in the model, albeit their own substantive meaningfulness is somewhat equivocal (Wheaton, 1987). Although correlated errors often fall into this latter category,[16] there are many situations—particularly with respect to social psychological research—in which these parameters can make strong

---

[16]Typically, the misuse in this instance arises from the incorporation of correlated errors into the model purely on the basis of statistical fit and to achieve a better-fitting model.

substantive sense and therefore should be included in the model (Jöreskog & Sörbom, 1993).

Having laboriously worked through the process involved in evaluating the fit of a hypothesized model, what can we conclude regarding the CFA model under scrutiny in this chapter? To answer this question, we must pool all the information gleaned from our study of the EQS text output. Considering (a) the feasibility and statistical significance of all parameter estimates; (b) the substantially good fit of the model, with particular reference to the CFI (.962) and RMSEA (.048) values; and (c) the lack of any substantial evidence of model misfit, I conclude that any further incorporation of parameters into the model would result in an overfitted model. Indeed, MacCallum et al. (1992, p. 501) cautioned that "when an initial model fits well, it is probably unwise to modify it to achieve even better fit because modifications may simply be fitting small idiosyncratic characteristics of the sample." Adhering to this caveat, I concluded that the four-factor model schematically portrayed in Fig. 3.1 represents an adequate description of self-concept structure for Grade 7 adolescents.

HYPOTHESIS 2:
Self-Concept Is a Two-Factor Structure

The model to be tested here postulates a priori that self-concept is a two-factor structure consisting of GSC and ASC. As such, it argues against the viability of subject-specific academic SC factors. As with the four-factor model, the four GSC measures load onto the General SC (GSC) factor; in contrast, all other measures load onto the Academic SC (ASC) factor. This hypothesized model is represented schematically in Figure 3.4; the EQS input file is shown in Table 3.8.

In reviewing these graphical and equation model specifications, two points relative to the modification of the input file are of interest. First, although the pattern of factor loadings remains the same for the GSC and ASC measures, it changes for both the English SC (ESC) and Math SC (MSC) measures in allowing them to load onto the ASC factor. Second, because only one of these eight ASC factor loadings needs to be fixed to 1.0, the two previously constrained parameters (i.e., SDQ2N10 [V33]; SDQ2N07 [V37]) are now freely estimated.

The EQS Output File

Because only the goodness-of-fit statistics are relevant to the present application, it is the only information provided in Table 3.9.

As indicated in the output, the $\chi^2_{(103)}$ value of 455.929 represents a poor fit to the data and a substantial decrement from the overall fit of the four-factor model ($\chi^2_{(98)}=158.512$). The gain of 5 degrees of freedom can be explained by the estimation of two fewer factor variances and five fewer factor covariances,

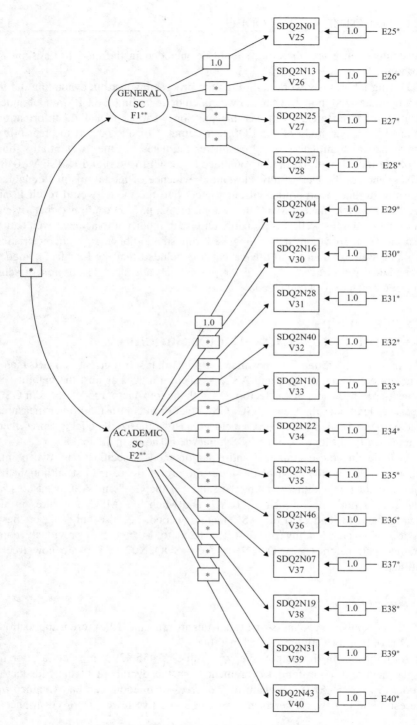

FIG. 3.4. Hypothesized two-factor model of self-concept.

TABLE 3.8
EQS Input for Two-Factor Model

/TITLE
 CFA OF ASC Structure - GRADE 7 "ASC7F2"
 2-Factor Model
/SPECIFICATIONS
 CASE=265; VAR=46; ME=ML; MA=RAW; FO= '(40F1.0,X,6F2.0)' ;
 DATA= 'C:\EQS61\Files\Books\Data\ASC7INDM.ess' ;
/LABELS
 V1=SPPCN08; V2=SPPCN18; V3=SPPCN28; V4=SPPCN38; V5=SPPCN48;
 V6=SPPCN58; V7=SPPCN01; V8=SPPCN11; V9=SPPCN21; V10=SPPCN31;
 V11=SPPCN41; V12=SPPCN51; V13=SPPCN06; V14=SPPCN16; V15=SPPCN26;
 V16=SPPCN36; V17=SPPCN46; V18=SPPCN56; V19=SPPCN03; V20=SPPCN13;
 V21=SPPCN23; V22=SPPCN33; V23=SPPCN43; V24=SPPCN53; V25=SDQ2N01;
 V26=SDQ2N13; V27=SDQ2N25; V28=SDQ2N37; V29=SDQ2N04; V30=SDQ2N16;
 V31=SDQ2N28; V32=SDQ2N40; V33=SDQ2N10; V34=SDQ2N22; V35=SDQ2N34;
 V36=SDQ2N46; V37=SDQ2N07; V38=SDQ2N19; V39=SDQ2N31; V40=SDQ2N43;
 V41=MASTENG1; V42=MASTMAT1; V43=TENG1; V44=TMAT1; V45=SENG1; V46=SMAT1;
/EQUATIONS
 V25= F1+E25;
 V26= *F1+E26;
 V27= *F1+E27;
 V28= *F1+E28;
   V29= F2+E29;
   V30= *F2+E30;
   V31= *F2+E31;
   V32= *F2+E32;
   V33= *F3+E33;
   V34= *F3+E34;
   V35= *F3+E35;
   V36= *F3+E36;
   V37= *F4+E37;
   V38= *F4+E38;
   V39= *F4+E39;
   V40= *F4+E40;
/VARIANCES
 F1 TO F2= *;
 E25 TO E40= *;
/CONSTRAINTS
 F1 TO F2= *;
/PRINT
 FIT=ALL;
/LMTEST
 SET=GVF, PEE;
/END

TABLE 3.9

EQS Output for Two-Factor Model: Goodness-of-Fit Statistics

GOODNESS OF FIT SUMMARY FOR METHOD = ML

INDEPENDENCE MODEL CHI-SQUARE   =   1696.728 ON   120 DEGREES OF FREEDOM

INDEPENDENCE AIC =   1456.72831   INDEPENDENCE CAIC =   907.16073
    MODEL AIC =   249.92879   MODEL CAIC =   -221.78339

CHI-SQUARE =   455.929 BASED ON   103 DEGREES OF FREEDOM
PROBABILITY VALUE FOR THE CHI-SQUARE STATISTIC IS   .00000
THE NORMAL THEORY RLS CHI-SQUARE FOR THIS ML SOLUTION IS   688.051.

FIT INDICES

BENTLER-BONETT NORMED FIT INDEX =   .731
BENTLER-BONETT NON-NORMED FIT INDEX =   .739
COMPARATIVE FIT INDEX (CFI)   =   .776
BOLLEN (IFI) FIT INDEX   =   .779
MCDONALD (MFI) FIT INDEX   =   .514
LISREL GFI FIT INDEX   =   .754
LISREL AGFI FIT INDEX   =   .676
ROOT MEAN-SQUARE RESIDUAL (RMR)   =   .182
STANDARDIZED RMR   =   .101
ROOT MEAN-SQUARE ERROR OF APPROXIMATION (RMSEA) =   .114
90% CONFIDENCE INTERVAL OF RMSEA (.103,   .124)

ITERATIVE SUMMARY

	PARAMETER		
ITERATION	ABS CHANGE	ALPHA	FUNCTION
1	.439992	1.00000	2.31433
2	.149129	1.00000	1.88294
3	.062831	1.00000	1.79004
4	.035740	1.00000	1.75530
5	.023792	1.00000	1.73949
6	.016281	1.00000	1.73238
7	.010849	1.00000	1.72927
8	.007131	1.00000	1.72794
9	.004625	1.00000	1.72738
10	.002978	1.00000	1.72715
11	.001907	1.00000	1.72706
12	.001217	1.00000	1.72702
13	.000775	1.00000	1.72700

albeit the estimation of two additional factor loadings (formerly SDQ2N10 [V33]; SDQ2N07 [V37]). As expected, all other indexes of fit reflect the fact that self-concept structure is not well represented by the hypothesized two-factor model. In particular, the CFI value of .776 and RMSEA value of .114 are strongly indicative of inferior goodness-of-fit between the hypothesized two-factor model and the sample data.

HYPOTHESIS 3:
Self-Concept Is a One-Factor Structure

Although it now seems obvious that a multidimensional model best represents the structure of SC for Grade 7 adolescents, some researchers still contend that self-concept is a unidimensional construct. Thus, for purposes of completeness and to address the issue of unidimensionality, Byrne and Worth Gavin (1996) proceeded in testing this hypothesis. However, because the one-factor model represents a restricted version of the two-factor model and thus cannot possibly represent a better-fitting model, these analyses are not presented herein due to space limitations.

In summary, it is evident from these analyses that both the two-factor and one-factor models of self-concept represent a misspecification of factorial structure for early adolescents. Based on these findings, Byrne and Worth Gavin (1996) concluded that self-concept is a multidimensional construct that, in their study, comprised the four facets of general, academic, English, and mathematics self-concepts.

4

Application 2: Testing for the Factorial Validity of Scores From a Measuring Instrument (First-Order CFA Model)

For the second application, we again examine a first-order CFA model. However, this time we test hypotheses bearing on a single measuring instrument, the Maslach Burnout Inventory (MBI; Maslach & Jackson, 1981, 1986), designed to measure three dimensions of burnout, which the authors term Emotional Exhaustion (EE), Depersonalization (DP), and Reduced Personal Accomplishment (PA). The term "burnout" denotes the inability to function effectively in one's job as a consequence of prolonged and extensive job-related stress; *emotional exhaustion* represents feelings of fatigue that develop as one's energies become drained; *depersonalization* is the development of negative and uncaring attitudes toward others; and *reduced personal accomplishment* is a deterioration of self-confidence and dissatisfaction in one's achievements.

The purpose of the original study (Byrne, 1994b), from which this example is taken, was to test for the validity and invariance of factorial structure within and across gender for elementary and secondary school teachers. In this chapter, however, only analyses bearing on the factorial validity of the MBI for a calibration sample of elementary male teachers ($n = 372$) are of interest.

Confirmatory factor analysis of a measuring instrument is most appropriately applied to measures that have been fully developed and their factor structures validated. The legitimacy of CFA use, of course, is tied to its conceptual rationale as a hypothesis-testing approach to data analysis. That is, based on theory, empirical

118

research, or a combination of both, the researcher postulates a model and then tests for its validity given the sample data. Thus, application of CFA procedures to assessment instruments still in the initial stages of development represents a serious misuse of this analytic strategy. In testing for the validity of factorial structure for an assessment measure, the researcher seeks to determine the extent to which items designed to measure a particular factor (i.e., latent construct) actually do so. In general, subscales of a measuring instrument are considered to represent the factors; all items in a particular subscale are therefore expected to load onto their related factor.

Given that the MBI has been commercially marketed since 1981, is the most widely used measure of occupational burnout, and has undergone substantial testing of its psychometric properties over the years (see, e.g., Byrne, 1991, 1993, 1994b), it certainly qualifies as a candidate for CFA research. Interestingly, until this is author's 1991 study of the MBI, virtually all previous factor analytic work had been based only on exploratory procedures. The next section describes this assessment instrument.

THE MEASURING INSTRUMENT UNDER STUDY

The MBI is a 22-item instrument structured on a seven-point Likert-type scale that ranges from 0 ("feeling has never been experienced") to 6 ("feeling experienced daily.") It is composed of three subscales, each measuring one facet of burnout: the EE subscale comprises nine items, the DP subscale five items, and the PA subscale eight items. The original version of the MBI (Maslach & Jackson, 1981) was constructed from data based on samples of workers from a wide range of human-service organizations. Subsequently, Maslach and Jackson (1986), in collaboration with Schwab, developed the Educators' Survey (i.e., MBI Form Ed), a version of the instrument specifically designed for use with teachers. The MBI Form Ed parallels the original version of the MBI except for the modified wording of certain items to make them more appropriate to a teacher's work environment.

THE HYPOTHESIZED MODEL

The CFA model of MBI structure hypothesizes a priori that (a) responses to the MBI can be explained by three factors: EE, DP, and PA; (b) each item has a nonzero loading on the burnout factor it was designed to measure and zero loadings on all other factors; (c) the three factors are correlated; and (d) the error–uniqueness terms associated with the item measurements are uncorrelated. A schematic representation of this model is shown in Fig. 4.1.

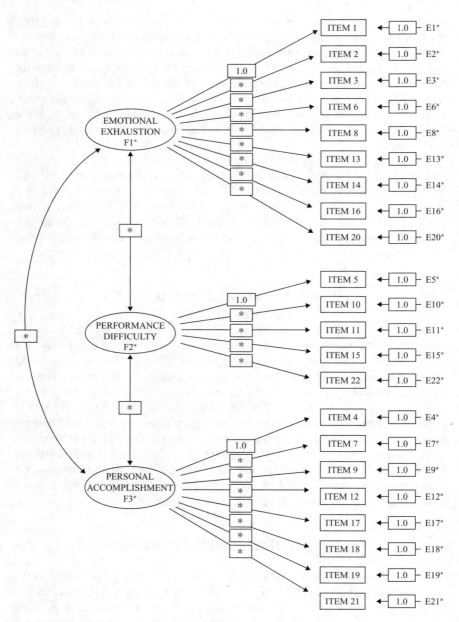

FIG. 4.1. Hypothesized model of factorial structure for the
Maslach Burnout Inventory.
Note: Item numbers correspond to variable numbers (e.g.,
ITEM 1 = V1).

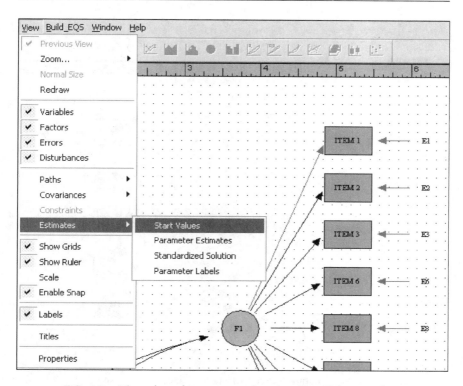

FIG. 4.2. View drop-down menu showing Start Values option.

Before reviewing the EQS input file for this model, I wish first to illustrate, two important and useful features of the DIAGRAMMER feature of the program. The first feature relates to the inclusion of start values on a figure should you wish to have them visible; the second addresses the question of modification to the component properties of a figure.

Inclusion of Start Values

In Fig. 4.1, the values of 1.0 are associated with fixed parameters in the model and asterisks (*) are associated with parameters to be freely estimated. In the initial structuring of a figure using the DIAGRAMMER, the first of each set of regression paths is considered fixed (by default) and, as such, is automatically displayed in a color different than that of the freely estimated paths; the value of 1.0 and the asterisks, however, are not automatically included. Nonetheless, these additions are easily made once the figure is complete. Chapter 2 describes how to include estimated parameter values in a model by dropping down the View menu

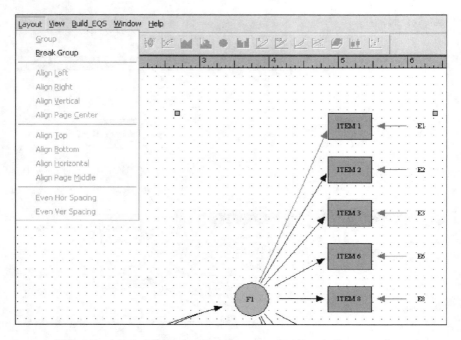

FIG. 4.3. Layout drop-down menu showing Break Group option.

and clicking on either unstandardized or standardized values (see Fig. 2.44). As illustrated in Fig. 4.2, the same procedure is used to make start values visible.[1]

Modification of Component Properties

With the DIAGRAMMER, particular colors are assigned by default to various components of a figure. Specifically, both the rectangles and ovals representing measured and latent variables, respectively, are a solid color (i.e., they contain fill). Because you will likely wish to remove this colored fill from a figure for purposes of publication, I now illustrate this process.

If you have constructed a figure using the DIAGRAMMER, all components of the finished product are automatically grouped as one object. The first step in the process, as shown in Fig. 4.3, is to separate the individual components by dropping down the Layout menu and clicking on Break Group; Fig. 4.4 illustrates the result of this action. To remove the fill, select one of the filled objects (the first measured variable is selected here, as shown in Fig. 4.5), right-click the mouse, and then select Properties, which yields the Components Properties dialog box

---

[1]Of course, had you assigned actual start values to the estimated parameters or selected an alternate regression path as the fixed parameter, these alternate values would appear on the diagram.

shown in Fig. 4.6. Other options are now available to modify lines, font, and/or size of various aspects of the figure. Clicking on Fill presents a selection of colors, with more selections, available by clicking the Other option. The bordered square shown within the Fill subdialog box represents the current color (i.e., green) of the rectangle. Clicking on the white square in the lower right-hand corner subsequently yields the selections shown in Fig. 4.7, and clicking OK results in the modification illustrated in Fig. 4.8. This process is repeated for the remaining measured and latent variables in the model.

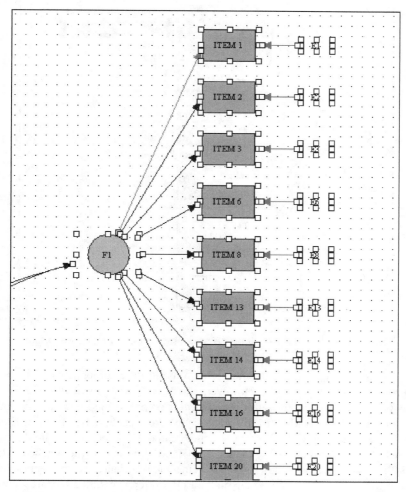

FIG. 4.4. Partial CFA model showing measured variables and latent factor as separate (i.e., ungrouped) objects.

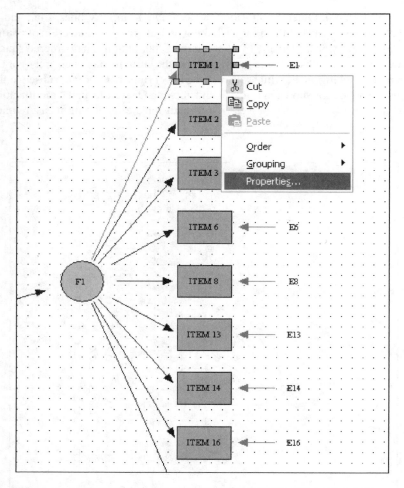

FIG. 4.5.   Mouse right-click menu showing variable Properties option.

Figures 4.3 through 4.8 illustrate how to modify the components of a single figure for a particular reason. However, should you wish always to work with figures devoid of color or with different color combinations, you can certainly customize the DIAGRAMMER by selecting the Preferences option from the drop-down Edit menu. However, these preferences can only be identified with the data file active and must precede use of the DIAGRAMMER in constructing the model. This three-step process is shown in Fig. 4.9, in which the data file in the background and the open EQS Diagrammer tab on the EQS Preference dialog box are shown. Clicking on the Dependent variable option (or any other object options) yields, the Color subdialog box. Figure 4.9 shows the wide variety of options available.

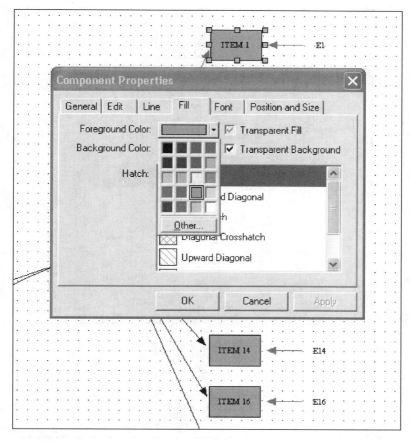

FIG. 4.6.   Component Properties dialog box showing open Fill tab
with color options.

THE EQS INPUT FILE

Now that you have learned a few tricks in using the DIAGRAMMER, let's preview
the input file in which translation of the hypothesized model of MBI structure into
EQS program language can be examined. As indicated in the /TITLE paragraph,
the input file shown in Table 4.1 represents the initially hypothesized model of
the MBI for the calibration sample of male elementary-school teachers. The first
line of the /SPECIFICATIONS paragraph identifies both the name of the data file
(elemm1.ess) and its location, within the context of the author's computer. The
second line of this paragraph states that the data (a) comprise 22 variables for each
of 372 cases, (b) are to be analyzed using maximum likelihood estimation (c) are

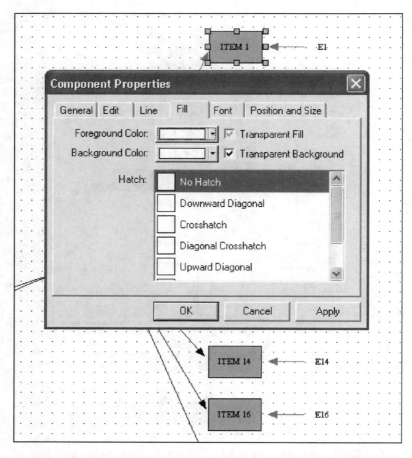

FIG. 4.7. Component Properties dialog box showing selected white Fill preference.

in the form of a raw data matrix, and (d) are formatted such that the score for each of the 22 variables occupies one column.[2] In the /LABELS paragraph, the labels for the observed variables, V1 through V22, are consistent with the item numbers composing the MBI; those for the unobserved variables, F1 through F3, represent the EE, DP, and PA factors, respectively.

We turn now to the model specifications. The /EQUATIONS paragraph, as presented herein, makes it easy to identify the pattern by which the items load onto each factor. As in the example reviewed in chapter 3, for purposes of model (statistical) identification and establishment of a metric for the latent variables, the

---

[2]In fact, given that the data reside in an .ess file, it is not necessary to specify its format to the program because this information is already known. However, I do so throughout the book solely as an aid to any readers who may wish to use the data (see preface) in working through the examples presented.

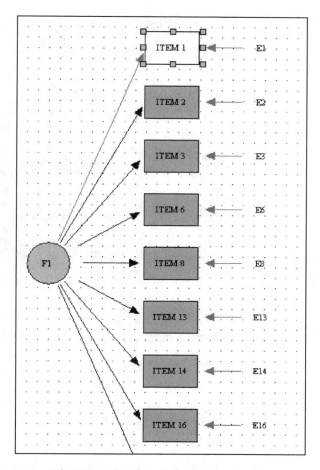

FIG. 4.8. Partial CFA model showing Item 1 rectangle with white fill.

first of each congeneric set of factor loadings is not estimated (i.e., no asterisk); as such, these parameters are automatically fixed to 1.00 by the program.[3] Likewise, the error–uniqueness term associated with each observed variable is specified as a fixed parameter. The /VARIANCES paragraph specifies that the variance of each factor and error term is to be estimated; the /COVARIANCES paragraph specifies that covariances among the three factors are to be estimated. Within the /PRINT paragraph, the command FIT=ALL assures that all available fit statistics are presented in the output file. Finally, the LM Test paragraph indicates that LM

---

[3]As noted in Chapter 2, these constraints need not be limited to the first of each congeneric set of loadings. Furthermore, if the reliability of the indicator variables is known, the constraint should be most appropriately assigned to the one exhibiting the highest reliability.

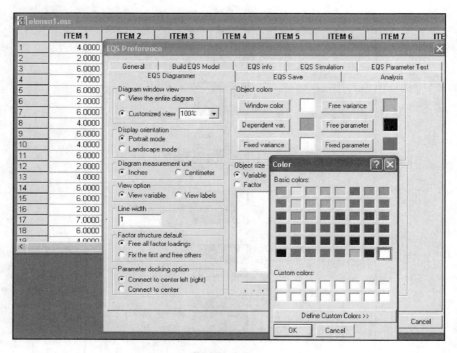

FIG. 4.9.   Preference dialog box showing options available for the
EQS DiaGRAMMER.

Test statistics bearing on misspecification related only to factor loadings (GVF)
and error–uniqueness terms (PEE) are provided in the output file.

THE EQS OUTPUT FILE

Although the lion's share of the EQS output file was reviewed in chapter 3, two
aspects of the analytic feedback were omitted to minimize information overload.
In this chapter, information related to the Sample Statistics and Reliability sections
of the output file are reviewed. In addition, I introduce you to the Robust Statistics
associated with the EQS program. We turn first to the sample statistics shown in
Table 4.2 as they relate to the initial test of MBI structure for elementary male
teachers.

Sample Statistics

Because the input data are in the form of a raw-score matrix, EQS automatically
provides an abundance of information related to univariate as well as multivariate

TABLE 4.1

EQS Input for Initially Hypothesized Model

/TITLE
CFA of MBI for Male Elementary Tchrs (Calbrn Grp) "MBIELM11"
Initial Model
/SPECIFICATIONS
DATA='c:\eqs61\files\books\runs\elemm1.ess';
VARIABLES=22; CASES=372;
METHOD=ML; ANALYSIS=COVARIANCE; MATRIX=RAW;
/LABELS
V1=ITEM 1; V2=ITEM 2; V3=ITEM 3; V4=ITEM 4; V5=ITEM 5;
V6=ITEM 6; V7=ITEM 7; V8=ITEM 8; V9=ITEM 9; V10=ITEM 10;
V11=ITEM 11; V12=ITEM 12; V13=ITEM 13; V14=ITEM 14; V15=ITEM 15;
V16=ITEM 16; V17=ITEM 17; V18=ITEM 18; V19=ITEM 19; V20=ITEM 20;
V21=ITEM 21; V22=ITEM 22;
F1=EE; F2=DP; F3=PA;
/EQUATIONS
V1 = 1F1 + E1;
V2 = *F1 + E2;
V3 = *F1 + E3;
V6 = *F1 + E6;
V8 = *F1 + E8;
V13 = *F1 + E13;
V14 = *F1 + E14;
V16 = *F1 + E16;
V20 = *F1 + E20;
      V5 = 1F2 + E5;
      V10 = *F2 + E10;
      V11 = *F2 + E11;
      V15 = *F2 + E15;
      V22 = *F2 + E22;
          V4 = 1F3 + E4;
          V7 = *F3 + E7;
          V9 = *F3 + E9;
          V12 = *F3 + E12;
          V17 = *F3 + E17;
          V18 = *F3 + E18;
          V19 = *F3 + E19;
          V21 = *F3 + E21;
/VARIANCES
F1 to F3 = *;
E1 to E22 = *;
/COVARIANCES
F1 to F3 = *;
/PRINT
FIT=ALL;
/LMTEST
SET=PEE,GVF;
/END

TABLE 4.2

EQS Output for Initially Hypothesized Model: Descriptive Statistics

UNIVARIATE STATISTICS

VARIABLE	ITEM1	ITEM2	ITEM3	ITEM4	ITEM5
MEAN	4.3656	4.8683	3.5269	6.2984	2.1989
SKEWNESS (G1)	-.1151	-.5070	.3169	-1.8111	1.3283
KURTOSIS (G2)	-1.1562	-.6926	-1.0997	3.6665	.9305
STANDARD DEV.	1.6616	1.5458	1.7334	.9985	1.4878

VARIABLE	ITEM6	ITEM7	ITEM8	ITEM9	ITEM10
MEAN	2.7070	6.3118	3.0430	6.0349	2.2043
SKEWNESS (G1)	.9238	-1.6490	.7407	-1.5422	1.2025
KURTOSIS (G2)	.0071	3.8021	-.5971	1.8694	.5827
STANDARD DEV.	1.5842	.8401	1.7276	1.3160	1.4467

VARIABLE	ITEM11	ITEM12	ITEM13	ITEM14	ITEM15
MEAN	2.2392	5.6989	3.5860	4.0269	1.7688
SKEWNESS (G1)	1.2731	-1.3195	.3472	.0309	2.0963
KURTOSIS (G2)	.8159	1.8669	-.7803	-.9253	4.2790
STANDARD DEV.	1.5293	1.1933	1.6825	1.7264	1.2991

VARIABLE	ITEM16	ITEM17	ITEM18	ITEM19	ITEM20
MEAN	2.4731	6.4059	5.7016	5.9462	2.2446
SKEWNESS (G1)	.9714	-1.9783	-1.2309	-1.4839	1.3001
KURTOSIS (G2)	.1735	5.1001	1.3641	2.2408	1.1929
STANDARD DEV.	1.4395	.8526	1.2737	1.1895	1.4149

VARIABLE	ITEM21	ITEM22			
MEAN	5.8522	2.5806			
SKEWNESS (G1)	-1.3000	1.0662			
KURTOSIS (G2)	1.1823	.1986			
STANDARD DEV.	1.2663	1.5804			

MULTIVARIATE KURTOSIS

MARDIA'S COEFFICIENT (G2,P) =	125.1437
NORMALIZED ESTIMATE =	37.1380

ELLIPTICAL THEORY KURTOSIS ESTIMATES

MARDIA-BASED KAPPA =   .2370 MEAN SCALED UNIVARIATE KURTOSIS =   .3640
MARDIA-BASED KAPPA IS USED IN COMPUTATION. KAPPA =   .2370

CASE NUMBERS WITH LARGEST CONTRIBUTION TO NORMALIZED MULTIVARIATE KURTOSIS:

CASE NUMBER	26	30	84	171	200
ESTIMATE	1194.8267	1446.5683	1221.4446	1136.6242	1078.3870

sample statistics. Given the strong underlying assumption of multivariate normality associated with SEM, such information is important to the interpretability of the findings. Turning first to the univariate statistics, we find mean, skewness, kurtosis, and standard-deviation coefficients printed for each MBI item. Although skewness values for all items can be considered satisfactory in general, kurtosis values for several items (in particular, Items 4, 7, 15, 17, and 19) bear serious consideration.

When variables demonstrate significant nonzero univariate kurtosis, it is certain that they will not be multivariately normally distributed. Although these aberrant items are not excessively kurtotic, they may be sufficiently non-normal to make interpretations based on the usual χ^2 statistic, the CFI and RMSEA problematic, an issue that is addressed in the specification of Model 2. (For elaboration on these problems, see Bentler, 2005; Curran, West, & Finch, 1996; and West, Finch, & Curran, 1995.)

The multivariate sample statistics all relate only to kurtosis and are variants of Mardia's (1970, 1974) coefficient. Elliptical theory estimates are also shown but are not typically relevant unless that theory is invoked. When the sample is very large and multivariately normal, the Mardia's normalized estimate is distributed as a unit normal variate such that large values reflect significant positive kurtosis and large negative values reflect significant negative kurtosis. Bentler (2005) has suggested that in practice, values >5.00 are indicative of data that are non-normally distributed. In this example, the Z-statistic of 37.1380, shown in Table 4.2, is highly suggestive of non-normality in the sample.

Multivariate Outliers

Another important aspect of the EQS program is its capability to identify extreme cases with respect to multivariate kurtosis. The program automatically prints out the five cases contributing most to the normalized multivariate kurtosis estimate. Nonetheless, it is entirely possible that none of the five cases is actually an outlier. Identification of an outlier is based on the estimate presented for one case relative to the estimate for the other four cases; there is no absolute value on which to make this judgment. In reviewing the output in Table 4.2, there apparently is no such evidence of an outlying case. This assessment is based on the observation that all five estimates fall approximately within the same range of values; typically, estimates for outlying cases are distinctively different from those representing the other cases. (For extensive discussion of the detection and treatment of outliers in SEM, see Berkane & Bentler, 1988; Bollen, 1989a; and Kline, 1998.)

Bentler–Weeks Structural Representation

Table 4.3 shows the Bentler–Weeks summary of the hypothesized model. It may be helpful to compare this summary with the graphic representation of the model in Fig. 4.1. Accordingly, we see first, that there are 22 dependent variables, which represent the observed indicator variables (i.e., MBI items). The number of independent variables is 25; 22 represent the error–uniqueness associated with each observed variable and three represent the underlying factors of EE, DP, and PA. From a different perspective, the summary concludes that the model has 47 free parameters and 25 nonzero fixed parameters. The free parameters represent 19

TABLE 4.3
Selected EQS Output for Initially Hypothesized Model: Bentler–Weeks Representation

```
BENTLER-WEEKS STRUCTURAL REPRESENTATION:

   NUMBER OF DEPENDENT VARIABLES = 22
       DEPENDENT V'S :    1    2    3    4    5    6    7    8    9   10
       DEPENDENT V'S :   11   12   13   14   15   16   17   18   19   20
       DEPENDENT V'S :   21   22

   NUMBER OF INDEPENDENT VARIABLES = 25
       INDEPENDENT F'S :    1    2    3
       INDEPENDENT E'S :    1    2    3    4    5    6    7    8    9   10
       INDEPENDENT E'S :   11   12   13   14   15   16   17   18   19   20
       INDEPENDENT E'S :   21   22

   NUMBER OF FREE PARAMETERS = 47
   NUMBER OF FIXED NONZERO PARAMETERS = 25

DETERMINANT OF INPUT MATRIX IS    .10275D+03

PARAMETER ESTIMATES APPEAR IN ORDER,
NO SPECIAL PROBLEMS WERE ENCOUNTERED DURING OPTIMIZATION.
```

factor loadings, 22 error variances, three factor variances, and three factor covariances. The 25 fixed parameters represent three factor loadings constrained to 1.00 for purposes of model identification and 22 error regression paths (known and fixed to 1.00).

Goodness-of-Fit Summary

Given the extensive description of available goodness-of-fit indexes in chapter 3, this evaluation is limited to only five criteria: the χ^2 statistic, the SRMR, CFI, RMSEA, and RMSEA 90% confidence interval (C.I.) in judging the adequacy of model fit; these values are listed in Table 4.4. (All remaining model-fit information was excluded due to space limitations.) Although both the SRMR (.073) and RMSEA (.080; 90% C.I. .073, .086) values are barely within the scope of adequate model fit, the CFI value of .848 clearly indicates, an ill-fitting model. Thus, it is apparent that some modification in specification is needed to determine a model that better represents the sample data. Clues to these modifications are derived from the LM Test statistics discussed in the Modification Indexes subsection.

Reliability Coefficients

As shown in Table 4.4, EQS computes several different reliability coefficients, each of which describes the internal consistency of a hypothetical composite of summed scores on the variables being analyzed. Although Conbach's (1951) Alpha (α) coefficient is undoubtedly the most widely known index of internal consistency

TABLE 4.4
Selected EQS Output for Initially Hypothesized Model: Goodness-of-Fit Statistics

GOODNESS OF FIT SUMMARY FOR METHOD = ML

CHI-SQUARE =   693.849 BASED ON   206 DEGREES OF FREEDOM
PROBABILITY VALUE FOR THE CHI-SQUARE STATISTIC IS   .00000

FIT INDICES

BENTLER-BONETT   NORMED FIT INDEX =   .798
BENTLER-BONETT NON-NORMED FIT INDEX =   .830
COMPARATIVE FIT INDEX (CFI)   =   .848
ROOT MEAN-SQUARE RESIDUAL (RMR)   =   .141
STANDARDIZED RMR   =   .073
ROOT MEAN-SQUARE ERROR OF APPROXIMATION (RMSEA)   =   .080
90% CONFIDENCE INTERVAL OF RMSEA (.073,   .086)

RELIABILITY COEFFICIENTS

CRONBACH'S ALPHA   =   .792
RELIABILITY COEFFICIENT RHO   =   .861
GREATEST LOWER BOUND RELIABILITY   =   .924
BENTLER'S DIMENSION-FREE LOWER BOUND RELIABILITY   =   .924
SHAPIRO'S LOWER BOUND RELIABILITY FOR A WEIGHTED COMPOSITE =   .963
WEIGHTS THAT ACHIEVE SHAPIRO'S LOWER BOUND:

ITEM1	ITEM2	ITEM3	ITEM4	ITEM5	ITEM6
.298	.294	.315	-.046	.158	.272
ITEM7	ITEM8	ITEM9	ITEM10	ITEM11	ITEM12
-.064	.358	-.103	.168	.205	-.183
ITEM13	ITEM14	ITEM15	ITEM16	ITEM17	ITEM18
.303	.246	.156	.271	-.103	-.119
ITEM19	ITEM20	ITEM21	ITEM22		
-.151	.235	-.079	.133		

reliability, its application to latent variable models—particularly those with a multidimensional structure—is questionable. This equivocal status of α arises from the fact that, theoretically, it is based on a very restrictive one-factor model that requires all factor loadings and error variances to be equal (Bentler, 2005). Thus, it is evident that unless a CFA model can meet these unrealistically stringent conditions, the related α value is not a good estimate of internal consistency of the composite. Given that the hypothesized model is a three-factor structure, the α coefficient value of .792 reported in Table 4.4 is not the best possible reliability estimate.

The remaining reliability values reported in the output file are all factor-based coefficients, thus making them appropriate for use with CFA models. When used with a multifactor model setup, the Rho coefficient provides a good estimate of internal consistency; here we find a value of .861 for our model. Furthermore, when a model contains correlated error terms and a user does not want such sources of variance to be considered as "true" variance, Rho is the most appropriate coefficient to use.

Three other reliability options are available to the researcher. In contrast to the Rho coefficient, which is a model-based statistic, these coefficients are not bound to the input model structure. Nonetheless, they do assume some type of factor structure with a large but unspecified number of latent factors and do consider all sources of covariance as true variance. The first, the Greatest Lower Bound Reliability, requires that all error variances be non-negative (i.e., they exhibit no Heywood cases).[4] The second option, Bentler's Dimension-Free Lower Bound Reliability does not have this restriction. As shown in Table 4.4, coefficients derived from each of these reliability computations were identical at a value of .924. The final reliability coefficient, Shapiro's Lower Bound Reliability, is based on a weighted sum of the variables (i.e., the variables are weighted differentially to achieve a higher reliability). Following the reported coefficient value of .963, the program then lists the weights that were applied in its computation. With respect to the present example, Bentler's Dimension-Free Lower Bound Reliability coefficient seems to be the most appropriate choice, with a value of .924 indicative of high internal consistency among the MBI items, regardless of the number of postulated factors of burnout. (For an extensive discussion of these reliability coefficients, see Bentler, 2005.)

Modification Indexes

Recall that in the initial EQS input file, the SET command was used to limit the search for misfitting parameters to only factor loadings (GVF) and error covariances (PEE); these parameters, then, are the only ones identified in the portion of the output bearing on the LM Test statistics shown in Table 4.5. Review of the ordered univariate test statistics in the upper portion of the table identifies two parameters (E16,E6; E2,E1) whose LM Test χ^2 values, at 91.038 and 82.228, stand apart from the rest; both represent error covariances. Under the Parameter Change column, we see that if an error covariance between Items 16 and 6 were specified and freely estimated in a subsequent run, the value of the resulting parameter would be approximately .735; for E2,E1, the value would be .614.

Turning to the multivariate portion of Table 4.5 and then to the multivariate χ^2 values under the heading Cumulative Multivariate Statistics, we observe that if both error covariances were freely estimated, the approximate drop in the overall χ^2

---

[4]Heywood cases are phenomena associated with CFA models that represent improper solutions in which the absolute value of an estimated error variance is negative or an estimated correlation is greater than 1.00. For an elaboration on the causes of Heywood cases, see Kline (1998) and Dillon, Kumar, and Mulani (1987).

TABLE 4.5

Selected EQS Output for Initially Hypothesized Model: Modification Indexes

LAGRANGE MULTIPLIER TEST (FOR ADDING PARAMETERS)
ORDERED UNIVARIATE TEST STATISTICS:

NO	CODE		PARAMETER	CHI-SQUARE	PROB.	HANCOCK 206 DF PROB.	PARAMETER CHANGE	STANDAR-DIZED CHANGE
1	2	6	E16,E6	91.038	.000	1.000	.735	.529
2	2	6	E2,E1	82.228	.000	1.000	.614	.549
3	2	12	V12,F1	41.402	.000	1.000	-.313	-.206
4	2	6	E11,E10	37.955	.000	1.000	.581	.524
5	2	6	E21,E7	33.441	.000	1.000	.264	.326
6	2	6	E7,E4	33.345	.000	1.000	.210	.324
7	2	12	V1,F3	28.654	.000	1.000	.871	1.193
8	2	6	E19,E18	18.558	.000	1.000	.250	;285
9	2	6	E6,E5	17.145	.000	1.000	.355	.232
•			•	•	•	•	•	•
•			•	•	•	•	•	•
•			•	•	•	•	•	•
•			•	•	•	•	•	•
274	2	12	V15,F1	.001	.976	1.000	-.002	-.001
275	2	6	E21,E2	.000	.991	1.000	-.001	-.001
276	2	0	V1,F1	.000	1.000	1.000	.000	.000

MULTIVARIATE LAGRANGE MULTIPLIER TEST BY SIMULTANEOUS PROCESS IN STAGE 1
PARAMETER SETS (SUBMATRICES) ACTIVE AT THIS STAGE ARE: PEE GVF

	CUMULATIVE MULTIVARIATE STATISTICS				UNIVARIATE INCREMENT			
STEP	PARAMETER	CHI-SQUARE	D.F.	PROB.	CHI-SQUARE	PROB.	HANCOCK'S SEQUENTIAL D.F.	PROB.
1	E16,E6	91.038	1	.000	91.038	.000	206	1.000
2	E2,E1	169.789	2	.000	78.751	.000	205	1.000
3	V12,F1	211.191	3	.000	41.402	.000	204	1.000
4	E11,E10	249.146	4	.000	37.955	.000	203	1.000
5	E21,E7	281.839	5	.000	32.692	.000	202	1.000
6	E7,E4	319.400	6	.000	37.561	.000	201	1.000
7	V1,F3	344.589	7	.000	25.189	.000	200	1.000
8	E21,E4	365.388	8	.000	20.798	.000	199	1.000
9	E6,E5	382.056	9	.000	16.668	.000	198	1.000
10	E3,E1	397.791	10	.000	15.735	.000	197	1.000
11	V2,F3	413.134	11	.000	15.344	.000	196	1.000
12	E13,E12	428.093	12	.000	14.959	.000	195	1.000
13	E14,E2	441.824	13	.000	13.731	.000	194	1.000
14	E19,E18	453.132	14	.000	11.308	.001	193	1.000
15	E19,E9	463.201	15	.000	10.069	.002	192	1.000
16	V14,F3	473.213	16	.000	10.012	.002	191	1.000
17	E20,E13	481.627	17	.000	8.414	.004	190	1.000
•	•	•	•	•	•	•	•	•
•	•	•	•	•	•	•	•	•
•	•	•	•	•	•	•	•	•
•	•	•	•	•	•	•	•	•
27	E15,E7	558.037	27	.000	5.357	.021	180	1.000
28	E17,E6	562.727	28	.000	4.690	.030	179	1.000
29	E12,E3	566.841	29	.000	4.114	.043	178	1.000

value for the model as a whole would be 169.789. To determine which parameters to free in the respecification of the model, turn to the Univariate Increment column and base the decision on the $LM\chi^2$ statistic and related probability value. Consistent with the ordered univariate statistics presented in the upper part of Table 4.5, values for the same two error covariances are substantially higher than those for the remaining parameters. That the value here for E2,E1 (78.751) differs from its univariate value (82.228) reported previously arises from its computation as a univariate increment based on the multivariate LM Test simultaneous analysis. Although the overall univariate LM Test results parallel those for the multivariate LM Test, decisions regarding which parameter(s) to freely estimate in subsequent respecification of a model should be based on the multivariate LM Test results.

These error covariances represent systematic rather than random measurement error in item responses, and they may derive from characteristics specific either to the items or the respondents (Aish & Jöreskog, 1990). For example, if these parameters reflect item characteristics, they may represent a small omitted factor. Conversely, if they represent respondent characteristics, they may reflect bias such as yea-/nay-saying, social desirability, and the like. Another type of method effect that can trigger correlated errors is a high degree of overlap in item content. Such redundancy occurs when an item, although worded differently, essentially asks the same question; the latter situation seems to be the case here. For example, Item 16 asks whether working directly with people puts too much stress on the respondent, whereas Item 6 asks whether working with people all day puts a real strain on the respondent. Likewise, Item 2 queries if the respondent feels used up at the end of the workday, whereas Item 1 queries if the respondent feels emotionally drained from his or her work.[5]

The question now, of course, is how to proceed from here? Having determined (a) inadequate fit of the hypothesized model to the sample data, and (b) at least two misspecified parameters in the model (i.e., the two error covariances were specified as zero), it seems both reasonable and logical to move into exploratory mode and attempt to modify this model in a sound and responsible manner. Model respecification that includes correlated errors, as with other parameters, must be supported by a strong substantive and/or empirical rationale (Jöreskog, 1993); it appears that this condition exists here. In light of (a) apparent item content overlap, (b) the replication of these same error covariances in previous MBI research (e.g., Byrne, 1991, 1993), and (c) Bentler and Chou's (1987) admonition that forcing large error terms to be uncorrelated is rarely appropriate with real data, I consider respecification of this initial model, with E16,E6 and E2,E1 freely estimated, to be justified. Testing of this respecified model (Model 2) now falls within the framework of post hoc analyses.

---

[5]Unfortunately, refusal of copyright permission by the MBI test publisher prevented the actual item statements from being presented.

Before moving on to these analyses, however, it is important to clarify two questions that may have been raised in the previous discussion: (a) Why respecify two parameters rather than just one in the respecification of Model 2?, and (b) Why not compute the difference in S-Bχ^2 values between Models 1 and 2? Answers to these queries follow.

Question 1: The reason that respecification of both error covariance parameters is possible with EQS is that the LM Test (see chap. 3) operates multivariately in the computation of modification indexes that point to misspecified parameters in the model. In contrast, modification indexes for both LISREL and AMOS are computed univariately, thereby dictating that only one fixed parameter can be freely estimated at a time in the search for optimal model fit.

Question 2: In working with EQS, there is no need to compute the χ^2 difference (D) value between nested models in determining fixed parameters to be freely estimated in the respecification of a model. The rationale in support of this claim derives from statistical theory that has verified the asymptotic equivalence of the D and LM Tests (see, e.g., Buse, 1982; Lee, 1985; and Satorra, 1989). What these statistical findings mean for the LM multivariate statistic is that its value can be interpreted as an approximate decrease in the χ^2 statistic of overall model fit resulting from the respecification of a model in which certain fixed parameters are instead freely estimated. As Bentler (2005, p. 163) has so cogently noted, it is not necessary to actually estimate alternative models to obtain statistics needed to compute the D test because, in principle, the D statistic "is no more accurate or meaningful as a test on the model-differentiating parameters than are the LM and W tests" (see also Yuan & Bentler, 2004a).

POST HOC ANALYSES

Model 2

The EQS Input File

The model specification portion of the input file for Model 2 is presented in Table 4.6, which shows only two differences between this input and the input for the initially hypothesized model. First, note a modification to the method, which now reads as METHOD=ML,ROBUST; second, note the addition of the two error covariance parameters (E16,E6; E2,E1) in the /COVARIANCES paragraph. While you will likely have no difficulty interpreting the specification of the error terms, modification to the Method command requires further explanation, which follows before proceeding with Model 2.

In reviewing the descriptive sample statistics presented previously, evidence of moderate kurtosis associated with five MBI items was noted. The effect of these

Table 4.6
Selected EQS Input for Model 2

/TITLE
CFA of MBI for Male Elementary Tchrs (Calbrn Grp) "MBIELM2
Model 2 - Added: 2 error covs (E16,E6; E2,E1)
/SPECIFICATIONS
DATA= 'c:\eqs61\files\books\data\elemm1.ess';
VARIABLES=22; CASES=372;
METHOD=ML,ROBUST; ANALYSIS=COVARIANCE; MATRIX=RAW;
    •
    •
    •
    •

/COVARIANCES
F1 to F3 = *;
E16,E6 = *; E2,E1 = *;
    •
    •
    •
    •

/END

---

kurtotic variables may be sufficient for the distribution to be multivariately non-normal, thereby violating the underlying assumption of normality associated with the maximum likelihood method of estimation. Violation of this assumption can seriously invalidate statistical hypothesis-testing with the result that the normal theory test statistic (χ^2) may not reflect an adequate evaluation of the model under study (Hu, Bentler, and Kano, 1992). Although other estimation methods were developed for use when the normality assumption does not hold (e.g., asymptotic distribution-free, elliptical, and heterogeneous kurtotic), Chou, Bentler, and Satorra (1991) and Hu et al. (1992) argued that it may be more appropriate to correct the test statistic rather than use a different mode of estimation.

Satorra and Bentler (1988) developed such a statistic that incorporates a scaling correction for the χ^2 statistic when distributional assumptions are violated; its computation takes into account the model, the estimation method, and the sample kurtosis values. The S-Bχ^2 has been shown to be the most reliable test statistic for evaluating mean and covariance structure models under various distributions and sample sizes (Hu et al., 1992; and Curran, West, & Finch, 1995). When the ROBUST option is invoked, the program automatically computes robust standard errors. In addition, however, robust versions of the CFI, RMSEA, and the 90% C.I. related to the latter are also computed.[6] Unquestionably, these robust statistics

---

[6]That the S-Bχ^2, its standard errors, CFI, and RMSEA are "robust" means that their computed values are valid, despite violation of the normality assumption underlying the estimation method.

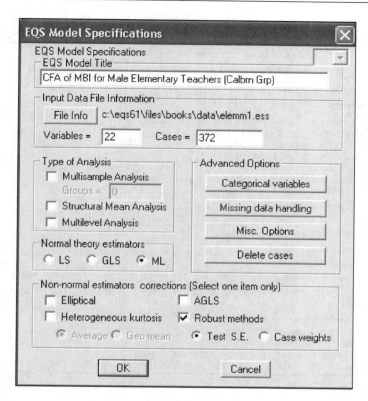

FIG. 4.10. EQS Model Specifications dialog box showing Robust Methods selected.

are worth their weight in gold when a researcher is faced with problems of non-normality in the data. At the time of writing this book, however, these invaluable fit statistics were available only with the EQS program. Fig. 4.10 illustrates how to specify the ROBUST option when constructing a model using BUILD EQS. As illustrated here, you simply select Robust Methods, as shown in the lower right-hand corner of Fig. 4.10.

The EQS Output File

Goodness-of-Fit Summary. The goodness-of-fit results for Model 2 are shown in Table 4.7. In reviewing this model-fit summary, observe two clearly delineated sections. Although the values reported in both sections derive from ML estimation, those for the Bentler–Bonett normed and non-normed fit indexes, the RMSEA and the RMSEA C.I.'s listed in the top half—are computed from the

Table 4.7
Selected EQS Output for Model 2: Goodness-of-Fit Statistics

GOODNESS OF FIT SUMMARY FOR METHOD = ML

```
CHI-SQUARE =      519.082 BASED ON      204 DEGREES OF FREEDOM
PROBABILITY VALUE FOR THE CHI-SQUARE STATISTIC IS            .00000
```

FIT INDICES

```
BENTLER-BONETT          NORMED FIT INDEX =       .849
BENTLER-BONETT NON-NORMED FIT INDEX    =       .889
COMPARATIVE FIT INDEX (CFI)            =       .902
ROOT MEAN-SQUARE RESIDUAL (RMR)        =       .130
STANDARDIZED RMR                       =       .069
ROOT MEAN-SQUARE ERROR OF APPROXIMATION (RMSEA)      =       .065
90% CONFIDENCE INTERVAL OF RMSEA    (        .058,         .071)
```

RELIABILITY COEFFICIENTS

```
CRONBACH'S ALPHA                       =       .792
RELIABILITY COEFFICIENT RHO            =       .844
```

GOODNESS OF FIT SUMMARY FOR METHOD = ROBUST

```
SATORRA-BENTLER SCALED CHI-SQUARE = 432.6538 ON 204 DEGREES OF FREEDOM
PROBABILITY VALUE FOR THE CHI-SQUARE STATISTIC IS            .00000
```

FIT INDICES

```
BENTLER-BONETT          NORMED FIT INDEX =       .852
BENTLER-BONETT NON-NORMED FIT INDEX    =       .904
COMPARATIVE FIT INDEX (CFI)            =       .915
ROOT MEAN-SQUARE ERROR OF APPROXIMATION (RMSEA)      =       .055
90% CONFIDENCE INTERVAL OF RMSEA    (        .048,         .062)
```

uncorrected χ^2 statistic; those in the bottom half are linked to the corrected value (i.e., the S-Bχ^2). Notice the difference between these two χ^2 values. Whereas the uncorrected value is 519.082[7] with 204 degrees of freedom, the S-Bχ^2 is 432.654; the size of this differential is evidence that the sample was indeed somewhat non-normally distributed.[8] The size of the discrepancy between these two values clearly indicates the extent to which the data are non-normally distributed. In light of such non-normality, then, we focus our attention on the Robust Statistics portion of the output.[9] Here, we observe substantial improvement in goodness-of-fit. Nonetheless, in keeping with the recommendations of Hu and Bentler (1999), Model 2 still

---

[7]This value is consistent with the approximate value predicted by the cumulative LM statistics provided in the EQS output reported for the initial model (see Fig. 4.5).

[8]Two degrees of freedom were used up in estimating the two error covariances, thereby accounting for a difference in degrees of freedom between the initial model and Model 2.

[9]Given that the standardized RMR is based on ML estimation, it is still appropriate to report this value in any related goodness-of-fit tables.

Table 4.8

Selected EQS Output for Model 2: Parameter Estimates

COVARIANCES AMONG INDEPENDENT VARIABLES

STATISTICS SIGNIFICANT AT THE 5% LEVEL ARE MARKED WITH @.

```
                                             E
                                            ---

E2 -ITEM2                                   .598*I
E1 -ITEM1                                   .083 I
                                           7.162@I
                                         (  .087)I
                                         ( 6.900@I
                                             I
E16-ITEM16                                  .709*I
E6 -ITEM6                                   .090 I
                                           7.856@I
                                         (  .122)I
                                         ( 5.812@I
                                             I
```

STANDARDIZED SOLUTION:

CORRELATIONS AMONG INDEPENDENT VARIABLES

```
                         E
                        ---

E2 -ITEM2               .473*I
E1 -ITEM1                   I
                            I
E16-ITEM16              .488*I
E6 -ITEM6                   I
                            I
```

must be considered only a marginally well-fitting model (CFI* = .915; RMSEA* = .055; 90% C.I. .048, .062). Thus, we need to review the related LM Test statistics to determine if there is any justification for additional modification to the model. Before turning to this portion of the output file, however, the estimates related to only the two error covariances are reviewed.

Selected Parameter Estimates.   Table 4.8 lists the unstandardized as well as standardized parameter estimates for the two error covariances. Turning first to the unstandardized estimates, you will see 5 rows of numbers associated with each of the two parameters. The first line represents the ML estimate. Values displayed on the second and third lines represent the uncorrected ML standard error and its related Z-statistic, respectively. Values on the fourth and fifth lines in parentheses represent the robust (i.e., corrected) standard errors and their resulting

Z-statistics, respectively. Focusing on the robust statistics, we determine that the error covariance between Items 2 and 1 has an estimated value of .598, a standard error of .087, and a Z-value of 6.900; the robust estimate for the error covariance between Items 16 and 6 is .709 with a standard error of .122, resulting in a Z-value of 5.812. Note that whereas both the uncorrected and corrected standard errors were fairly close for Items 1 and 2, they were substantially different for Items 6 and 16, again illustrating how the two values can differ in light of non-normality in the data. Overall, however, both error covariance parameters were found to be statistically significant. Finally, review of the standardized solution shows the strength of these error correlations. With values of .473 (E2,E1) and .488 (E16,E6), we must conclude that these values are indeed substantial.

Modification Indexes.   An abbreviated summary of modification indexes related to Model 2 is presented in Table 4.9. Review of these values related to the multivariate portion of the output shows that the parameter with the highest LM Test incremental univariate χ^2 value represents a cross-loading (V12,F1) and has a probability < .05. In the initial model, Item 12 was specified as loading on Factor 3 (Reduced Personal Accomplishment), yet the LM Test is telling us that this item should additionally load on Factor 1 (Emotional Exhaustion). To understand why this cross-loading might be occurring, let's look at the actual item content, which asks for a level of agreement or disagreement with the statement that the respondent "feels very energetic."

Although this item was deemed by Maslach and Jackson (1981, 1986) to measure a sense of personal accomplishment, it seems both evident and logical that it also taps a respondent's feelings of emotional exhaustion. Ideally, items on a measuring instrument should clearly target only one of its underlying constructs (or factors). The question in this analysis of the MBI, however, is whether to include this parameter in a second respecified model. Provided with some justification for the double-loading effect, together with evidence from the literature that this same cross-loading has been noted in other research, I consider it appropriate to respecify (Model 3) with this parameter freely estimated.

Given the close proximity of the LM Test χ^2 values for the next three error covariance parameters (before the drop-off at Step 5), you are undoubtedly wondering why I did not include them also in Model 3. In selecting which parameters to free in subsequent models, the researcher walks a thin line between adequately fitting and overfitting the model; this is the same dilemma with respect to the next three parameters. Thus, in light of (a) the existing Model 2 fit, (b) the fact that these subsequent parameters represent error covariances, and (c) the importance of parsimony, I prefer to estimate only one additional parameter in Model 3 at this time. Findings from this test of Model 3 will determine if further respecification of the MBI structure is justified.

Table 4.9

Selected EQS Output for Model 2: Modification Indexes

LAGRANGE MULTIPLIER TEST (FOR ADDING PARAMETERS)
ORDERED UNIVARIATE TEST STATISTICS:

NO	CODE		PARAMETER	CHI-SQUARE	PROB.	HANCOCK 206 DF PROB.	PARAMETER CHANGE	STANDAR- DIZED CHANGE
1	2	12	V12,F1	40.912	.000	1.000	-.332	-.229
2	2	6	E11,E10	37.068	.000	1.000	.576	.522
3	2	6	E21,E7	33.548	.000	1.000	.264	.327
4	2	6	E7,E4	33.436	.000	1.000	.210	.324
5	2	6	E19,E18	18.543	.000	1.000	.250	.285
•		•	•	•	•	•	•	•
•		•	•	•	•	•	•	•
•		•	•	•	•	•	•	•
•		•	•	•	•	•	•	•
272	2	6	E13,E10	.001	.978	1.000	-.002	-.002
273	2	6	E5,E2	.000	.997	1.000	.000	.000
274	2	0	V1,F1	.000	1.000	1.000	.000	.000

MULTIVARIATE LAGRANGE MULTIPLIER TEST BY SIMULTANEOUS PROCESS IN STAGE 1
PARAMETER SETS (SUBMATRICES) ACTIVE AT THIS STAGE ARE: PEE GVF

	CUMULATIVE MULTIVARIATE STATISTICS				UNIVARIATE INCREMENT		HANCOCK'S SEQUENTIAL	
STEP	PARAMETER	CHI-SQUARE	D.F.	PROB.	CHI-SQUARE	PROB.	D.F.	PROB.
1	V12,F1	40.912	1	.000	40.912	.000	204	1.000
2	E11,E10	77.981	2	.000	37.068	.000	203	1.000
3	E21,E7	110.737	3	.000	32.756	.000	202	1.000
4	E7,E4	148.334	4	.000	37.597	.000	201	1.000
5	E21,E4	169.122	5	.000	20.788	.000	200	1.000
•	•	•	•	•	•	•	•	•
•	•	•	•	•	•	•	•	•
•	•	•	•	•	•	•	•	•
•	•	•	•	•	•	•	•	•
24	E15,E7	343.483	24	.000	5.425	.020	181	1.000
25	E17,E6	347.951	25	.000	4.468	.035	180	1.000
26	E14,E2	352.109	26	.000	4.157	.041	179	1.000

Model 3

The EQS Input File

An abbreviated version of the Model 3 input file is included so readers can visualize how to specify an item that loads on two factors. Accordingly, in Table 4.10, Item 12 (V12) is shown as loading on both F3 and F1, and both of these regression paths are freely estimated. Of course, the two error covariances specified in Model 2 are also estimated as shown in the /COVARIANCES paragraph.

Table 4.10

Selected EQS Input for Model 3

/TITLE

CFA of MBI for Male Elementary Tchrs (Calbrn Grp) "MBIELM3

Model 2 - Added: 2 error covs (E16,E6; E2,E1)

Model 3 - Added: 1 cross-loading (V12,F1)

/SPECIFICATIONS

DATA= 'c:\eqs61\files\books\data\elemm1.ess' ;

VARIABLES=22; CASES=372;

METHOD=ML,ROBUST; ANALYSIS=COVARIANCE; MATRIX=RAW;

-
-
-
-

/EQUATIONS

V1 = 1F1 + E1;

V2 = *F1 + E2;

V3 = *F1 + E3;

V4 = 1F3 + E4;

V5 = 1F2 + E5;

V6 = *F1 + E6;

V7 = *F3 + E7;

V8 = *F1 + E8;

V9 = *F3 + E9;

V10 = *F2 + E10;

V11 = *F2 + E11;

V12 = *F3 + *F1 + E12;

V13 = *F1 + E13;

V14 = *F1 + E14;

V15 = *F2 + E15;

V16 = *F1 + E16;

V17 = *F3 + E17;

V18 = *F3 + E18;

V19 = *F3 + E19;

V20 = *F1 + E20;

V21 = *F3 + E21;

V22 = *F2 + E22;

-
-
-
-

/COVARIANCES

F1 to F3 = *;

E16,E6 = *; E2,E1 = *;

/END

Table 4.11

Selected EQS Output for Model 3: Goodness-of-Fit Statistics

GOODNESS OF FIT SUMMARY FOR METHOD = ML

```
CHI-SQUARE =           477.298 BASED ON        203 DEGREES OF FREEDOM
PROBABILITY VALUE FOR THE CHI-SQUARE STATISTIC IS           .00000
```

FIT INDICES

```
BENTLER-BONETT       NORMED FIT INDEX =        .861
BENTLER-BONETT NON-NORMED FIT INDEX   =        .903
COMPARATIVE FIT INDEX (CFI)           =        .915
ROOT MEAN-SQUARE RESIDUAL (RMR)       =        .109
STANDARDIZED RMR                      =        .058
ROOT MEAN-SQUARE ERROR OF APPROXIMATION (RMSEA)        =        .060
90% CONFIDENCE INTERVAL OF RMSEA     (        .053,        .067)
```

RELIABILITY COEFFICIENTS

```
CRONBACH'S ALPHA                      =        .792
RELIABILITY COEFFICIENT RHO           =        .843
```

GOODNESS OF FIT SUMMARY FOR METHOD = ROBUST

```
SATORRA-BENTLER SCALED CHI-SQUARE =      399.1564 ON 203 DEGREES OF FREEDOM
PROBABILITY VALUE FOR THE CHI-SQUARE STATISTIC IS .00000
```

FIT INDICES

```
BENTLER-BONETT       NORMED FIT INDEX =        .863
BENTLER-BONETT NON-NORMED FIT INDEX   =        .917
COMPARATIVE FIT INDEX (CFI)           =        .927
ROOT MEAN-SQUARE ERROR OF APPROXIMATION (RMSEA)        =        .051
90% CONFIDENCE INTERVAL OF RMSEA     (        .044,        .058)
```

The EQS Output File

Goodness-of-Fit Summary. A review of goodness-of-fit statistics in Table 4.11 related to Model 3 reveals only a modest increase in the robust CFI value from Model 2 (CFI* = .915) to Model 3 (CFI* = .927), with only minimally better values for both the SRMR (from .069 to .060) and RMSEA (from .055 to .051).

Selected Parameter Estimates. Due to space limitations, only a few regression path estimates are presented in Table 4.12. Most important among these estimates are those related to Item 12. As you will readily observe, the loading of this item on both factors is not only statistically significant but also basically of the same degree of intensity. Nonetheless, the standardized estimates show the original loading of Item 12 on Factor 3 (Personal Accomplishment) to be slightly higher (.425) than its cross-loading (−.324) on Factor 1 (Emotional Exhaustion). Also of note is the negative sign associated with the cross-loading, which, of course, makes sense substantively.

Table 4.12
Selected EQS Output for Model 3: Parameter Estimates

**MEASUREMENT EQUATIONS WITH STANDARD ERRORS AND TEST STATISTICS
   STATISTICS SIGNIFICANT AT THE 5% LEVEL ARE MARKED WITH @.
                (ROBUST STATISTICS IN PARENTHESES)**

```
ITEM1    =V1  =        1.000 F1   + 1.000 E1
ITEM2    =V2  =         .877*F1   + 1.000 E2
                        .049
                       17.942@
                   (   .041)
                   (  21.345@
ITEM3    =V3  =        1.074*F1   + 1.000 E3  .
                        .075
                       14.287@
                   (   .058)
                   (  18.434@
ITEM12   =V12 =        -.317*F1   + 1.134*F3   + 1.000 E12
                        .050          .188
                       -6.389@       6.037@
                   (   .054)     (   .202)
                   (  -5.911@    (   5.618@
```

        •
        •
        •

STANDARDIZED SOLUTION:

```
ITEM1    =V1  =     .735 F1    + .679 E1
ITEM2    =V2  =     .693*F1    + .721 E2
ITEM3    =V3  =     .756*F1    + .655 E3
ITEM4    =V4  =     .448 F3    + .894 E4
ITEM5    =V5  =     .561 F2    + .828 E5
ITEM6    =V6  =     .586*F1    + .810 E6
ITEM7    =V7  =     .515*F3    + .857 E7
ITEM8    =V8  =     .860*F1    + .511 E8
ITEM9    =V9  =     .599*F3    + .801 E9
ITEM10   =V10 =     .665*F2    + .747 E10
ITEM11   =V11 =     .746*F2    + .666 E11
ITEM12   =V12 =    -.324*F1    + .425*F3    + .793 E12
ITEM13   =V13 =     .778*F1    + .629 E13
ITEM14   =V14 =     .621*F1    + .784 E14
ITEM15   =V15 =     .586*F2    + .811 E15
ITEM16   =V16 =     .616*F1    + .788 E16
ITEM17   =V17 =     .697*F3    + .717 E17
ITEM18   =V18 =     .664*F3    + .747 E18
ITEM19   =V19 =     .635*F3    + .773 E19
ITEM20   =V20 =     .695*F1    + .719 E20
ITEM21   =V21 =     .474*F3    + .880 E21
ITEM22   =V22 =     .406*F2    + .914 E22
```

Maintaining a watchful eye on parsimony, it behooves the researcher to test a model in which the aberrant item is specified as loading on the alternate factor rather than the one on which it was originally designed to load. Within the context of the present example, this model would specify Item 12 as loading on F1 (Emotional Exhaustion) rather than F3 (Personal Accomplishment); in other words, there is no specified cross-loading. In the interest of space, once again, I simply report the most important criteria determined from this model compared with those of Model 2 in which Item 12 was specified as loading on F3 (its original targeted factor). Accordingly, findings from the estimation of this alternative model revealed (a) model fit to be poorer (CFI* = .907) than for Model 2 (CFI* = .915), and (b) the standardized estimate to be weaker (−.468) than for Model 2 (0.554). As might be expected, the LM Test identified parameter V12,F3 (loading of Item 12 on Factor 3) to be the top candidate considered for specification in a subsequent model (LMχ^2 = 58.507) compared with 37.364 for the parameter with the next largest LMχ^2 value (E11,E10).

It seems evident that Item 12 is problematic and definitely in need of content revision, a task beyond the scope of this chapter. However, provided with evidence of no clear loading of this item, it seems most appropriate to leave the cross-loading in place and to continue reviewing the EQS output related to Model 3. As such, we turn now to the modification indexes which are presented in Table 4.13.

Modification Indexes. Review of the values displayed in Table 4.13 shows that the error covariance, E11,E10, exhibits the highest incremental univariate LMχ^2 value. Two items bear on this error covariance: Items 10 and 11. Item 10 asks if the teacher has become more callous toward people since taking this job; Item 11 asks if the teacher worries that the job is hardening him emotionally.

Again, content overlap is apparently generating these error covariances. In light of this rationale, together with evidence of the same error covariance parameters found in previous studies of the MBI (e.g., Byrne, 1991, 1993), Model 3 was respecified with this error covariance specified as a freely estimated parameter.

Model 4

The EQS Input File

Table 4.14 shows an abbreviated version of the input file for Model 4. Basically, the only changes are in the /TITLE and /COVARIANCES paragraphs. Note that the cross-loading of Item 12 on both F3 and F1 remains specified.

The EQS Output File

Goodness-of-Fit Summary. Review of the robust statistics in Table 4.15 reveals a substantial increase in model fit (CFI* = .937) following incorporation into the model of error covariance E11, E10. This index is supported by an

Table 4.13
Selected EQS Output for Model 3: Modification Indexes

LAGRANGE MULTIPLIER TEST (FOR ADDING PARAMETERS)
ORDERED UNIVARIATE TEST STATISTICS:

NO	CODE		PARAMETER	CHI-SQUARE	PROB.	HANCOCK 206 DF PROB.	PARAMETER CHANGE	STANDAR-DIZED CHANGE
1	2	6	E11,E10	36.569	.000	1.000	.573	.521
2	2	6	E21,E7	32.640	.000	1.000	.260	.324
3	2	6	E7,E4	32.119	.000	1.000	.205	.320
4	2	6	E19,E18	18.393	.000	1.000	.252	.288
5	2	6	E15,E5	16.083	.000	1.000	.319	.246
•			•	•	•	•	•	•
•			•	•	•	•	•	•
•			•	•	•	•	•	•
•			•	•	•	•	•	•
270	2	12	V3,F2	.001	.975	1.000	.004	.003
271	2	6	E13,E10	.001	.976	1.000	-.002	-.002
272	2	6	E17,E1	.000	.997	1.000	.000	.000

MULTIVARIATE LAGRANGE MULTIPLIER TEST BY SIMULTANEOUS PROCESS IN STAGE 1
PARAMETER SETS (SUBMATRICES) ACTIVE AT THIS STAGE ARE: PEE GVF

	CUMULATIVE MULTIVARIATE STATISTICS				UNIVARIATE INCREMENT			
STEP	PARAMETER	CHI-SQUARE	D.F.	PROB.	CHI-SQUARE	PROB.	D.F.	HANCOCK'S SEQUENTIAL PROB.
1	E11,E10	36.569	1	.000	36.569	.000	203	1.000
2	E21,E7	69.209	2	.000	32.640	.000	202	1.000
3	E7,E4	106.570	3	.000	37.361	.000	201	1.000
4	E21,E4	127.710	4	.000	21.140	.000	200	1.000
•	•	•	•	•	•	•	•	•
•	•	•	•	•	•	•	•	•
•	•	•	•	•	•	•	•	•
•	•	•	•	•	•	•	•	•
23	E15,E7	301.498	23	.000	5.412	.020	181	1.000
24	E17,E6	306.032	24	.000	4.534	.033	180	1.000
25	E14,E2	310.308	25	.000	4.276	.039	179	1.000

acceptable RMSEA* value of .047, with a 90% C.I. of .040, .055. Given these findings, we can consider this model to adequately represent the sample data. The parameter estimates derived from this final model are discussed in the following subsection and their values are reported in Table 4.16.

Parameter Estimates.   Again, for each estimated variable, the ML estimate is presented first, followed by the standard error and Z-value; the robust statistics follow on Lines 4 and 5 in parentheses. All estimates are statistically significant including the one cross-loading and the three error covariances. Although the standardized estimates are not reported herein, due to space restrictions, they are all substantial; of particular interest are the values for the correlated errors, which

Table 4.14
Selected EQS Input for Final Model

/TITLE
CFA of MBI for Male Elementary Tchrs (Calbrn Grp) "MBIELMF"
Model 2 - Added: 2 error covs (E16,E6; E2,E1)
Model 3 - Added: 1 cross-loading (V12,F1)
Final Model: Added 1 error cov (E11,E10)
/SPECIFICATIONS
DATA='c:\eqs61\files\books\data\elemm1.ess';
VARIABLES=22; CASES=372;
METHOD=ML,ROBUST; ANALYSIS=COVARIANCE; MATRIX=RAW;
-
-
-
-

/EQUATIONS
V1 =   1F1 + E1;
V2 = *F1 + E2;
V3 = *F1 + E3;
V4 = 1F3 + E4;
V5 = 1F2 + E5;
V6 = *F1 + E6;
V7 = *F3 + E7;
V8 = *F1 + E8;
V9 = *F3 + E9;
V10 = *F2 + E10;
V11 = *F2 + E11;
V12 = *F3 + *F1 + E12;
V13 = *F1 + E13;
V14 = *F1 + E14;
V15 = *F2 + E15;
V16 = *F1 + E16;
V17 = *F3 + E17;
V18 = *F3 + E18;
V19 = *F3 + E19;
V20 = *F1 + E20;
V21 = *F3 + E21;
V22 = *F2 + E22;
-
-
-

/COVARIANCES
F1 to F3 = *;
E16,E6 = *; E2,E1 = *; E11,E10 = *;
/END

Table 4.15

Selected EQS Output for Final Model: Goodness-of-Fit Statistics

---

GOODNESS OF FIT SUMMARY FOR METHOD = ML

CHI-SQUARE =   445.220 BASED ON   202 DEGREES OF FREEDOM
PROBABILITY VALUE FOR THE CHI-SQUARE STATISTIC IS   .00000

FIT INDICES

BENTLER-BONETT   NORMED FIT INDEX =   .871
BENTLER-BONETT NON-NORMED FIT INDEX   =   .913
COMPARATIVE FIT INDEX (CFI)   =   .924
ROOT MEAN-SQUARE RESIDUAL (RMR)   =   .105
STANDARDIZED RMR   =   .057
ROOT MEAN-SQUARE ERROR OF APPROXIMATION (RMSEA)   =   .057
90% CONFIDENCE INTERVAL OF RMSEA   (.050,   .064)

RELIABILITY COEFFICIENTS

CRONBACH'S ALPHA   =   .792
RELIABILITY COEFFICIENT RHO   =   .836

GOODNESS OF FIT SUMMARY FOR METHOD = ROBUST

SATORRA-BENTLER SCALED CHI-SQUARE =   370.9958 ON   202 DEGREES OF FREEDOM
PROBABILITY VALUE FOR THE CHI-SQUARE STATISTIC IS   .00000

FIT INDICES

BENTLER-BONETT   NORMED FIT INDEX =   .873
BENTLER-BONETT NON-NORMED FIT INDEX   =   .928
COMPARATIVE FIT INDEX (CFI)   =   .937
BOLLEN (IFT) FIT INDEX   =   .938
MCDONALD (MFT) FIT INDEX   =   .797
ROOT MEAN-SQUARE ERROR OF APPROXIMATION (RMSEA)   =   .047
90% CONFIDENCE INTERVAL OF RMSEA   (.040,   .055)

---

are .469, .488, and .368 for Items 2 and 1, Items 16 and 6, and Items 11 and 10, respectively. These findings are suggestive of redundant content.

Modification Indexes.   Not surprisingly, the LM Test statistics shown in Table 4.17 suggest that additional misspecification in the model is mostly due to error covariances among MBI items. Although from a statistical perspective respecification that includes the first two parameters is justified, substantive considerations do not support this decision. Thus, for reasons described earlier, I consider it inappropriate to continue fitting the model beyond this point. Therefore, Model 4 represents the final model of MBI structure.

Historically, one of the major concerns associated with post hoc model-fitting has been the potential for capitalization on chance factors in the respecification of alternate models. Recently, procedures were developed that address this issue of Type I errors. In chapter 3, Hancock's (1999) Scheffé-type adjustment procedure was introduced and is now implemented in EQS. However, this approach to controlling for Type I errors is conservative, leading Bentler (2005) to caution that,

Table 4.16

Selected EQS Output for Final Model: Parameter Estimates

MEASUREMENT EQUATIONS WITH STANDARD ERRORS AND TEST STATISTICS STATISTICS SIGNIFICANT AT THE 5% LEVEL ARE MARKED WITH @. (ROBUST STATISTICS IN PARENTHESES)

```
ITEM1    =V1  =    1.000 F1   + 1.000 E1
ITEM2    =V2  =     .878*F1   + 1.000 E2
                    .049
                  17.945@
                 (  .041)
                 ( 21.345@
ITEM3    =V3  =    1.073*F1   + 1.000 E3
                    .075
                  14.284@
                 (  .058)
                 ( 18.484@
ITEM4    =V4  =    1.000 F3   + 1.000 E4
ITEM5    =V5  =    1.000 F2   + 1.000 E5
ITEM6    =V6  =     .764*F1   + 1.000 E6
                    .069
                  10.996@
                 (  .076)
                 ( 10.005@
ITEM7    =V7  =     .973*F3   + 1.000 E7
                    .147
                   6.607@
                 (  .128)
                 (  7.616@
ITEM8    =V8  =    1.215*F1   + 1.000 E8
                    .075
                  16.277@
                 (  .066)
                 ( 18.407@
ITEM9    =V9  =    1.762*F3   + 1.000 E9
                    .248
                   7.098@
                 (  .316)
                 (  5.570@
ITEM10   =V10 =     .889*F2   + 1.000 E10
                    .114
                   7.819@
                 (  .124)
                 (  7.187@
ITEM11   =V11 =    1.105*F2   + 1.000 E11
                    .125
                   8.808@
                 (  .129)
                 (  8.542@
```

(Continued)

Table 4.16
(Continued)

ITEM12   =V12 =   -.316*F1   + 1.130*F3   + 1.000 E12
                    .050   .188
                  -6.358@   6.016@
                 (.054)   (.201)
                 (-5.899@   (5.616@

ITEM13   =V13 =   1.072*F1   + 1.000 E13
                    .073
                  14.719@
                 (.069)
                 (15.436@

ITEM14   =V14 =   .880*F1   + 1.000 E14
                    .075
                  11.657@
                 (.062)
                 (14.089@

ITEM15   =V15 =   .921*F2   + 1.000 E15
                    .105
                   8.780@
                 (.120)
                 (7.681@

ITEM16   =V16 =   .727*F1   + 1.000 E16
                    .063
                  11.541@
                 (.072)
                 (10.045@

ITEM17   =V17 =   1.326*F3   + 1.000 E17
                    .176
                   7.549@
                 (.197)
                 (6.728@

ITEM18   =V18 =   1.888*F3   + 1.000 E18
                    .255
                   7.414@
                 (.290)
                 (6.508@

ITEM19   =V19 =   1.694*F3   + 1.000 E19
                    .232
                   7.294@
                 (.285)
                 (5.942@

ITEM20   =V20 =   .806*F1   + 1.000 E20
                    .062
                  13.095@
                 (.066)
                 (12.144@

Table 4.16
(Continued)

```
ITEM21   =V21 =   1.342*F3     + 1.000 E21
                   .213
                  6.286@
                (  .223)
                ( 6.004@
ITEM22   =V22 =    .776*F2     + 1.000 E22
                   .116
                  6.721@
                (  .116)
                ( 6.677@
```

VARIANCES OF INDEPENDENT VARIABLES

```
              V                              F
             ---                            ---
                      I F1 - F1        1.490*I
                      I                  .187 I
                      I                 7.971@I
                      I               (  .150)I
                      I               ( 9.946@I
                      I                      I
                      I F2 - F2         .803*I
                      I                  .144 I
                      I                 5.560@I
                      I               (  .171)I
                      I               ( 4.691@I
                      I                      I
                      I F3 - F3         .200*I
                      I                  .049 I
                      I                 4.110@I
                      I               (  .051)I
                      I               ( 3.904@I
```

VARIANCES OF INDEPENDENT VARIABLES

```
              E
             ---
E1  -ITEM1          1.271*I
                     .106 I
                   11.976@I
                 (   .103)I
                 ( 12.285@I
                          I
E2  -ITEM2          1.242*I
                     .101 I
                   12.293@I
                 (   .098)I
                 ( 12.648@I
     •              •
     •              •
     •              •
     •              •
```

(Continued)

Table 4.16
(Continued)

```
E22   -ITEM22              2.014*I
                            .160 I
                          12.614@I
                       (   .182)I
                       ( 11.036@I
                               I
```

COVARIANCES AMONG INDEPENDENT VARIABLES

```
                E                            F
               ---                          ---
                            I F2 - F2            .749*I
                            I F1 - F1            .104 I
                            I                   7.188@I
                            I               (   .106)I
                            I               ( 7.048@I
                            I                        I
                            I F3 - F3           -.167*I
                            I F1 - F1            .040 I
                            I                  -4.163@I
                            I               (   .038)I
                            I               ( -4.362@I
                            I                        I
                            I F3 - F3           -.182*I
                            I F2 - F2            .038 I
                            I                  -4.762@I
                            I               (   .038)I
                            I               ( -4.796@I
```

COVARIANCES AMONG INDEPENDENT VARIABLES

```
                E
               ---
E2    -ITEM2               .590*I
E1    -ITEM1               .083 I
                          7.122@I
                       (   .086)I
                       ( 6.879@I
                               I
E16   -ITEM16              .708*I
E6    -ITEM6               .090 I
                          7.858@I
                       (   .122)I
                       ( 5.781@I
                               I
E11   -ITEM11              .518*I
E10   -ITEM10             .102 I
                          5.099@I
                       (   .110)I
                       ( 4.726@I
                               I
```

Table 4.17

Selected EQS Output for Final Model: Modification Indexes

LAGRANGE MULTIPLIER TEST (FOR ADDING PARAMETERS)
ORDERED UNIVARIATE TEST STATISTICS:

NO	CODE		PARAMETER	CHI-SQUARE	PROB.	HANCOCK 206 DF PROB.	PARAMETER CHANGE	STANDAR- DIZED CHANGE
1	2	6	E21,E7	32.419	.000	1.000	.259	.324
2	2	6	E7,E4	31.926	.000	1.000	.205	.319
3	2	6	E19,E18	18.231	.000	1.000	.251	.287
4	2	12	V1,F3	14.609	.000	1.000	.540	.727
5	2	6	E18,E7	14.375	.000	1.000	-.161	-.236
•			•	•	•	•	•	•
•			•	•	•	•	•	•
•			•	•	•	•	•	•
•			•	•	•	•	•	•
268	2	6	E14,E3	.001	.977	1.000	.003	.002
269	2	6	E22,E11	.000	.991	1.000	.001	.001
270	2	6	E16,E7	.000	.993	1.000	.000	.000

MULTIVARIATE LAGRANGE MULTIPLIER TEST BY SIMULTANEOUS PROCESS IN STAGE 1
PARAMETER SETS (SUBMATRICES) ACTIVE AT THIS STAGE ARE: PEE GVF

		CUMULATIVE MULTIVARIATE STATISTICS			UNIVARIATE INCREMENT		HANCOCK'S SEQUENTIAL	
STEP	PARAMETER	CHI-SQUARE	D.F.	PROB.	CHI-SQUARE	PROB.	D.F.	PROB.
1	E21,E7	32.419	1	.000	32.419	.000	202	1.000
2	E7,E4	69.556	2	.000	37.138	.000	201	1.000
3	E21,E4	90.806	3	.000	21.250	.000	200	1.000
4	V1,F3	105.415	4	.000	14.608	.000	199	1.000
5	E13,E12	118.674	5	.000	13.259	.000	198	1.000
•	•	•	•	•	•	•	•	•
•	•	•	•	•	•	•	•	•
•	•	•	•	•	•	•	•	•
•	•	•	•	•	•	•	•	•
20	E14,E10	252.892	20	.000	4.967	.026	183	1.000
21	E17,E6	257.192	21	.000	4.300	.038	182	1.000
22	E14,E2	261.379	22	.000	4.187	.041	181	1.000

Table 4.18

Selected EQS Output for Final Model: The Wald Test

WALD TEST (FOR DROPPING PARAMETERS)
ROBUST INFORMATION MATRIX USED IN THIS WALD TEST
MULTIVARIATE WALD TEST BY SIMULTANEOUS PROCESS

		CUMULATIVE MULTIVARIATE STATISTICS			UNIVARIATE INCREMENT	
STEP	PARAMETER	CHI-SQUARE	D.F.	PROBABILITY	CHI-SQUARE	PROBABILITY

* * * * * * * * * * * *

    NONE OF THE FREE PARAMETERS IS DROPPED IN THIS PROCESS.

in practice, this criterion will likely be helpful only in situations in which there are huge misspecifications in a model (i.e., $\chi^2/df = $ or >5). Indeed, this was the case with the present work. Although results for the multivariate LM Test pointed to obvious misspecification in the model, the Hancock criterion considered these misspecified parameters unimportant to the model ($p = 1.000$).

Taking a different approach to the problem of Type I errors in SEM, Green and associates (Green & Babyak, 1997; and Green, Thompson, & Poirier, 2001) proposed a Bonferroni-type correction to the number of parameters added to a respecified model during post hoc analyses. Although a third approach to controlling for Type I errors was originally suggested informally by Chou and Bentler (1990), it was regenerated and presented in a more formal manner by Green, Thompson, and Poirier (1999). This strategy is based on a two-step process in which parameters are first added to the model in the process of optimizing model fit and then subsequently tested and deleted from the model if they cease to contribute importantly to model fit. Another approach to the problem of chance factors is to cross-validate the final model in a second independent new or split sample. This issue of cross-validation is addressed in chapter 8.

With four new parameters (i.e., three error covariances and one cross-loading) added to the respecified model of MBI structure (i.e., Step 1), we now test for their validity (i.e., Step 2). EQS works well in this approach through use of the LM Test and Wald test (WTest) capabilities. Whereas the LM Test focuses on the freeing up of parameters specified as fixed in a given model, the WTest focuses on the fixing of parameters specified as free in the model. The task now is to test the final model of MBI structure using the WTest. In specifying this command, it is only necessary to replace /LM Test with /WTest and delete the SET=GVF,PEE; statement. Results stemming from this WTest of the final model are presented in Table 4.18; as clearly indicated, all parameters were considered important to the specified model.

CONCLUSION

In this chapter, the validity of scores derived from the MBI for a sample of male elementary-school teachers was tested. Based on sound statistical and theoretical rationales, we can be confident of the modified model of MBI structure as determined through post hoc model-fitting procedures based on the LM Test and subsequent testing for their validity in the model based on the WTest. Figure 4.11 is a schematic summary of this final well-fitting model.

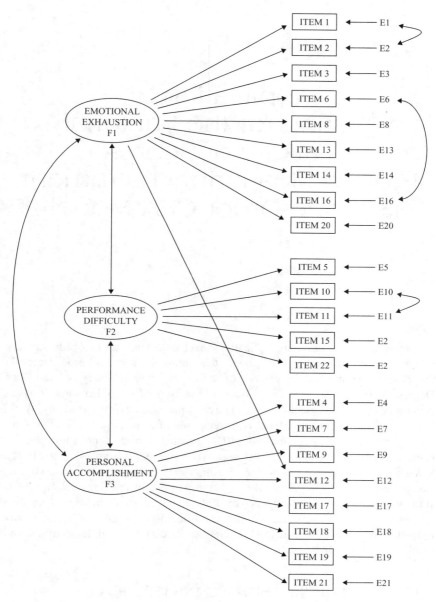

FIG. 4.11. Final model of factorial structure for the Maslach Burnout Inventory.
Note: Item numbers correspond to variable numbers (e.g., ITEM 1 = V1).

5

Application 3:
Testing for the Factorial
Validity of Scores
From a Measuring Instrument
(Second-Order CFA Model)

In contrast to the two previous applications that focused on CFA first-order models, this application examines a CFA model that comprises a second-order factor. In this chapter, we test for the validity of scores on a hierarchically ordered Beck Depression Inventory (BDI; Beck, Ward, Mendelson, Mock, & Erbaugh, 1961) as they relate to nonclinical adolescents. The example is taken from a study by Byrne, Baron, and Campbell (1993) and represents one of a series of studies that have tested for the validity of second-order BDI structure for high school adolescents in Canada (Byrne & Baron, 1993, 1994; and Byrne, Baron, & Campbell, 1993, 1994), Sweden (Byrne, Baron, Larsson, & Melin, 1995, 1996), and Bulgaria (Byrne, Baron, & Balev, 1996, 1998). Although the purpose of the Byrne et al. (1993) study was to test for the equivalence of BDI structure across gender for Canadian high school students, this chapter focuses on factorial validity as it relates only to the female sample ($n = 321$). (For details regarding the sample, analyses, and results, see the original article.)

THE MEASURING INSTRUMENT
UNDER STUDY

The BDI is a 21-item scale that measures symptoms related to cognitive, behavioral, affective, and somatic components of depression. Although originally designed for use by trained interviewers, it is now typically used as a self-report measure. For each item, respondents are presented with four statements rated from 0 to 3 in terms of intensity and asked to select the one that most accurately describes their own feelings; higher scores represent a more severe level of reported depression. For the study from which the current application is taken, scores were recoded such that their scale points ranged from 1 through 4 rather than from 0 through 3. As discussed in chapter 4, the CFA of a measuring instrument is most appropriately conducted with fully developed assessment measures that have demonstrated satisfactory factorial validity. Justification for CFA procedures in this instance is based on evidence provided by Tanaka and Huba (1984) and replicated studies by Byrne and associates (cited previously) that have shown BDI score data to be most adequately represented by a hierarchical factorial structure. As such, it is argued that the three first-order factors are explained by some higher order factor that, in the case of the BDI, represents a single second-order factor of general depression.

The Hypothesized Model

The model to be tested in this application derives from the work of Byrne et al. (1993). As such, the CFA model hypothesized a priori that (a) responses to the BDI could be explained by three first-order factors (i.e., Negative Attitude, Performance Difficulty, and Somatic Elements) and one second-order factor (i.e., General Depression); (b) each item would have a nonzero loading on the first-order factor it was designed to measure and zero loadings on the other two first-order factors; (c) error terms associated with each item would be uncorrelated; and (d) covariation among the three first-order factors would be explained fully by their regression on the second-order factor. A diagrammatic representation of this model is presented in Fig. 5.1.

Before reviewing the EQS input file for this hypothesized model, I wish, once again, to provide you with additional information that I hope you will find helpful in your own SEM applications using the EQS program. Thus let us take a brief digression here in order that I can (a) illustrate the process used by EQS in converting a raw data file into a system .ess file, and (b) review various considerations bearing on the analysis of categorical data in SEM.

Creating an .ess file.   In EQS, system files carry the extension ".ess" and thus are colloquially termed "ESS files." Although these files can be thought of as data files, they actually go beyond the usual score-only data because they store additional information including number of variables, variable labels, and sample size. Because ESS files are the most convenient files with which to work, users may consider converting a given data set into an ESS file. This process is relatively straightforward and begins by asking EQS to open the raw data set to be converted. As soon as EQS detects that it is a non-ESS file, it presents the Raw Data File

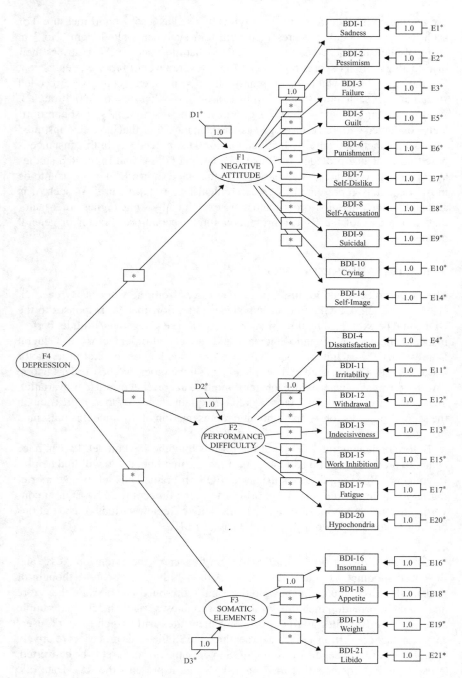

FIG. 5.1.   Hypothesized model of second-order factorial structure for the Back Depression Inventory.

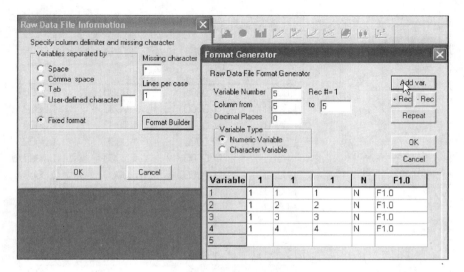

FIG. 5.2. Raw Data File Information dialog box with Format Generator box.

Information dialog box, shown on the left-hand side of Fig. 5.2. Here, the program asks for details that describe the format of the raw data file. In the case of the BDI data used in this application, Fixed Format (shown with a highlighted dot) was selected, which then activated the Format Builder tab. The program requires the user to specify the number of lines of data per subject and allows the user to code missing data in any way desired. Given that we have selected Fixed Format, we now click on the Format Builder tab, which triggers the Format Generator dialog box illustrated on the right-hand side of Fig. 5.2. Each row at the bottom of this dialog box specifies the format for a given variable; four have been completed and the fifth is being specified. If we are satisfied that it is in column 5, we click "Add var.", which is located at the cursor in the upper right-hand side of the figure. Each click of this tab adds one variable to the ESS file. In the case of the BDI data, there are 21 variables, each occupying only one column. A portion of the final ESS file is shown in Fig. 5.3.

Review of the data file in Fig. 5.3 shows that the variables are all labeled with the program format (e.g., V4, V5, and so on). Because you will likely want to identify each variable by its proper label. I now show you how to accomplish this task. With the ESS file open, as shown in Fig. 5.3; drop down the Data menu and select the Information option. This action initiates the Define Variables and Group Names dialog box displayed on the left-hand side of Fig. 5.4. To change the variable name from the EQS labeling to your own set of labels, simply highlight and double-click each variable separately. As you double click, the Variable and Code Name Editing dialog box (shown on the right-hand side of Fig. 5.4) appears with the selected variable listed under Variable Name; then simply edit the variable

| Data | Analysis | Data Plot | Build_EQS | Window | Help |

	V4	V5	V6
Information			
Use Data	.0000	2.0000	1.0000	1.0000
Missing Values	.0000	1.0000	1.0000	1.0000
Join	.0000	1.0000	1.0000	1.0000
Merge	.0000	2.0000	1.0000	1.0000
Contract Variables	.0000	1.0000	1.0000	1.0000
Expand Variables	.0000	1.0000	4.0000	3.0000
Transformation	.0000	1.0000	1.0000	1.0000
Group	.0000	2.0000	1.0000	3.0000
Sort	2.0000	1.0000	1.0000	4.0000
Reverse	2.0000	2.0000	1.0000	4.0000
	.0000	1.0000	2.0000	1.0000
Moving Average	.0000	2.0000	2.0000	1.0000
Differences	.0000	2.0000	1.0000	1.0000

FIG. 5.3. Open .ess file with Data drop-down menu showing Information option.

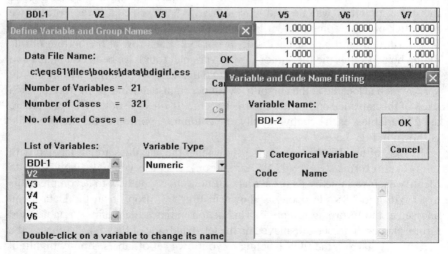

FIG. 5.4. Define Variables and Group Names dialog box with Variable and Code Name Editing dialog box.

name. For example, review of Fig. 5.4 shows that the variable V1 label has already been changed to BDI-1. The variable undergoing change in Fig. 5.4 is V2, and the label has already been edited to read as BDI-2. This process continues until all variables in the complete data set have been relabeled. The ESS. file is saved using Save As with a meaningful file name.

Analysis of Categorical Data.   Thus far in this book, analyses have been based on maximum likelihood (ML) estimation (see chap. 3) and Robust ML estimation (see chap. 4). An important assumption underlying both estimation procedures is that the scale of the observed variables is continuous. In both chapters, however, the observed variables were Likert-scaled items that realistically represent categorical data of an ordinal scale, albeit they were treated as if they were continuous. Indeed, such practice has been the norm for many years and applies to traditional statistical techniques (e.g., ANOVA and MANOVA) as well as SEM analyses. Paralleling this widespread practice of treating ordinal data as if they were continuous, however, has been ongoing debate concerning the pros and cons of doing so. Given (a) the prevalence of this practice in the SEM field, (b) the importance of acquiring an understanding of the issues involved, and (c) the intent, in this chapter, to illustrate analysis of data based on categorically coded variables, it is important to address these issues before examining the input file related to the hypothesized model of BDI structure (see Fig. 5.1).

Categorical Variables Analyzed as Continuous Variables

Review of SEM applications during the past 15 years (in psychological research, at least) reveals most to be based on Likert-type scaled data with estimation of parameters using ML procedures (see, e.g., Breckler, 1990). Given the known limitations associated with available alternative estimation strategies (described later), however, this common finding is not surprising. The primary issues associated with this customary practice are briefly reviewed in the next subsection.

The Issues.   From a review of Monte Carlo studies that addressed this issue (see, e.g., Babakus, Ferguson, & Jöreskog, 1987; Boomsma, 1982; and Muthén & Kaplan, 1985), West and colleagues (1995) reported several important findings. First, Pearson correlation coefficients appear to be higher when computed between two continuous variables than when computed between the same two variables restructured with an ordered categorical scale. However, the greatest attenuation occurs with variables having fewer than five categories and those exhibiting a high degree of skewness—the latter condition being made worse by variables skewed in opposite directions (i.e., one variable positively skewed, the other negatively skewed; see Bollen & Barb, 1981). Second, when categorical variables approximate a normal distribution, (a) the number of categories has little effect on the χ^2 likelihood ratio test of model fit. Nonetheless, increasing skewness—particularly differential skewness (i.e., variables skewed in opposite directions)—leads to increasingly inflated χ^2 values: (b) factor loadings and factor correlations are only modestly underestimated. However, underestimation becomes more critical when there are fewer than three categories, skewness is greater than 1.0, and differential skewness occurs across variables; (c) error variance estimates, more so than other parameters, appear to be most sensitive to the categorical and skewness issues noted in (b); and (d) standard error estimates for all parameters tend to be too low, with this result being more so when the distributions are highly and differentially skewed (see Finch, West, & MacKinnon, 1997).

In summary, the literature to date appears to support the notion that when the number of categories is large and the data approximate a normal distribution, failure to address the ordinality of the data is likely to be negligible (Atkinson, 1988; Babakus et al., 1987; and Muthén & Kaplan, 1985). Indeed, Bentler and Chou (1987, p. 88) argued that given normally distributed categorical variables, "continuous methods can be used with little worry when a variable has four or more categories." More recent findings support these earlier contentions and have further shown that the χ^2 statistic is influenced most by the two-category response format and becomes less so as the number of categories increases (Green, Akey, Fleming, Hershberger, & Marquis, 1997).

Categorical Variables Analyzed as Categorical Variables

The Theory.   In addressing the categorical nature of observed variables, the researcher automatically assumes that each has an underlying continuous scale. As such, the categories can be regarded as only crude measurements of an unobserved variable that, in truth, has a continuous scale (Jöreskog & Sörbom, 1993) with each pair of thresholds (or initial scale points) representing a portion of the continuous scale. The crudeness of these measurements arises from the splitting of the continuous scale of the construct into a fixed number of ordered categories (DiStefano, 2002). Indeed, this categorization process led O'Brien (1985) to argue that the analysis of Likert-scaled data actually contributes to two types of error: (a) categorization error resulting from the splitting of the continuous scale into categorical scale, and (b) transformation error resulting from categories of unequal widths.

For purposes of illustration, let's consider the measuring instrument under study in this chapter in which each item is structured on a four-point scale. The work of Jöreskog and Sörbom (1993) is drawn upon to describe the decomposition of these categorical variables. Let z represent the ordinal variable (the item) and z^* the unobserved continuous variable. The threshold values can then be conceptualized as follows:

If $z^* <$ or $= \tau_1$, z is scored 1.
If $\tau_1 < z^* <$ or $= \tau_2$, z is scored 2.
If $\tau_2 < z^* <$ or $= \tau_3$, z is scored 3.
If $\tau_3 < z^*$, z is scored 4.

Where $\tau_1 < \tau_2 < \tau_3$ represent threshold values for z^*.

In conducting SEM with categorical data, analyses must be based on the correct correlation matrix. Where the correlated variables are both of an ordinal scale, the resulting matrix comprises, *polychoric correlations*; where one variable is of an ordinal scale and the other is of a continuous scale, the resulting matrix comprises *polyserial correlations*. If two variables are dichotomous, this special case of a polychoric correlation is called a *tetrachoric correlation*. If a polyserial correlation involves a dichotomous rather than a more general ordinal variable, the polyserial correlation is also called a *biserial correlation*.

The Assumptions. Applications involving the use of categorical data are based on three critically important assumptions: (a) underlying each categorical observed variable is an unobserved latent counterpart, the scale of which is both continuous and normally distributed; (b) sample size is sufficiently large to enable reliable estimation of the related correlation matrix; and (c) the number of observed variables is kept to a minimum. As Bentler (2005) cogently notes, however, it is this very set of assumptions that essentially epitomizes the primary weakness in this methodology. Let's now take a brief look at why this should be so.

That each categorical variable has an underlying continuous and normally distributed scale is undoubtedly a difficult criterion to meet and, in fact, may be totally unrealistic. For example, in this chapter, scores tapping aspects of depression for nonclinical adolescents are examined. Clearly, we would expect such item scores for normal adolescents to be low, thereby reflecting no incidence of depressive symptoms. As a consequence, we can expect to find evidence of kurtosis and possibly skewness related to these variables, with this pattern being reflected in their presumed underlying continuous distribution. Consequently, in the event that the model under test is deemed to be less than adequate, it may well be that the normality assumption is unreasonable in this instance.

The rationale underlying the latter two assumptions stems from the fact that in working with categorical variables, analyses must proceed from a frequency table comprising number of thresholds x number of observed variables to an estimation of the correlation matrix. The problem lies with the occurrence of cells having zero or near-zero cases, which can subsequently lead to estimation difficulties (Bentler, 2005). This problem can arise because (a) sample size is small relative to the number of response categories (i.e., specific category scores across all categorical variables); (b) the number of variables is excessively large; and/or (c) the number of thresholds is large. Taken in combination, the larger the number of observed variables and/or number of thresholds for these variables and the smaller the sample size, the greater the chance of having cells comprising zero to near-zero cases.

General Analytic Strategies.   Until recently, two primary approaches to the analysis of categorical data (Jöreskog, 1990, 1994; and Muthén, 1984) have dominated this area of research. Both methodologies use standard estimates of polychoric and polyserial correlations followed by a type of asymptotic distribution-free (ADF) methodology for the structured model. Unfortunately, the positive aspects of these categorical variable methodologies have been offset by the ultra restrictive assumptions noted previously and which, for most practical researchers, are both impractical and difficult to meet. In particular, conducting ADF estimation has the same problem of requiring huge sample sizes as in Browne's (1984a) ADF method for continuous variables. Attempts to resolve these difficulties in recent years have resulted in the development of several different approaches to modeling categorical data (see, e.g., Bentler, 2005; Coenders, Satorra, & Saris, 1997; Moustaki, 2001; and Muthén & Muthén, 2004). One of these newer strategies is incorporated in the EQS 6.1 program described in the following subsection.

The EQS Strategy.   Given both the stringency and dubious appropriateness of assumptions underpinning the analysis of categorical data, Bentler (2005) argued that it may make more sense to correct the test statistic while using a mode of estimation that works well with not-too-large samples. Using a normal theory-based method such as ML followed by Satorra-Bentler corrections (Satorra & Bentler, 1988) yields a reliable procedure (see, e.g., DiStefano, 2002). The use of an improved estimator of polychoric and polyserial correlations (Lee, Poon, & Bentler, 1995), together with ROBUST methodologies, distinguishes the EQS approach to the analysis of categorical data from that of other SEM programs.

Consistent with the traditions of Muthén (1984), Jöreskog (1994), and Lee, Poon, and Bentler (1990, 1992), EQS follows a three-step sequential approach to estimation. Univariate statistics such as thresholds are estimated first, followed by estimation of bivariate statistics such as correlations. Estimation of the SEM model is completed using a method like ML followed by ROBUST computations based on an appropriate weight matrix. (For technical details related to this three-stage approach, see Bentler, 2005, and the original articles.) It is important to note that although the correlation estimates and weight matrices in EQS are similar to those of Muthén (1984) and Jöreskog (1994), they are not identical.

From the perspective of sample size, at least, the EQS approach to analysis of categorical data is more practical than the one based on full estimation. Whereas sample size requirements for both the Muthén (1984) and Jöreskog (1994) methodological strategies have been reported as substantial (see, e.g., Dolan, 1994; and

Lee, Poon, & Bentler, 1995), those associated with the ML ROBUST approach in EQS are much less so. Indeed, Bentler (2005) contends that the ROBUST methodology allows for the attainment of correct statistics, which are quite stable even in relatively small samples. Although the ML estimator (or another simpler estimator—e.g., GLS) is not asymptotically optimal when used with categorical variables, the inefficiency is small and certainly offset by improved performance in smaller samples. The Satorra–Bentler scaled χ^2 and ROBUST standard errors provide trustworthy statistics. Of course, if sample size is huge, ME=AGLS can always be used, which, in EQS, gives the asymptotically optimal solution.

With an understanding of the issues involved in the analysis of categorical variables, we move to an application based on the BDI data described at the beginning of this chapter.

ANALYSES BASED ON DATA REGARDED AS CATEGORICAL

The EQS Input File

By now, you will be fairly familiar with the EQS input file setup so details related to all aspects of the file shown in Table 5.1 are not reiterated; my explanation is to therefore limited model specifications not previously addressed. Two features of the current application are of particular interest: (a) that the ordinality of the data is being taken into account and (b) that the model under study is a higher order CFA model.

We turn first to /SPECIFICATIONS and, in particular, the first line of this paragraph. Here we see that the score data are based on 321 cases, an adequate sample to use with the ML estimator but certainly not large enough to use with AGLS, the distribution-free estimator (see Bentler, 2005). Thus, the next specification of note is the method to be used in analyzing the data; here we see ME=ML, ROBUST. This specification conveys two important pieces of information: (a) that ML estimation is to be used in analyzing the correlation matrix, and (b) that the χ^2 and standard errors are to be corrected (i.e., made robust) through use of a large optimal weight matrix appropriate for analysis of categorical data. Given that ML estimation assumes the variables under study are continuous, it is important to acknowledge this obvious misspecification. Bentler (2005) notes that although the estimates will be good, it is essential to follow up with the ROBUST option to obtain the correct S-Bχ^2 and Yuan–Bentler tests and standard errors. As a final point, analyses are based on a raw matrix (MA=RAW)—another necessary requirement in the analysis of categorical data.

Line 2 contains commands that must be specified to perform analyses that include categorical variables. The CATEGORY specification identifies which variables are of a categorical nature. In this case, all 21 variables have an ordinal

TABLE 5.1

EQS Input for Initially Hypothesized Model

/TITLE
CFA OF 2nd-order BDI Structure for Adolescent Females "BDIGIRL1"
Treated as Categorical Variables
/SPECIFICATIONS
CASE=321; VAR=21; ME=ML,ROBUST; MA=RAW; FO='(21F1.0)';
CATEGORY=V1 to V21; ANALYSIS=CORRELATION;
DATA='C:\EQS61\Files\Books\Data\bdigirl.ess';
/LABELS
V1=I1SAD; V2=I2PESS; V3=I3FAIL; V4=I4DISSAT; V5=I5GUILT;
V6=I6PUNISH; V7=I7SDISL; V8=I8SACCUS; V9=I9SUI; V10=I10CRY;
V11=I11IRRIT; V12=I12WDRL; V13=I13INDEC; V14=I14SIMAGE; V15=I15WINHIB;
V16=I16INSOM; V17=I17FATIG; V18=I18ALOSS; V19=I19WLOSS; V20=I20HYPOC;
V21=I21LLOSS;

F1=NEGATT; F2=PERFDIFF; F3=SOMELEM; F4=DEPRESS;
/EQUATIONS
V1 =   F1 + E1 ;
V2 = *F1 + E2 ;
V3 = *F1 + E3 ;
V5 = *F1 + E5 ;
V6 = *F1 + E6 ;
V7 = *F1 + E7 ;
V8 = *F1 + E8 ;
V9 = *F1 + E9 ;
V10 = *F1 + E10 ;
V14 = *F1 + E14 ;
       V4 =   F2 + E4;
       V11 = *F2 + E11;
       V12 = *F2 + E12 ;
       V13 = *F2 + E13 ;
       V15 = *F2 + E15 ;
       V17 = *F2 + E17 ;
       V20 = *F2 + E20 ;
            V16 = F3 + E16 ;
            V18 = *F3 + E18 ;
            V19 = *F3 + E19 ;
            V21 = *F3 + E21 ;
F1= *F4 + D1;
F2= *F4 + D2;
F3= *F4 + D3;
/VARIANCES
   F4= 1.0;
   D1= *;
   D2= *;
   D3= *;
   E1 to E21 = *;
/CONSTRAINTS
(D2,D2) = (D3,D3);
/PRINT
FIT = ALL;
/LMTEST
SET=PEE,GVF;
/END

scale; hence, the specification of V1 to V21. However, it may well be that in some other data set, the number of categorical variables may only be a subset of otherwise continuous variables. In such a case, only these categorical variables need be identified. In EQS, there is no need to specify the number of scale points associated with categorical variables because the program automatically determines this information as you will see later (demonstrated when the output is reviewed). The second specification on this line advises the program that analyses are to be based on a correlation rather than the default covariance structure. Finally, Line 3 of the /SPECIFICATION paragraph specifies the filename and location of the data, which is the bdigirl.ess file created from raw data at the beginning of this chapter.

In the /VARIANCES paragraph, the variance associated with each of the measurement errors (E1 to E21) as well as with the disturbance terms (D1 to D3) is to be estimated. However, variance related to each of the first-order factors is not estimated. These factors represent dependent variables in the model and, as discussed in chapter 1, dependent variables and their covariances (in the Bentler–Weeks sense) cannot be estimated; they remain to be explained by the model. Finally, you may wonder why the variance for Factor 4 (F4; Depression) is fixed to a value of 1.0. This specification derives from an important corollary in SEM, which states that either a regression path or a variance can be estimated but not both. Before relating this corollary to Factor 4 (i.e., the second-order factor that explains correlations among the first-order factors F1–F3), allow me to first illustrate its application using a simple example. Let's turn to Fig. 5.1 and review the error terms. In each case, the variance is estimated, whereas the related regression path is fixed to 1.0. In this instance, a choice had to be made: either estimate the variance or the regression path. The error variance, of course, is of greater interest and, therefore, the regression path must be fixed to 1.0. However, if we want to estimate the regression path rather than the variance (which does not make much sense but is possible nonetheless), we need to fix the variance to 1.0. Returning to the input file in Table 5.1, note that each of the higher order factor loadings (i.e., F1 = *F4 + D1; F2 = *F4 + D2; F3 = *F4 + D3) is estimated; as a result, the variance of Factor 4 must be fixed to 1.0. Had we elected to fix one of these second-order paths to 1.0, the variance of Factor 4 could be freely estimated. However, typically with higher order models, the loadings rather than the variance of the higher order factor are of interest.

The final specification of note lies within the /CONSTRAINTS paragraph. The information being conveyed is that the variance of the disturbance term associated with Factor 2 (D2,D2) is to be constrained equal to that for Factor 3 (D3,D3). What is the rationale for such specification? Recall that in Chapter 2, I emphasized the importance of computing the degrees of freedom associated with hypothesized models to ascertain their status with respect to statistical identification. With hierarchical models, it is additionally critical to check the identification status of the higher order portion of the model. In the current case, given the specification of only three first-order factors, the higher order structure is just-identified unless a constraint is placed on at least one parameter in this upper level of the model (see, e.g., Bentler, 2005; and Rindskopf & Rose, 1988). More specifically, with three first-order factors, there are six (i.e., [4 × 3]/2) pieces of information; the number of estimable parameters is also six (i.e., three factor loadings and three residual variances), thereby resulting in a just-identified model. This result is acceptable; but if we wish also to resolve this condition of just-identification, equality constraints can be placed on particular parameters known to yield estimates that are approximately equal. An initial test of the hypothesized model shown in Fig. 5.1 revealed the estimated values for D2 and D3 to be very close. For this reason, the variance of D3 was equated with that of D2, thereby providing 1 degree of freedom at the higher order level of the model.

The EQS Output File

Table 5.2 presents the first citation from the output related to the hypothesized model. Here we see that the program has identified 21 variables, with all but one (V12) consisting of four categories. Although Item 12 actually had four categories,

TABLE 5.2
Selected EQS Output for Initially Hypothesized Model: Categorical Variable Summary

YOUR MODEL HAS SPECIFIED CATEGORICAL VARIABLES

TOTAL NUMBER OF VARIABLES ARE   21

NUMBER OF CONTINUOUS VARIABLES ARE   0

NUMBER OF DISCRETE   VARIABLES ARE   21

INFORMATION ON DISCRETE VARIABLES

V1   WITH   4 CATEGORIES
V2   WITH   4 CATEGORIES
V3   WITH   4 CATEGORIES
V4   WITH   4 CATEGORIES
V5   WITH   4 CATEGORIES
V6   WITH   4 CATEGORIES
V7   WITH   4 CATEGORIES
V8   WITH   4 CATEGORIES
V9   WITH   4 CATEGORIES
V10 WITH   4 CATEGORIES
V11 WITH   4 CATEGORIES
V12 WITH   3 CATEGORIES
V13 WITH   4 CATEGORIES
V14 WITH   4 CATEGORIES
V15 WITH   4 CATEGORIES
V16 WITH   4 CATEGORIES
V17 WITH   4 CATEGORIES
V18 WITH   4 CATEGORIES
V19 WITH   4 CATEGORIES
V20 WITH   4 CATEGORIES
V21 WITH   4 CATEGORIES

TABLE 5.3
Selected EQS Output for Initially Hypothesized Model: Polychoric Thresholds and Matrix

RESULTS OF POLYCHORIC PARTITION

AVERAGE THRESHOLDS

V 1	.2354	1.2766	1.7013
V 2	.3924	1.1114	1.9264
V 3	.5438	1.1877	1.9875
V 4	-.0559	.9789	1.3744
V 5	.4835	1.6311	2.0618
V 6	.3134	.8468	1.1581
V 7	.0634	1.3318	1.6990
V 8	-.1990	1.0297	1.5416
V 9	.1531	1.6638	2.1366
V10	.1095	.7752	.9779
V11	-.4173	.8731	1.1118
V12	.6826	1.7347	
V13	.0044	.5114	1.8171
V14	.1520	.5708	1.1428
V15	-.0631	.9901	2.2324
V16	.0565	1.0979	1.5381
V17	-.3536	1.2066	1.6979
V18	.2054	.9647	1.4175
V19	1.0154	1.5975	1.8670
V20	.3853	1.2065	1.9227
V21	1.0692	1.5396	1.9816

POLYCHORIC CORRELATION MATRIX BETWEEN DISCRETE VARIABLES

	V 1	V 2	V 3	V 4	V 5
V 1	1.000				
V 2	.357	1.000			
V 3	.444	.486	1.000		
V 4	.381	.284	.322	1.000	
V 5	.336	.345	.409	.282	1.000
V 6	.428	.383	.436	.312	.468
V 7	.475	.499	.631	.420	.431
V 8	.321	.332	.385	.316	.339
V 9	.546	.411	.381	.369	.226
V 10	.477	.244	.467	.284	.289

no subject responded to the fourth category; as a result, EQS assumed that this item had only three categories. Appearing next in the output are the average thresholds for each categorical variable, followed by the polychoric correlation matrix, shown in Table 5.3. Note that Variables with four categories have three thresholds, whereas V12 (Item 12) has two thresholds for its three categories (i.e., there were no response scores in Category 4). Only a portion of this matrix is presented here to give you a flavor of the type of information that EQS provides when the variables under study are categorical.

TABLE 5.4

Selected EQS Output for Initially Hypothesized Model: Warning Messages

SAMPLE STATISTICS BASED ON COMPLETE CASES

*** NOTE *** CATEGORICAL VARIABLES LISTED ABOVE ARE INDICATORS OF LATENT
              CONTINUOUS VARIABLES.   THEIR UNIVARIATE AND JOINT STATISTICS
              MAY NOT BE MEANINGFUL.

UNIVARIATE STATISTICS

VARIABLE	BDI1SAD	BDI2PESS	BDI3FAIL	BDI4DISSAT	BDI5GUILT
MEAN	1.5296	1.4829	1.4081	1.7508	1.3645
SKEWNESS (G1)	1.5320	1.4757	1.7337	1.1455	1.8754
KURTOSIS (G2)	2.0716	1.3265	2.1816	.6015	3.9313
STANDARD DEV.	.7623	.7627	.7279	.8910	.6184

*** WARNING *** NORMAL THEORY STATISTICS MAY NOT BE
                MEANINGFUL DUE TO ANALYZING CORRELATION MATRIX

			BDI1SAD	BDI2PESS	BDI3FAIL	BDI4DISSAT	BDI5GUILT
			V 1	V 2	V 3	V 4	V 5
BDI1SAD	V	1	1.000				
BDI2PESS	V	2	.357	1.000			
BDI3FAIL	V	3	.444	.486	1.000		
BDI4DISSAT	V	4	.381	.284	.322	1.000	
BDI5GUILT	V	5	.336	.345	.409	.282	1.000
BDI6PUNISH	V	6	.428	.383	.436	.312	.468
BDI7SDISL	V	7	.475	.499	.631	.420	.431
BDI8SACCUS	V	8	.321	.332	.385	.316	.339
BDI9SUI	V	9	.546	.411	.381	.369	.226
BDI10CRY	V	10	.477	.244	.467	.284	.289

Consistent with output related to continuous variables, EQS presents the sample univariate statistics, which represent statistics for the data file. Because the scores 1, 2, 3, and 4 in the data file are not of interest, the program presents the warning messages shown in Table 5.4 advising that the univariate statistics may not be meaningful—and they are not; therefore, this output should be ignored. Thereafter, the program presents the polychoric correlation matrix to be analyzed, but it prints a message reminding the user that normal theory statistics such as ML (which follow) should be scrutinized for relevance. The ML $\chi 2$ test and standard errors should be ignored in favor of their ROBUST counterparts; this reminder is shown in the top line of Table 5.5. The table presents information related to the standardized residuals: the discrepancy between the sample polychoric correlations and those estimated from the factor model. Appearing first is an excerpt from the standardized residual matrix followed by values for the average residual estimate, ignoring their signs (.0528; over both diagonal and off-diagonal elements) and average off-diagonal residual estimate (.0581; over cross-diagonal elements only). In the largest of these standardized residuals, we see that the largest misspecification

TABLE 5.5

Selected EQS Output for Initially Hypothesized Model: Standardized Residuals

---

```
MAXIMUM LIKELIHOOD SOLUTION (NORMAL DISTRIBUTION THEORY)
WITH ROBUST STATISTICS (LEE, POON, AND BENTLER OPTIMAL WEIGHT MATRIX)

STANDARDIZED RESIDUAL MATRIX:
                         BDI1SAD   BDI2PESS  BDI3FAIL  BDI4DISSAT  BDI5GUILT
                          V  1      V  2      V  3       V  4        V  5
    BDI1SAD     V  1       .000
    BDI2PESS    V  2      -.045      .000
    BDI3FAIL    V  3      -.042      .045      .000
    BDI4DISSAT  V  4       .014     -.048     -.081       .002
    BDI5GUILT   V  5      -.028      .014      .008      -.020        .000
    BDI6PUNISH  V  6       .022      .014     -.011      -.024        .133
    BDI7SDISL   V  7      -.045      .028      .060      -.011        .002
    BDI8SACCUS  V  8      -.037      .007     -.009       .019        .043
    BDI9SUI     V  9       .103      .009     -.106       .002       -.140
    BDI10CRY    V 10       .096     -.101      .049      -.031       -.025
```

```
                    AVERAGE ABSOLUTE STANDARDIZED RESIDUALS      =      .0528
        AVERAGE OFF-DIAGONAL ABSOLUTE STANDARDIZED RESIDUALS     =      .0581
```

```
LARGEST STANDARDIZED RESIDUALS:

    NO.   PARAMETER   ESTIMATE    NO.   PARAMETER   ESTIMATE
    ---   ---------   --------    ---   ---------   --------
     1    V21, V20      .278      11    V19, V7      -.155
     2    V11, V10      .209      12    V9,  V5      -.140
     3    V19, V14     -.193      13    V12, V11     -.137
     4    V19, V8       .192      14    V6,  V5       .133
     5    V21, V19      .189      15    V15, V6      -.132
     6    V19, V3      -.183      16    V19, V18      .130
     7    V11, V2      -.178      17    V18, V10      .129
     8    V19, V2      -.175      18    V20, V4      -.128
     9    V20, V6       .162      19    V18, V9       .128
    10    V13, V8       .161      20    V17, V2      -.124
```

```
DISTRIBUTION OF STANDARDIZED RESIDUALS
```

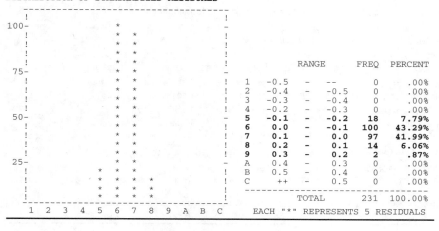

```
      !                                       !
 100-                  *                       -
      !                 *   *                  !
      !                 *   *                  !
      !                 *   *                  !
      !                 *   *                  !      RANGE      FREQ   PERCENT
  75-                   *   *                  -
      !                 *   *                  !   1  -0.5  -   --      0     .00%
      !                 *   *                  !   2  -0.4  -  -0.5     0     .00%
      !                 *   *                  !   3  -0.3  -  -0.4     0     .00%
      !                 *   *                  !   4  -0.2  -  -0.3     0     .00%
  50-                   *   *                  -   5  -0.1  -  -0.2    18    7.79%
      !                 *   *                  !   6   0.0  -  -0.1   100   43.29%
      !                 *   *                  !   7   0.1  -   0.0    97   41.99%
      !                 *   *                  !   8   0.2  -   0.1    14    6.06%
      !                 *   *                  !   9   0.3  -   0.2     2     .87%
  25-                   *   *                  -   A   0.4  -   0.3     0     .00%
      !           *     *   *                  !   B   0.5  -   0.4     0     .00%
      !           *     *   *   *              !   C   ++   -   0.5     0     .00%
      !           *     *   *   *              !  ----------------------------------
      !           *     *   *   *              !        TOTAL        231  100.00%
      --------------------------------------
       1   2   3   4   5   6   7   8   9   A   B   C    EACH "*" REPRESENTS 5 RESIDUALS
```

in the model appears to involve Items 21 and 20 (V21,V20). Finally, a distribution table summarizes the spread of these residuals. Ideally, this distribution should be symmetric with residual values clustered around the zero point. Although the distribution shown in Table 5.5 shows the bulk of these residuals falling into this category, with values ranging from −.1 to 1.0 (85.28%), there is nonetheless some indication of misfit, with 7.79% of residual values ranging from −.1 to −.2 and 6.06% ranging from .1 to .3. The LM Test statistics will shed more light on this possible model misspecification.

Turning to the goodness-of-fit statistics presented in Table 5.6, we observe a vast difference in values derived from ML normal theory estimation versus those based

TABLE 5.6

Selected EQS Output for Initially Hypothesized Model: Goodness-of-Fit Statistics

GOODNESS OF FIT SUMMARY FOR METHOD = ML

CHI-SQUARE =   766.221 BASED ON   187 DEGREES OF FREEDOM
PROBABILITY VALUE FOR THE CHI-SQUARE STATISTIC IS   .00000

THE NORMAL THEORY RLS CHI-SQUARE FOR THIS ML SOLUTION IS   698.784.

FIT INDICES

BENTLER-BONETT   NORMED FIT INDEX =   .709
BENTLER-BONETT NON-NORMED FIT INDEX =   .732
COMPARATIVE FIT INDEX (CFI)   =   .761
ROOT MEAN-SQUARE RESIDUAL (RMR)   =   .071
STANDARDIZED RMR   =   .071
ROOT MEAN-SQUARE ERROR OF APPROXIMATION (RMSEA)   =   .098
90% CONFIDENCE INTERVAL OF RMSEA (.091,   .105)

RELIABILITY COEFFICIENTS

CRONBACH'S ALPHA   =   .889
RELIABILITY COEFFICIENT RHO   =   .898

GOODNESS OF FIT SUMMARY FOR METHOD = ROBUST

SATORRA-BENTLER SCALED CHI-SQUARE =   264.5675 ON   187 DEGREES OF FREEDOM
PROBABILITY VALUE FOR THE CHI-SQUARE STATISTIC IS   .00016

RESIDUAL-BASED TEST STATISTIC   =   784.402
PROBABILITY VALUE FOR THE CHI-SQUARE STATISTIC IS   .00000

YUAN-BENTLER RESIDUAL-BASED TEST STATISTIC   =   227.784
PROBABILITY VALUE FOR THE CHI-SQUARE STATISTIC IS   .02240

YUAN-BENTLER RESIDUAL-BASED F-STATISTIC   =   1.757
DEGREES OF FREEDOM =   187,   134
PROBABILITY VALUE FOR THE F-STATISTIC IS   .00030

FIT INDICES

BENTLER-BONETT   NORMED FIT INDEX =   .798
BENTLER-BONETT NON-NORMED FIT INDEX =   .921
COMPARATIVE FIT INDEX (CFI)   =   .930
ROOT MEAN-SQUARE ERROR OF APPROXIMATION (RMSEA)   =   .036
90% CONFIDENCE INTERVAL OF RMSEA (.025,   .046)

on the robust statistics; these appear to be particularly discrepant with respect to the Fit Indexes. For example, whereas the CFI is .76 with uncorrected ML estimation, it is .93 with corrected robust estimation. However, it is important to emphasize again, that when EQS analyses are based on categorical data, interpretation of model fit must be based on the ROBUST statistical output.

In the ROBUST goodness-of-fit statistics, we see that, in addition to the S-Bχ^2 value (264.57 with 187 df) there are three statistics that have not been addressed. These distribution-free statistics are based on the distribution of residuals, and each is included in the output when ROBUST statistics are requested. These are new statistics (Bentler, 2005). The first, the RESIDUAL-BASED STATISTIC, is of a type developed by Browne (1982, 1984a). The use of this statistic, however, is curtailed by the fact that its interpretation is meaningful only when sample size is very large. The YUAN-BENTLER RESIDUAL-BASED STATISTIC (based on the work of Yuan & Bentler, 1998; and Bentler & Yuan, 1999) represents an extension of Browne's residual-based test such that it can be used with smaller samples. In this regard, Bentler (2005) notes that in addition to performing better in smaller samples than the original RESIDUAL-BASED STATISTIC, it does so without any loss of its large-sample properties. Finally, the YUAN-BENTLER RESIDUAL-BASED F-STATISTIC (Yuan & Bentler, 1998), designed to take sample size into account more adequately, represents a more extensive modification of Browne's (1984a) statistic and is considered by Bentler (2005) to be the best available residual-based test at this time. (For technical details related to these residual-based tests, see Bentler, 2005). In this input, all test statistics imply some degree of misfit in the model.

We now turn to an evaluation of the hypothesized BDI structure shown in Fig. 5.1 using fit indexes. Focusing on the ROBUST fit indexes, we find a CFI value of .93 and a RMSEA value of .036, with a 90% C.I. ranging from .025 to .046. On the basis of these indexes, this model exemplifies a relatively good fit to the data, although, admittedly, it does not reach the CFI value of .95 recommended by Hu and Bentler (1999). However, recall that the standardized residuals indicated some degree of misfit with respect to Items 20 and 21. To further assess this situation, we turn now to the results of the LM Test presented in Table 5.7.

As expected, review of the LM Test univariate incremental values reveals an error covariance between Items 21 and 20 to contribute most to any misfit in the model. Item 21 is concerned with loss of interest in sex, whereas Item 20 targets health concerns. It is interesting that in the original study (Byrne et al., 1993), which focused on a comparison of the BDI structure across gender, this error covariance did not exist for boys. In light of the degree of social attention accorded sexually transmitted diseases in general and AIDS in particular, we argued that it is not surprising that female adolescents develop health concerns related to sexual activity. Given that the content of Items 20 and 21 appears to elicit responses reflective of the same mind set, we argued that specification of an error covariance

TABLE 5.7
Selected EQS Output for Initially Hypothesized Model: Modification Indexes

MULTIVARIATE LAGRANGE MULTIPLIER TEST BY SIMULTANEOUS PROCESS IN STAGE 1

PARAMETER SETS (SUBMATRICES) ACTIVE AT THIS STAGE ARE: PEE GVF

		CUMULATIVE MULTIVARIATE STATISTICS			UNIVARIATE INCREMENT			
							HANCOCK'S SEQUENTIAL	
STEP	PARAMETER	CHI-SQUARE	D.F.	PROB.	CHI-SQUARE	PROB.	D.F.	PROB.
1	E21,E20	41.006	1	.000	41.006	.000	187	1.000
2	V19,F4	77.172	2	.000	36.166	.000	186	1.000
3	E19,E8	108.537	3	.000	31.365	.000	185	1.000
4	V20,F4	129.980	4	.000	21.443	.000	184	1.000
5	E11,E10	150.814	5	.000	20.834	.000	183	1.000
6	E9,E5	169.776	6	.000	18.962	.000	182	1.000
7	E9,E3	192.556	7	.000	22.780	.000	181	1.000
8	E13,E8	209.477	8	.000	16.921	.000	180	1.000
9	E11,E2	226.103	9	.000	16.626	.000	179	1.000
10	E11,E7	242.605	10	.000	16.502	.000	178	1.000
11	E12,E11	257.768	11	.000	15.163	.000	177	1.000
12	E20,E6	271.329	12	.000	13.561	.000	176	1.000
13	E13,E12	284.842	13	.000	13.514	.000	175	1.000
14	E17,E13	299.161	14	.000	14.319	.000	174	1.000
15	V10,F4	312.412	15	.000	13.251	.000	173	1.000

between these two items was substantively reasonable. In contrast, it is difficult to substantiate estimation of the two subsequent parameters (i.e., V19,F4 and E19,E8), the only two worthy of consideration. Although the loading of Item 19 (i.e., measuring weight loss) on the higher order factor of Depression might seem reasonable substantively, it is not realistic psychometrically. With respect to the third parameter, specification of an error covariance between Item 19 (weight loss) and Item 8 (self-accusation) is substantively unjustified. Keeping a watchful eye on parsimony, then, I consider only the error covariance between Items 20 and 21 to be a reasonable addition to the model, for two reasons: (a) the specification is substantively reasonable, and (b) the model already represents a fairly adequate fit to the data. We now move into exploratory mode and peruse EQS output related to Model 2.

POST HOC ANALYSES: MODEL 2

The EQS Output File

Goodness-of-fit statistics related to Model 2 are presented in Table 5.8. With the inclusion of the one error covariance between Items 20 and 21 and a CFI of .944

TABLE 5.8

Selected EQS Output for Model 2: Goodness-of-Fit Statistics

```
GOODNESS OF FIT SUMMARY FOR METHOD = ML

CHI-SQUARE =        723.505 BASED ON       186 DEGREES OF FREEDOM
PROBABILITY VALUE FOR THE CHI-SQUARE STATISTIC IS        .00000

FIT INDICES
-----------
BENTLER-BONETT      NORMED FIT INDEX =        .725
BENTLER-BONETT NON-NORMED FIT INDEX =        .750
COMPARATIVE FIT INDEX (CFI)         =        .778
ROOT MEAN-SQUARE RESIDUAL (RMR)     =        .068
STANDARDIZED RMR                    =        .068
ROOT MEAN-SQUARE ERROR OF APPROXIMATION (RMSEA)     =        .095
90% CONFIDENCE INTERVAL OF RMSEA (        .088,        .102)

GOODNESS OF FIT SUMMARY FOR METHOD = ROBUST

SATORRA-BENTLER SCALED CHI-SQUARE =      247.1578 ON       186 DEGREES OF FREEDOM
PROBABILITY VALUE FOR THE CHI-SQUARE STATISTIC IS        .00180

YUAN-BENTLER RESIDUAL-BASED TEST STATISTIC      =    225.840
PROBABILITY VALUE FOR THE CHI-SQUARE STATISTIC IS        .02452

YUAN-BENTLER RESIDUAL-BASED F-STATISTIC       =      1.728
DEGREES OF FREEDOM   =                      186,   135
PROBABILITY VALUE FOR THE F-STATISTIC IS          .00042

FIT INDICES
-----------
BENTLER-BONETT      NORMED FIT INDEX =        .811
BENTLER-BONETT NON-NORMED FIT INDEX =        .937
COMPARATIVE FIT INDEX (CFI)         =        .944
ROOT MEAN-SQUARE ERROR OF APPROXIMATION (RMSEA)     =        .032
90% CONFIDENCE INTERVAL OF RMSEA (        .020,        .042)
```

and RMSEA of .032, the BDI structure as specified in Model 2 represents a very adequate fit to the data.

In Table 5.9, only a few parameter estimates are again included to provide an overview of the printout when analyses are based on categorical data. Note first the reminder that results based on the normal theory standard errors are not to be used; only the categorical variable ROBUST statistics (in parentheses) should be interpreted. As seen in the last set of estimates, the error covariance between Items 20 and 21 was statistically significant ($Z = 3.553$). The standardized estimates are presented in Table 5.10, which shows the error correlation between these two items to be quite high, considering that this correlation represents similarity in responses to items with different content.

Before we close this chapter, I thought it would be interesting to test the original model again but, rather than honoring the categorical nature of the variables, we treat them as if they were continuous. Let's see how much difference this change in approach really makes.

TABLE 5.9

Selected EQS Output for Model 2: Parameter Estimates

*** WARNING *** WITH CATEGORICAL DATA, NORMAL THEORY RESULTS WITHOUT
CORRECTION SHOULD NOT BE TRUSTED.

**MEASUREMENT EQUATIONS WITH STANDARD ERRORS AND TEST STATISTICS
STATISTICS SIGNIFICANT AT THE 5% LEVEL ARE MARKED WITH @.
(CATEGORICAL-VARIABLE ROBUST STATISTICS IN PARENTHESES)**

```
I1SAD    =V1 =   1.000 F1    + 1.000 E1

I2PESS   =V2 =    .907*F1    + 1.000 E2
                  .093
                 9.709@
                (  .109)
                ( 8.291@

I3FAIL   =V3 =   1.095*F1    + 1.000 E3
                  .096
                11.450@
                (  .104)
                (10.487@
```

CONSTRUCT EQUATIONS WITH STANDARD ERRORS AND TEST STATISTICS

```
NEGATT   =F1 =    .588*F4    + 1.000 D1
                  .052
                11.407@
                (  .055)
                (10.625@

PERFDIFF =F2 =    .633*F4    + 1.000 D2
                  .054
                11.608@
                (  .050)
                (12.691@

SOMELEM  =F3 =    .504*F4    + 1.000 D3
                  .056
                 8.951@
                (  .064)
                ( 7.905@
```

COVARIANCES AMONG INDEPENDENT VARIABLES

```
                        E
                       ---
E21 -I21LLOSS          .291*
E20 -I20HYPOC          .050
                      5.838@
                     (  .082)
                     ( 3.553@
```

TABLE 5.10

Selected EQS Output for Model 2: Standardized Solution

STANDARDIZED SOLUTION:						R-SQUARED
I1SAD =V1 =	.666	F1	+ .746	E1		.444
I2PESS =V2 =	.604*	F1	+ .797	E2		.365
I3FAIL =V3 =	.730*	F1	+ .684	E3		.532
I4DISSAT=V4 =	.645	F2	+ .764	E4		.416
I5GUILT =V5 =	.547*	F1	+ .837	E5		.299
I6PUNISH=V6 =	.610*	F1	+ .793	E6		.372
I7SDISL =V7 =	.782*	F1	+ .623	E7		.612
I8SACCUS=V8 =	.540*	F1	+ .842	E8		.292
I9SUI =V9 =	.669*	F1	+ .744	E9		.447
I10CRY =V10 =	.571*	F1	+ .821	E10		.326
I11IRRIT=V11 =	.402*	F2	+ .916	E11		.161
I12WDRL =V12 =	.555*	F2	+ .832	E12		.308
I13INDEC=V13 =	.684*	F2	+ .729	E13		.468
I14SIMAG=V14 =	.511*	F1	+ .859	E14		.261
I15WINHI=V15 =	.556*	F2	+ .831	E15		.309
I16INSOM=V16 =	.519	F3	+ .854	E16		.270
I17FATIG=V17 =	.622*	F2	+ .783	E17		.387
I18ALOSS=V18 =	.533*	F3	+ .846	E18		.284
I19WLOSS=V19 =	-.155*	F3	+ .988	E19		.024
I20HYPOC=V20 =	.503*	F2	+ .864	E20		.253
I21LLOSS=V21 =	.386*	F3	+ .922	E21		.149
NEGATT =F1 =	.882*	F4	+ .471	D1		.778
PERFDIFF=F2 =	.981*	F4	+ .195	D2		.962
SOMELEM =F3 =	.970*	F4	+ .242	D3		.941

```
   CORRELATIONS AMONG INDEPENDENT VARIABLES
   -----------------------------------------

                        E
                       ---
E21 -I21LLOSS                    .367*
E20 -I20HYPOC
```

ANALYSES BASED ON DATA REGARDED AS CONTINUOUS

The EQS Output File

Table 5.11 presents a summary of the standardized residuals related to the hypothesized model. You will quickly recognize that the format of this table is consistent with Table 5.5, in which the values were based on categorical data. Comparing the results in these two tables reveals at least two interesting points: (1) in general, standardized residuals derived from the categorical methodology were larger than those derived from the continuous methodology; and (2) although the distributional pattern remained the same, the extent to which the standardized residuals spread

TABLE 5.11

Selected EQS Output for Initially Hypothesized Model: Standardized Residuals

MAXIMUM LIKELIHOOD SOLUTION (NORMAL DISTRIBUTION THEORY)

STANDARDIZED RESIDUAL MATRIX:

		BDI1SAD V 1	BDI2PESS V 2	BDI3FAIL V 3	BDI4DISSAT V 4	BDI5GUILT V 5
BDI1SAD	V 1	.000				
BDI2PESS	V 2	-.031	.000			
BDI3FAIL	V 3	.000	.027	.000		
BDI4DISSAT	V 4	.005	-.029	-.072	-.002	
BDI5GUILT	V 5	-.044	.018	.037	-.020	.000
BDI6PUNISH	V 6	.019	.032	-.019	-.004	.073
BDI7SDISL	V 7	-.036	.038	.047	-.019	-.010
BDI8SACCUS	V 8	-.013	-.007	-.024	.039	.035
BDI9SUI	V 9	.048	-.004	-.090	.017	-.089
BDI10CRY	V 10	.075	-.090	.041	-.053	-.013

AVERAGE ABSOLUTE STANDARDIZED RESIDUALS	=	.0420
AVERAGE OFF-DIAGONAL ABSOLUTE STANDARDIZED RESIDUALS	=	.0462

LARGEST STANDARDIZED RESIDUALS:

NO.	PARAMETER	ESTIMATE	NO.	PARAMETER	ESTIMATE
1	V21, V20	.246	11	V15, V6	-.101
2	V11, V10	.163	12	V14, V2	.099
3	V13, V8	.152	13	V19, V14	-.098
4	V20, V6	.151	14	V17, V2	-.096
5	V11, V2	-.135	15	V15, V8	.095
6	V20, V4	-.126	16	V18, V4	-.094
7	V18, V9	.112	17	V20, V3	.094
8	V12, V11	-.108	18	V19, V16	.092
9	V17, V1	.106	19	V19, V8	.092
10	V20, V10	.102	20	V19, V2	-.090

DISTRIBUTION OF STANDARDIZED RESIDUALS

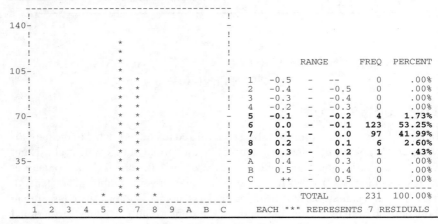

```
    ---------------------------------------
    !                               !
140-                               -
    !                               !
    !           *                   !
    !           *                   !
    !           *                   !        RANGE       FREQ    PERCENT
105-           *                   -
    !           *   *               !   1  -0.5  -   --      0     .00%
    !           *   *               !   2  -0.4  -  -0.5     0     .00%
    !           *   *               !   3  -0.3  -  -0.4     0     .00%
    !           *   *               !   4  -0.2  -  -0.3     0     .00%
 70-           *   *               -   5  -0.1  -  -0.2     4    1.73%
    !           *   *               !   6   0.0  -  -0.1   123   53.25%
    !           *   *               !   7   0.1  -   0.0    97   41.99%
    !           *   *               !   8   0.2  -   0.1     6    2.60%
    !           *   *               !   9   0.3  -   0.2     1     .43%
 35-           *   *               -   A   0.4  -   0.3     0     .00%
    !           *   *               !   B   0.5  -   0.4     0     .00%
    !           *   *               !   C   ++   -   0.5     0     .00%
    !           *   *               !      ---------------------------------
    !       *   *   *   *           !          TOTAL       231  100.00%
    ---------------------------------------
     1   2   3   4   5   6   7   8   9   A   B   C    EACH "*" REPRESENTS 7 RESIDUALS
```

TABLE 5.12

Selected EQS Output for Initially Hypothesized Model: Goodness-of-Fit Statistics

```
        GOODNESS OF FIT SUMMARY FOR METHOD = ML

CHI-SQUARE =       340.157 BASED ON      187 DEGREES OF FREEDOM
PROBABILITY VALUE FOR THE CHI-SQUARE STATISTIC IS        .00000

THE NORMAL THEORY RLS CHI-SQUARE FOR THIS ML SOLUTION IS          341.950.

FIT INDICES
-----------
BENTLER-BONETT      NORMED FIT INDEX =       .778
BENTLER-BONETT NON-NORMED FIT INDEX =       .870
COMPARATIVE FIT INDEX (CFI)         =       .884
ROOT MEAN-SQUARE RESIDUAL (RMR)     =       .036
STANDARDIZED RMR                    =       .055
ROOT MEAN-SQUARE ERROR OF APPROXIMATION (RMSEA)     =      .051
90% CONFIDENCE INTERVAL OF RMSEA  (        .042,        .059)

RELIABILITY COEFFICIENTS
------------------------
CRONBACH'S ALPHA                    =       .844
RELIABILITY COEFFICIENT RHO         =       .855

        GOODNESS OF FIT SUMMARY FOR METHOD = ROBUST

SATORRA-BENTLER SCALED CHI-SQUARE =      266.6617 ON      187 DEGREES OF FREEDOM
PROBABILITY VALUE FOR THE CHI-SQUARE STATISTIC IS        .00012

RESIDUAL-BASED TEST STATISTIC                   =    695.619
PROBABILITY VALUE FOR THE CHI-SQUARE STATISTIC IS        .00000

YUAN-BENTLER RESIDUAL-BASED TEST STATISTIC      =    219.643
PROBABILITY VALUE FOR THE CHI-SQUARE STATISTIC IS        .05127

YUAN-BENTLER RESIDUAL-BASED F-STATISTIC    =      1.558
DEGREES OF FREEDOM   =                    187,   134
PROBABILITY VALUE FOR THE F-STATISTIC IS         .00334

FIT INDICES
-----------
BENTLER-BONETT      NORMED FIT INDEX =       .765
BENTLER-BONETT NON-NORMED FIT INDEX =       .903
COMPARATIVE FIT INDEX (CFI)         =       .914
ROOT MEAN-SQUARE ERROR OF APPROXIMATION (RMSEA)     =      .036
90% CONFIDENCE INTERVAL OF RMSEA  (        .026,        .046)
```

across the zero point for the categorical variables was much greater than when the variables were treated as continuous. For example, whereas 85.28% of the residuals ranged between −0.1 and 0.1 for variables treated as categorical, this range occurred for 95.24% of the residuals associated with variables treated as continuous. Although these results suggest that the degree of misfit was less when the ordinal variables were treated as if they were continuous, this conclusion does not bear out with review of the goodness-of-fit statistics in Table 5.12. Clearly, the information provided in this table reveals that the model is extremely poor-fitting under normal theory estimation and is only slightly better when estimates are derived from the robust methodology. It is evident from comparing this table with Table 5.6 that the model was best fitted to the data when the categorical nature of the variables was taken into account.

TABLE 5.13

Selected EQS Output for Initially Hypothesized Model: Modification Indexes

MULTIVARIATE LAGRANGE MULTIPLIER TEST BY SIMULTANEOUS PROCESS IN STAGE 1

PARAMETER SETS (SUBMATRICES) ACTIVE AT THIS STAGE ARE: PEE GVF

		CUMULATIVE MULTIVARIATE STATISTICS			UNIVARIATE INCREMENT		HANCOCK'S SEQUENTIAL	
STEP	PARAMETER	CHI-SQUARE	D.F.	PROB.	CHI-SQUARE	PROB.	D.F.	PROB.
1	E21,E20	22.594	1	.000	22.594	.000	187	1.000
2	V20,F4	38.406	2	.000	15.813	.000	186	1.000
3	E13,E8	50.682	3	.000	12.275	.000	185	1.000
4	E11,E10	61.896	4	.000	11.214	.001	184	1.000
5	E17,E1	72.375	5	.000	10.479	.001	183	1.000
6	V19,F4	82.404	6	.000	10.029	.002	182	1.000
7	E18,E9	91.763	7	.000	9.360	.002	181	1.000
8	E11,E2	100.179	8	.000	8.416	.004	180	1.000
9	E9,E3	107.903	9	.000	7.723	.005	179	1.000
10	E20,E6	114.735	10	.000	6.832	.009	178	1.000
11	E19,E8	121.538	11	.000	6.803	.009	177	1.000
12	E9,E5	128.296	12	.000	6.759	.009	176	1.000
13	E15,E8	134.915	13	.000	6.619	.010	175	1.000
14	E12,E11	141.293	14	.000	6.378	.012	174	1.000
15	E11,E7	148.032	15	.000	6.738	.009	173	1.000

In comparing the LM Test statistics in Table 5.13 with those in Table 5.7, it is evident that, overall, the ordering of the parameters tagged for inclusion in the model differed across the two analytic approaches. However, the identification of the error covariance between Items 20 and 21 was consistent, albeit the size of the univariate chi-square value was substantially different.

Model 2

The EQS Output File

Let's turn first to the goodness-of-fit statistics in Table 5.14 where we see that model fit is higher within the framework of the ROBUST statistics (CFI = .930) than within the framework of ML estimation (e.g., CFI = .901). Now, if we compare the statistics in this table with those in Table 5.8, we see that the same pattern holds with respect to ML fit indexes being lower (e.g., CFI = .778) than the ROBUST fit indexes (e.g., CFI = .944). Conversely, if we compare values across Tables 5.8 and 5.14, we see that whereas the ML fit indexes for the categorical data (e.g., CFI = .778) are less than those for continuous data (e.g., CFI = .901), the ROBUST fit indexes for the categorical data are higher (e.g., CFI = .944) than those for the continuous data (e.g., CFI = .930). Overall, it appears that model fit is optimal when the four-category variables are treated as categorical data.

TABLE 5.14

Selected EQS Output for Model 2: Goodness-of-Fit Statistics

GOODNESS OF FIT SUMMARY FOR METHOD = ML

CHI-SQUARE = 316.797 BASED ON 186 DEGREES OF FREEDOM
PROBABILITY VALUE FOR THE CHI-SQUARE STATISTIC IS .00000

FIT INDICES

BENTLER-BONETT NORMED FIT INDEX = .793
BENTLER-BONETT NON-NORMED FIT INDEX = .888
COMPARATIVE FIT INDEX (CFI) = .901
ROOT MEAN-SQUARE RESIDUAL (RMR) = .036
STANDARDIZED RMR = .053
ROOT MEAN-SQUARE ERROR OF APPROXIMATION (RMSEA) = .047
90% CONFIDENCE INTERVAL OF RMSEA (.038, .055)

RELIABILITY COEFFICIENTS

CRONBACH'S ALPHA = .844
RELIABILITY COEFFICIENT RHO = .851

GOODNESS OF FIT SUMMARY FOR METHOD = ROBUST

ROBUST INDEPENDENCE MODEL CHI-SQUARE = 1136.751 ON 210 DEGREES OF FREEDOM

SATORRA-BENTLER SCALED CHI-SQUARE = 251.1182 ON 186 DEGREES OF FREEDOM
PROBABILITY VALUE FOR THE CHI-SQUARE STATISTIC IS .00103

RESIDUAL-BASED TEST STATISTIC = 697.296
PROBABILITY VALUE FOR THE CHI-SQUARE STATISTIC IS .00000

YUAN-BENTLER RESIDUAL-BASED TEST STATISTIC = 219.810
PROBABILITY VALUE FOR THE CHI-SQUARE STATISTIC IS .04543

YUAN-BENTLER RESIDUAL-BASED F-STATISTIC = 1.582
DEGREES OF FREEDOM = 186, 135
PROBABILITY VALUE FOR THE F-STATISTIC IS .00249

FIT INDICES

BENTLER-BONETT NORMED FIT INDEX = .779
BENTLER-BONETT NON-NORMED FIT INDEX = .921
COMPARATIVE FIT INDEX (CFI) = .930
ROOT MEAN-SQUARE ERROR OF APPROXIMATION (RMSEA) = .033
90% CONFIDENCE INTERVAL OF RMSEA (.022, .043)

Table 5.15 presents partial parameter estimates and standard errors related to variables treated as continuous data. Robust standard errors are somewhat larger than those for ML. Consistent with the pattern found for the standardized residuals, the parameter estimates are somewhat lower than those produced when the variables are treated as categorical data (see Table 5.9). However, a direct comparison is not possible without going to the standardized solution. In general, the factor loadings are smaller in Table 5.16 than the corresponding ones in Table 5.10. These findings support those of West and colleagues (1995) (discussed previously) that with fewer than five categories and data that exhibit evidence of non-normality, parameter estimates tend to be attenuated. Nonetheless, the bottom-line results regarding statistical significance remain across the two sets of analyses.

TABLE 5.15
Selected EQS Output for Model 2: Parameter Estimates

MEASUREMENT EQUATIONS WITH STANDARD ERRORS AND TEST STATISTICS
STATISTICS SIGNIFICANT AT THE 5% LEVEL ARE MARKED WITH @.
(ROBUST STATISTICS IN PARENTHESES)

```
I1SAD   =V1 =  1.000 F1   + 1.000 E1

I2PESS  =V2 =   .888*F1   + 1.000 E2
                .112
               7.898@
              (  .150)
              ( 5.898@

I3FAIL  =V3 =  1.003*F1   + 1.000 E3
                .112
               8.984@
              (  .132)
              ( 7.622@
```

CONSTRUCT EQUATIONS WITH STANDARD ERRORS AND TEST STATISTICS

```
NEGATT   =F1 =   .424*F4   + 1.000 D1
                 .044
                9.737@
               (  .054)
               ( 7.781@

PERFDIFF =F2 =   .479*F4   + 1.000 D2
                 .052
                9.172@
               (  .053)
               ( 8.952@

SOMELEM  =F3 =   .346*F4   + 1.000 D3
                 .049
                7.059@
               (  .055)
               ( 6.291@
```

COVARIANCES AMONG INDEPENDENT VARIABLES

```
                      E
                      ---
E21 -I21LLOSS         .104*
E20 -I20HYPOC         .023
                     4.583@
                    (  .038)
                    ( 2.773@
```

TABLE 5.16

Selected EQS Output for Model 2: Standardized Solution

STANDARDIZED SOLUTION:					R-SQUARED
I1SAD =V1 =	.602 F1	+	.799 E1		.362
I2PESS =V2 =	.534*F1	+	.845 E2		.285
I3FAIL =V3 =	.632*F1	+	.775 E3		.400
I4DISSAT=V4 =	.586 F2	+	.810 E4		.344
I5GUILT =V5 =	.469*F1	+	.883 E5		.220
I6PUNISH=V6 =	.535*F1	+	.845 E6		.286
I7SDISL =V7 =	.695*F1	+	.719 E7		.483
I8SACCUS=V8 =	.482*F1	+	.876 E8		.232
I9SUI =V9 =	.571*F1	+	.821 E9		.326
I10CRY =V10 =	.495*F1	+	.869 E10		.246
I11IRRIT=V11 =	.293*F2	+	.956 E11		.086
I12WDRL =V12 =	.442*F2	+	.897 E12		.196
I13INDEC=V13 =	.618*F2	+	.786 E13		.382
I14SIMAG=V14 =	.443*F1	+	.897 E14		.196
I15WINHI=V15 =	.494*F2	+	.869 E15		.244
I16INSOM=V16 =	.490 F3	+	.872 E16		.240
I17FATIG=V17 =	.541*F2	+	.841 E17		.293
I18ALOSS=V18 =	.548*F3	+	.837 E18		.300
I19WLOSS=V19 =	-.046*F3	+	.999 E19		.002
I20HYPOC=V20 =	.414*F2	+	.910 E20		.172
I21LLOSS=V21 =	.235*F3	+	.972 E21		.055
NEGATT =F1 =	.923*F4	+	.384 D1		.852
PERFDIFF=F2 =	.915*F4	+	.404 D2		.837
SOMELEM =F3 =	.853*F4	+	.522 D3		.728

CORRELATIONS AMONG INDEPENDENT VARIABLES

```
                          E
                          ---
E21 -I21LLOSS             .275*
E20 -I20HYPOC
```

Overall, in the case of the current data, it appears that analyses for which the ordinality of the data was considered yielded the best fit to the data and was ultimately the most appropriate approach to follow. Nonetheless, Hutchinson and Olmos (1998) admonish that when assessment of model fit is based on data that are both categorical and non-normally distributed, researchers must realize that external artifacts such as model complexity, sample size, type of estimator, and degree of non-normality are all important to this goodness-of-fit criterion.

In conclusion, I leave you with one further caveat regarding this topic of categorical data. Because there is no way as yet to evaluate whether the assumption underlying polychoric and polyserial correlations is reasonable, we may be unaware that we are misusing this methodology. What would we do if we really doubted normality of the latent traits? Bentler (2005, p. 150) suggests that "in practice, we should do the technically wrong thing and treat the ordinal variables as continuous."

6

Application 4:
Testing for the Validity
of a Causal Structure

In this chapter, we take our first look at a full structural equation model (SEM). The hypothesis to be tested relates to the pattern of causal structure linking several stressor variables that bear on the construct of burnout. The original study from which this application is taken (Byrne, 1994c) tested and cross-validated the impact of organizational and personality variables on three dimensions of burnout for elementary, intermediate, and secondary school teachers. For purposes of illustration here, however, the application is limited to the calibration sample of secondary school teachers only.

As was the case with the factor analytic applications illustrated in chapters 3 through 5, those structured as full SEMs are presumed to be of a confirmatory nature. That is, postulated causal relations among all variables in the hypothesized model must be grounded in theory and/or empirical research. Typically, the hypothesis to be tested argues for the validity of specified causal linkages among the variables of interest. Let's turn now to an in-depth examination of the hypothesized model under study in this chapter.

THE HYPOTHESIZED MODEL

Formulation of the hypothesized model shown in Fig. 6.1 derived from the consensus of findings from a review of the burnout literature as it relates to the teaching

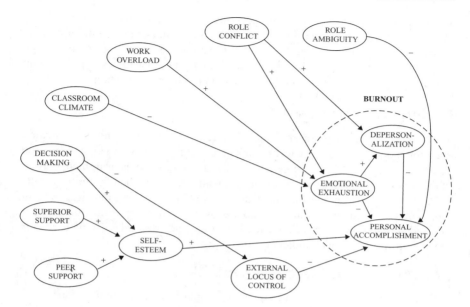

FIG. 6.1. Hypothesized model of causal structure depicting determinants of teacher burnout. Reprinted from Byrne (1994). Burnout:
testing for the validity, replication, and invariance of causal structure across elementary, intermediate, and secondary teachers.
American Educational Research Journal, 31, pp. 645–73 (Fig. 1,
p. 656). Copyright (1994) by the American Educational Research
Association. Reprinted by permission of the publisher.

profession. (For a more detailed summary of this research, see Byrne, 1994c,
1999.) Review of this model shows that burnout is represented as a multidimensional construct with Emotional Exhaustion (EE), Depersonalization (DP),
and Personal Accomplishment (PA) operating as conceptually distinct factors.
This part of the model is based on the work of Leiter (1991) in conceptualizing burnout as a cognitive-emotional reaction to chronic stress. The paradigm
argues that EE holds the central position because it is considered the most re-
sponsive of the three facets to various stressors in a teacher's work environment. DP and reduced PA, on the other hand, represent the cognitive aspects
of burnout in that they indicate the extent to which teachers' perceptions of their
students, their colleagues, and themselves become diminished. As indicated by
the signs associated with each path in the model, EE is hypothesized to impact
positively on DP but negatively on PA; DP is hypothesized to impact negatively
on PA.

The paths (and their associated signs) leading from the organizational (i.e.,
role ambiguity, role conflict, work overload, classroom climate, decisionmaking,

superior support, peer support) and personality (i.e., self-esteem, external locus of control) variables to the three dimensions of burnout reflect findings in the literature.[1] For example, high levels of role conflict are expected to cause high levels of emotional exhaustion; in contrast, high (i.e., good) levels of classroom climate are expected to generate low levels of emotional exhaustion.

Preliminary Analyses

The model in Fig. 6.1 represents only the structural portion of the full structural equation model. Thus, before testing this model, it is necessary to know how each construct in this model is to be measured. In other words, the measurement portion of the structural equation model (see chap. 1) must be established. In contrast to the CFA models studied previously, the task involved in developing the measurement model of a full structural equation model is twofold: (a) to determine the number of indicators to use in measuring each construct, and (b) to identify which items to use in formulating each indicator.

Formulation of Indicator Variables

In the applications examined in chapters 3 through 5, the formulation of measurement indicators was relatively straightforward; all examples involved CFA models and, therefore consisted of only measurement models. In the measurement of multidimensional facets of self-concept (see chap. 3), each indicator represented a subscale score (i.e., the sum of all items designed to measure a particular self-concept facet). In chapters 4 and 5, the factorial validity of a measuring instrument was the focus of interest. As such, we were concerned with the extent to which items loaded onto their targeted factor. Adequate assessment of this phenomenon demanded that each item be included in the model. Thus, the indicator variables in these cases each represented one item in the measuring instrument under study.

In contrast to these previous examples, formulation of the indicator variables in the present application is somewhat more complex. Specifically, multiple indicators of each construct were formulated through the judicious combination of particular items to comprise item parcels. Items were carefully grouped according to content to equalize the measurement weighting across the set of indicators measuring the same construct (Hagtvet & Nasser, 2004). For example, the Classroom Environment Scale (Bacharach, Bauer, & Conley, 1986) used to measure Classroom Climate consists of items that tap classroom size, ability/interest of students, and various types of abuse by students. Indicators of this construct were formed so that each item in the composite measured a different aspect of classroom climate.

---

[1]To facilitate interpretation, particular items were reflected such that high scores on role ambiguity, role conflict, work overload, EE, DP, and external locus of control represented negative perceptions; high scores on the remaining constructs represented positive perceptions.

In the measurement of classroom climate, self-esteem, and external locus of control, indicator variables consisted of items from a single unidimensional scale; all other indicators comprised items from subscales of multidimensional scales. (For an extensive description of all measuring instruments used in construction of this model, see Byrne, 1994c.) In total, 32 item-parcel indicator variables were used to measure the hypothesized structural model; Fig. 6.2 is a schematic presentation of this model.

Since the current study was conducted (1994), there has been growing interest in the question of item-parceling. Research has focused on such issues as method of parceling (Bandalos & Finney, 2001; Hagtvet & Nasser, 2004; Kim & Hagtvet, 2003; Kishton & Widaman, 1994; Little, Cunningham, Shahar, & Widaman, 2002; and Rogers & Schmitt, 2004), number of items to include in a parcel (Marsh, Hau, Balla, & Grayson, 1998), extent to which item parcels affect model fit (Bandalos, 2002), and, more generally, whether researchers should even engage in item-parceling at all (Little et al., 2002). The latter article is an excellent summary of the pros and cons of using item-parceling, and the Bandalos and Finney (2001) chapter, a thorough review of the related issues. (For details related to each of these aspects of item parceling, readers are advised to consult these references directly.)

Confirmatory Factor Analyses

Because (a) the structural portion of a full structural equation model involves relations among only latent variables, and (b) the primary concern in working with a full model is to assess the extent to which these relations are valid, it is critical that the measurement of each latent variable be psychometrically sound. Thus, an important preliminary step in the analysis of full latent variable models is to first test for the validity of the measurement model before attempting to evaluate the structural model. Accordingly, CFA procedures are used in testing the validity of the indicator variables. Once it is known that the measurement model is operating adequately, researchers can have more confidence in findings related to assessment of the hypothesized structural model.

In this case, CFAs were conducted for indicator variables derived from each of the two multidimensional scales: the Teacher Stress Scale (TSS; Pettegrew & Wolf, 1982) and the MBI (Maslach & Jackson, 1986). The TSS comprises six subscales, with items designed to measure Role Ambiguity, Role Conflict, Work Overload, Decision-making, Superior Support, and Peer Support. The MBI (see chap. 4) comprises three subscales, with items designed to measure three facets of burnout: Emotional Exhaustion, Depersonalization, and Personal Accomplishment.

As with all analyses conducted in this chapter, CFA testing of these two measurement models was based on Robust ML estimation. Although both the TSS (*CFI = .96; *RMSEA = .069) and the MBI (*CFI = .97; *RMSEA = .075) were found to be reasonably well fitting, the LM Test univariate incremental

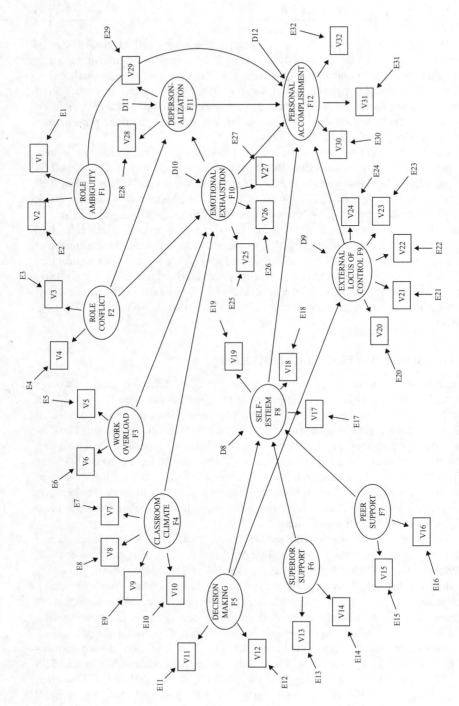

FIG. 6.2. Hypothesized model of teacher burnout: Initially specified measurement and structural components.

190

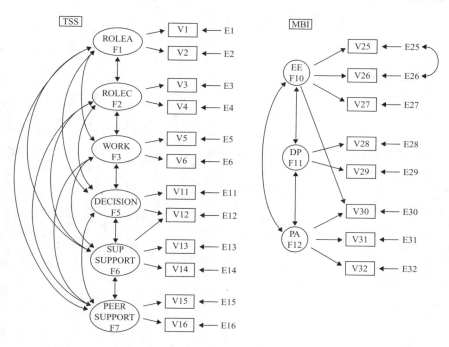

FIG. 6.3.   Final CFA models of indicator variables representing the TSS and the MBI.

χ^2 statistic revealed sharp evidence of misspecification with respect to three parameters overall. These suggested misspecifications included one cross-loading for the TSS (V12 on F6) and one cross-loading (V30 on F1) and one error covariance (E26,E25) for the MBI. Both models were respecified to include these parameters, as schematically portrayed in Fig. 6.3. The final measurement model retained this revised specification throughout all analyses of the full causal model, the modification of which is shown in Fig. 6.4.

THE EQS INPUT FILE

With the measurement model fully established, certain aspects of the input file for the initially hypothesized model are highlighted, as shown in Table 6.1. Turning first to the /SPECIFICATIONS paragraph, we see that this calibration sample of secondary school teachers comprises 716 cases and the model includes 32 indicator variables. In the /EQUATIONS paragraph, it will appear that there are two sections. The first set of equations, easily identified by their augmenting indentation, defines the measurement model; as such, each equation is specified in terms of the indicator

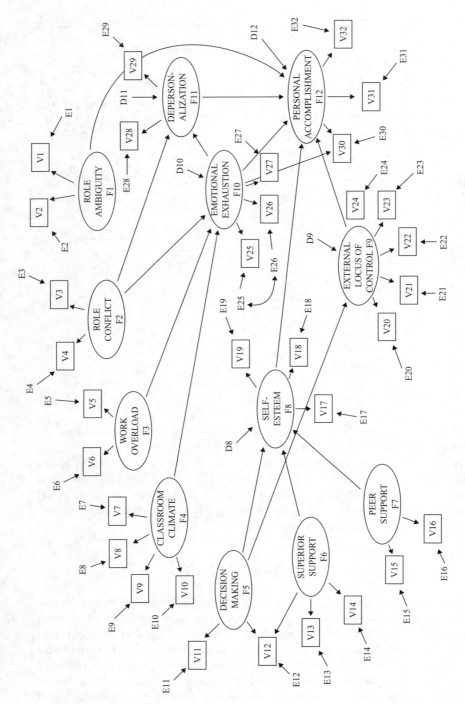

FIG. 6.4. Hypothesized model of teacher burnout: Revised measurement model.

TABLE 6.1
EQS Input for Hypothesized Model of Burnout

/TITLE
FULL BURNOUT MODEL FOR SECONDARY TCHRS (GRP1); "BURNHS1I.EQS"
INITIAL MODEL
CROSS-LOADINGS: F6 TO V12 (SSUP TO DEC2); F10 TO V30 (EE TO PA1)
ERROR COV: E26,E25 (EE)

/SPECIFICATION
CASE=716; VAR=32; ME=ML,ROBUST; MA=RAW; FO=' (19F4.2/13F4.2) ';
DATA=' C:\EQS61\Files\Books\Data\secind1.ess ';

/LABELS
V1=ROLEA1;   V2=ROLEA2;   V3=ROLEC1;   V4=ROLEC2;   V5=WORK1;
V6=WORK2;   V7=CLIMATE1;   V8=CLIMATE2;   V9=CLIMATE3;   V10=CLIMATE4;
V11=DEC1;   V12=DEC2;   V13=SSUP1;   V14=SSUP2;   V15=PSUP1;
V16=PSUP2;   V17=SELF1;   V18=SELF2;   V19=SELF3;   V20=XLOC1;
V21=XLOC2;   V22=XLOC3;   V23=XLOC4;   V24=XLOC5;   V25=EE1;
V26=EE2;   V27=EE3;   V28=DP1;   V29=DP2;   V30=PA1;
V31=PA2;   V32=PA3;
F1=ROLEA; F2=ROLEC; F3=WORK; F4=CLIMATE; F5=DEC; F6=SSUP; F7=PSUP;
F8=SELF; F9=XLOC; F10=EE; F11=DP; F12=PA;

/EQUATIONS
V1= F1+E1;
V2= *F1+E2;
    V3= F2+E3;
    V4= *F2+E4;
        V5= F3+E5;
        V6= *F3+E6;
            V7= F4+E7;
            V8= *F4+E8;
            V9= *F4+E9;
            V10= *F4+E10; .
                V11= F5+E11;
                V12= *F5+*F6+E12;
                    V13= F6+E13;
                    V14= *F6+E14;
                        V15= F7+E15;
                        V16= *F7+E16;
                            V17= F8+E17;
                            V18= *F8+E18;
                            V19= *F8+E19;
                                V20= F9+E20;
                                V21= *F9+E21;
                                V22= *F9+E22;
                                V23= *F9+E23;
                                V24= *F9+E24;
                                    V25= F10+E25;
                                    V26= *F10+E26;
                                    V27= *F10+E27;
                                        V28= F11+E28;
                                        V29= *F11+E29;
                                            V30= F12+*F10+E30;
                                            V31= *F12+E31;
                                            V32= *F12+E32;

(Continued)

TABLE 6.1
(Continued)

F8= *F5+ *F6+*F7+D8;
F9= *F5+D9;
F10= *F2+ *F3+ *F4+D10;
F11= *F2+ *F10+D11;
F12= *F1+ *F8+ *F9+ *F10+ *F11+D12;
/VARIANCES
 F1 TO F7 = *;
 E1 to E32 = *;
 D8 TO D12=*;
/COVARIANCES
 F1 to F7 =*;
 E26,E25 = *;
/PRINT
 FIT=ALL;
/LMTEST
 SET=GFF, BFF, PDD;
/END

---

variables (i.e., the V's). In particular, note the cross-loadings associated with V12 and V30. The second set of equations defines the model in terms of the latent variables; as such, it describes the structural model or causal network encompassing these variables, as depicted in Fig. 6.1.

The /VARIANCES paragraph specifies the estimation of variances for the independent factors (F1 to F7), error terms associated with each indicator variable (E1 through E32), and disturbance terms associated with each dependent factor (D8 through D12). Estimated covariances in the/COVARIANCES paragraph are specified for all factor pairs involving the independent Factors 1 through 7.[2] Also included is the error covariance (E26,E25) specified for the MBI component of the measurement model.

Finally, the /LMTEST paragraph incorporates, the SET command to limit LM Test statistics to (a) misspecified structural paths (i.e., paths that are not specified but should be)—these paths can flow from either independent to dependent factors (GFF) or one dependent factor to another (BFF); and (b) misspecified covariances among the disturbance terms (PDD).

The input file just reviewed was created manually; however, it is likely that you may prefer to build it interactively using the Build EQS option. Thus, before proceeding to the output file, let's walk through the process of building this same file using Build EQS. As outlined in chapter 2, the first step is to open the data file upon which the analyses will be based; in this case, the data file is labeled

---

[2]Recall that variances and covariances can be estimated only for independent variables (observed or latent) in a model.

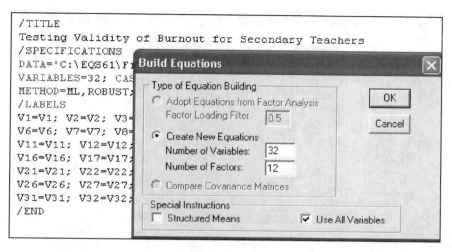

```
/TITLE
Testing Validity of Burnout for Secondary Teachers
/SPECIFICATIONS
DATA='C:\EQS61\F
VARIABLES=32; CA
METHOD=ML,ROBUST;
/LABELS
V1=V1; V2=V2; V3=
V6=V6; V7=V7; V8=
V11=V11; V12=V12;
V16=V16; V17=V17;
V21=V21; V22=V22;
V26=V26; V27=V27;
V31=V31; V32=V32;
/END
```

Build Equations   ⊠

Type of Equation Building

○ Adopt Equations from Factor Analysis
   Factor Loading Filter [0.5]

● Create New Equations
   Number of Variables: [32]
   Number of Factors: [12]

○ Compare Covariance Matrices

Special Instructions
☐ Structured Means   ☑ Use All Variables

[OK]   [Cancel]

FIG. 6.5. Build Equations dialog box to create an EQS input file using BUILD EQS.

"secind1.ess".[3] After dropping down the Build EQS menu, the first step is to click the Title/Specification tab and complete the required information. This portion of the completed file is shown in the background of Fig. 6.5. Superimposed on this part of the input file is the Build Equations dialog box, which was obtained by clicking the Build Equations tab of the menu. In this box, we note that the model comprises 32 variables and 12 factors; additionally, it is noted that all variables are to be used in the analyses. Clicking OK yields the first of two dialog boxes in which the user specifies the model. The first dialog box relates to the measurement model, the second relates to the structural model. Fig. 6.6 shows the portion of the measurement model involving complete specification for Factors 9 through 12 (note the cross-loading of V30 onto Factor 10 highlighted within the rectangle). Specifications pertinent to the structural model are shown in Fig. 6.7. The location of the asterisks, however, requires explanation. To interpret these specifications, the user reads down from the factor listed at the top of the column and then across to the factor in the far left column. For example, the asterisk appearing in column 1 indicates that F1 causes F12; those in column 2 indicate, first, that F2 causes F10 and, second, that F2 causes F11.

The final step in building the full structural equation model file concerns specifications related to the variances and covariances. Fig. 6.8 shows partial specification for the factors with respect to their variances, albeit full specification regarding

---

[3]The data file used for all analyses in this chapter is based on raw data and thus carries the .dat extension (i.e., secind1.dat). However, to build the file using Build EQS, the data file must be in the .ess format. The procedure used in converting files in this manner is described in chapter 5.

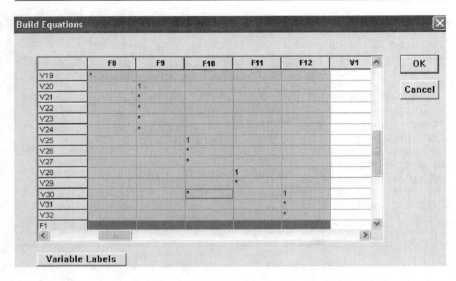

FIG. 6.6. Build Equations dialog box showing partial measurement model specification.

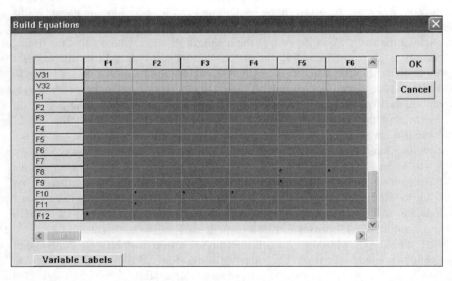

FIG. 6.7. Build Equations dialog box showing structural model specification.

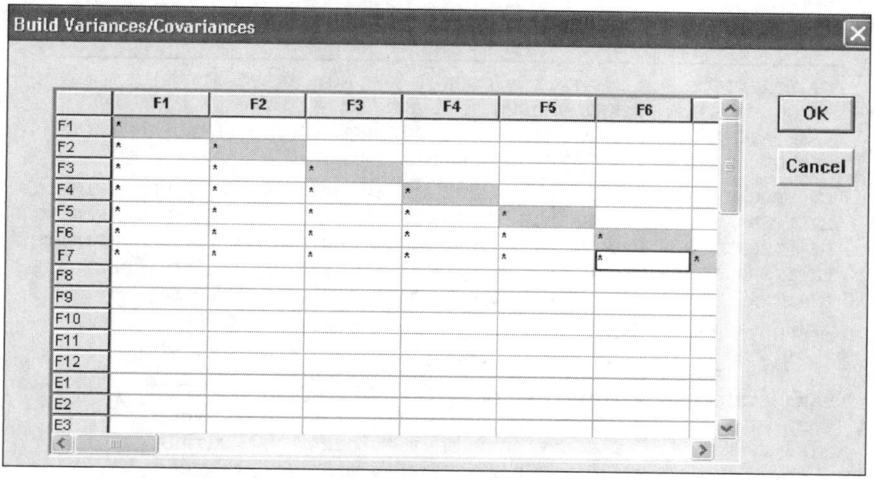

FIG. 6.8. Build Variances and Covariances dialog box showing partial specification of factor variances, albeit full specification of their covariances.

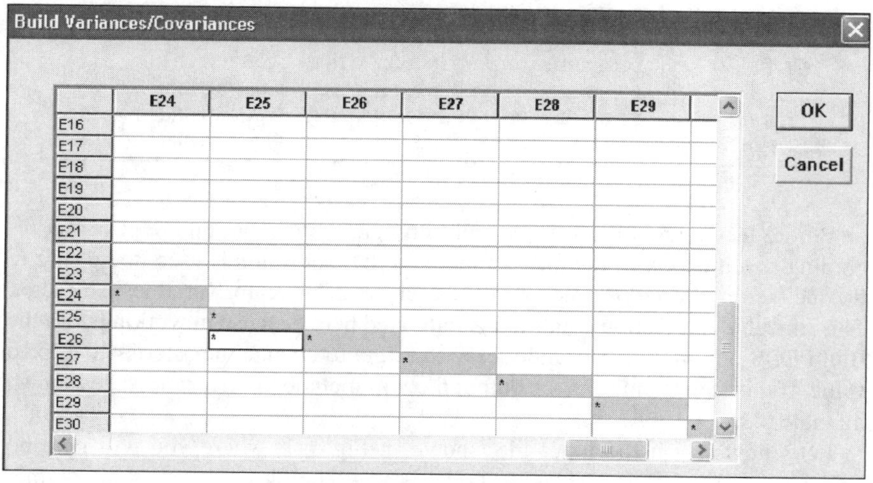

FIG. 6.9. Build Variances and Covariances dialog box showing partial specification of error variances as well as error covariance between E26,E25.

their covariances. As seen in this dialog box, covariances are specified only for the independent factors in the model (F1–F7) and all factors are specified as being intercorrelated. Fig. 6.9 shows the specification of variances for error terms associated with Variables 24 through 29 (E24–E29) as well as the error covariance (boxed) between E25 and E26.

TABLE 6.2

Hypothetical EQS Output: Failure to Address Model Identification

---

IN ITERATION # 1, MATRIX W-CFUNCT MAY NOT BE POSITIVE DEFINITE.
  YOU HAVE BAD START VALUES TO BEGIN WITH.
  IF ABOVE MESSAGE APPEARS ON EVERY ITERATION, PLEASE PROVIDE
BETTER START VALUES AND RE-RUN THE JOB.

IN ITERATION # 2, MATRIX W-CFUNCT MAY NOT BE POSITIVE DEFINITE.
IN ITERATION # 3, MATRIX W-CFUNCT MAY NOT BE POSITIVE DEFINITE.
IN ITERATION # 4, MATRIX W-CFUNCT MAY NOT BE POSITIVE DEFINITE.
IN ITERATION # 5, MATRIX W-CFUNCT MAY NOT BE POSITIVE DEFINITE.
IN ITERATION # 6, MATRIX W-CFUNCT MAY NOT BE POSITIVE DEFINITE.

*** NOTE *** RESIDUAL-BASED STATISTICS CANNOT BE
             CALCULATED BECAUSE OF PIVOTING PROBLEMS.

PARAMETER	CONDITION CODE
F2,F1	LINEARLY DEPENDENT ON OTHER PARAMETERS
F3,F2	LINEARLY DEPENDENT ON OTHER PARAMETERS
F4,F1	LINEARLY DEPENDENT ON OTHER PARAMETERS
F7,F3	LINEARLY DEPENDENT ON OTHER PARAMETERS
F7,F4	LINEARLY DEPENDENT ON OTHER PARAMETERS
D10,D10	CONSTRAINED AT LOWER BOUND
D12,D12	LINEARLY DEPENDENT ON OTHER PARAMETERS
V12,F5	LINEARLY DEPENDENT ON OTHER PARAMETERS
V13,F6	LINEARLY DEPENDENT ON OTHER PARAMETERS
F10,F3	LINEARLY DEPENDENT ON OTHER PARAMETERS
V17,F8	LINEARLY DEPENDENT ON OTHER PARAMETERS
V21,F9	LINEARLY DEPENDENT ON OTHER PARAMETERS
V29,F11	LINEARLY DEPENDENT ON OTHER PARAMETERS

Before leaving this Build EQS walk-through, there is an important caveat regarding specification of the measurement model that reminds users to be sure to fix one factor-loading parameter within each set of indicator variables per factor. This model identification condition is reiterated here because in working with the Build EQS option, it is especially easy to forget to change the asterisk to a fixed value. If this step is omitted, the output file will include the error messages shown in Table 6.2.

Let's now revisit the input file, shown in Fig. 6.1, where you will note no evidence of start values. Unless a model is very complex or the actual parameter estimates are far from the initial EQS start values used in the iterative process, typically it is not necessary to be concerned about inserting these values. If the program is having difficulty with the minimization process, all action stops after 30 iterations and users are presented with a message about bad start values. However, this situation is easily rectified within the EQS program by using the extremely valuable RETEST option.

Admittedly, the input file shown in Fig. 6.1 runs quite satisfactorily without the addition of start values. However, because the RETEST feature of EQS is a remarkable option that can save hours of frustration if start values must be provided, its implementation is demonstrated with the present causal model. To begin, the command RETEST = 'filename.out' is included within the /PRINT paragraph. In the present file, for example, this paragraph would appear as follows:

```
/PRINT
  FIT = ALL;
  RETEST = 'HSSTART.OUT';
```

With invocation of the RETEST command, EQS executes the input file and simultaneously creates a separate output file (as labeled) in which the start values are included for all estimated parameters. The user simply cuts and pastes this section into the input file. A reduced version of this section of the output is shown in Table 6.3.[4]

THE EQS OUTPUT FILE

Reviewing the output file related to the hypothesized causal model, we look first at the univariate statistics shown in Table 6.4, where relatively high kurtosis values for four indicator variables are circled. (Of the remaining 22 indicator variables, kurtosis values were all less than 1.00 except for ROLEA2, which had a value of 1.29.) Overall, Mardia's normalized estimate was 40.7136, thereby indicating some degree of non-normality for the data. Hence, estimation based on the Robust statistics was considered appropriate.

At the bottom of Table 6.4 is a listing of case numbers that EQS identified as making the largest contribution to normalized multivariate kurtosis. In determining possible multivariate outliers in the data, we compare the size of these estimates relative to one another; the absolute values of these estimates are meaningless. What a user looks for in the determination of outliers is the extent to which the estimate for one case is strikingly different from all the rest. In Table 6.4, I would consider the value estimate for Case #440 to be substantially different from those for all other cases.

In addressing this data problem, the same input file was estimated again but with Case #440 deleted from the analyses. This analysis again revealed one multivariate outlier (#77). No additional outliers were identified in the subsequent run in which both Cases #440 and #77 were deleted from the analyses; thus, all subsequent tests of the model specified deletion of these two cases. This input specification is shown in Table 6.5 and the resulting output is shown in Table 6.6.

---

[4]Due to space limitations, only a few values were included in the /VARIANCES and /COVARIANCES paragraphs.

TABLE 6.3
EQS Output for Restart Option: Start Values

```
!
! FOLLOWING LISTS ARE GENERATED FROM RETEST
!
/EQUATIONS
    V1  =   1.000 F1   +   1.000 E1   ;
    V2  =   1.308*F1   +   1.000 E2   ;
    V3  =   1.000 F2   +   1.000 E3   ;
    V4  =   1.253*F2   +   1.000 E4   ;
    V5  =   1.000 F3   +   1.000 E5   ;
    V6  =    .708*F3   +   1.000 E6   ;
    V7  =   1.000 F4   +   1.000 E7   ;
    V8  =   1.664*F4   +   1.000 E8   ;
    V9  =    .987*F4   +   1.000 E9   ;
    V10 =   1.385*F4   +   1.000 E10  ;
    V11 =   1.000 F5   +   1.000 E11  ;
    V12 =    .242*F5   +    .898*F6   +   1.000 E12  ;
    V13 =   1.000 F6   +   1.000 E13  ;
    V14 =   1.101*F6   +   1.000 E14  ;
    V15 =   1.000 F7   +   1.000 E15  ;
    V16 =   1.060*F7   +   1.000 E16  ;
    V17 =   1.000 F8   +   1.000 E17  ;
    V18 =   1.263*F8   +   1.000 E18  ;
    V19 =   1.417*F8   +   1.000 E19  ;
    V20 =   1.000 F9   +   1.000 E20  ;
    V21 =    .911*F9   +   1.000 E21  ;
    V22 =   1.060*F9   +   1.000 E22  ;
    V23 =    .957*F9   +   1.000 E23  ;
    V24 =   1.246*F9   +   1.000 E24  ;
    V25 =   1.000 F10  +   1.000 E25  ;
    V26 =   1.052*F10  +   1.000 E26  ;
    V27 =   1.219*F10  +   1.000 E27  ;
    V28 =   1.000 F11  +   1.000 E28  ;
    V29 =    .920*F11  +   1.000 E29  ;
    V30 =   -.171*F10  +   1.000 F12  +   1.000 E30  ;
    V31 =   1.234*F12  +   1.000 E31  ;
    V32 =   1.179*F12  +   1.000 E32  ;
    F8  =    .363*F5       -.114* F6       -.044*F7   +   1.000 D8   ;
    F9  =   -.262*F5   +   1.000 D9   ;
    F10 =   -.128*F2   +    .745* F3       -.898*F4   +   1.000 D10  ;
    F11 =    .549*F10  +    .147* F2   +   1.000 D11  ;
    F12 =    .512*F8       -.188* F9   +    .019*F10      -.195*F11      -.041*F1
        +   1.000 D12  ;
/VARIANCES
    F1=    .388* ;


    .

    F7=    .622* ;
    E1=    .446* ;

    .

    .

    E32=   .382* ;
    D8=    .077* ;

    .

    .

    D12=   .270*  ;
```

(Continued)

TABLE 6.3

(Continued)

```
/COVARIANCES
    F2,F1  =     .389* ;
    .
    .
    F7,F6  =     .391* ;
    E26,E25 =    .259* ;
/END
```

TABLE 6.4

Selected EQS Output for Initially Hypothesized Model:
Descriptive Statistics and Outliers

UNIVARIATE STATISTICS

VARIABLE	PSUP2	SELF1	SELF2	SELF3	XLOC1
MEAN	4.6056	3.6286	3.6367	3.4988	2.9263
SKEWNESS (G1)	-.7470	-1.7292	-1.8829	-1.3731	-.0946
KURTOSIS (G2)	.8260	5.1611	4.3166	2.3505	-.0574
STANDARD DEV.	.9392	.4439	.5076	.5522	.6143

VARIABLE	EE2	EE3	DP1	DP2	PA1
MEAN	3.5354	3.1362	2.3842	2.1684	5.7729
SKEWNESS (G1)	.3811	.6495	1.1237	1.4611	-.8599
KURTOSIS (G2)	-.3170	-.1712	1.2063	2.0608	.6924
STANDARD DEV.	1.2536	1.3205	1.1369	1.2427	.8983

MULTIVARIATE KURTOSIS

```
MARDIA'S COEFFICIENT (G2,P) =    141.9525
NORMALIZED ESTIMATE =             40.7136
```

CASE NUMBERS WITH LARGEST CONTRIBUTION TO NORMALIZED MULTIVARIATE KURTOSIS:

CASE NUMBER	77	297	306	316	440
ESTIMATE	1945.8853	1838.9729	1769.1764	1733.7342	3037.6603

TABLE 6.5

Selected EQS Input for Hypothesized Model of Burnout: Deleted Cases

```
/TITLE
FULL BURNOUT MODEL FOR SECONDARY TCHRS (GRP1); "BURNHS1ID.EQS"
INITIAL MODEL
Two Cases Deleted
CROSS-LOADINGS: F6 TO V12 (SSUP TO DEC2); F10 TO V30 (EE TO PA1)
ERROR COV: E26,E25 (EE)
/SPECIFICATIONS
CASE=716; VAR=32; ME=ML, ROBUST; MA=RAW; FO='(19F4.2/13F4.2)'; DEL=440,77;
DATA='C:\EQS61\Files\Books\Data\secind1.dat';
/EQUATIONS
```

TABLE 6.6

Selected EQS Output for Initially Hypothesized Model: Possible Outlying Cases

```
                        MULTIVARIATE KURTOSIS
                        ----------------------

MARDIA'S COEFFICIENT (G2,P) =    132.2515
NORMALIZED ESTIMATE =             37.8783
```

CASE NUMBERS WITH LARGEST CONTRIBUTION TO NORMALIZED MULTIVARIATE KURTOSIS:

CASE NUMBER	297	298	306	316	570
ESTIMATE	1829.5197	1645.9204	1934.5730	1732.5257	1692.0514

TABLE 6.7

Selected EQS Output for Initially Hypothesized Model: Bentler–Weeks Representation

```
BENTLER-WEEKS STRUCTURAL REPRESENTATION:

    NUMBER OF DEPENDENT VARIABLES = 37
         DEPENDENT V'S :     1    2    3    4    5    6    7    8    9   10
         DEPENDENT V'S :    11   12   13   14   15   16   17   18   19   20
         DEPENDENT V'S :    21   22   23   24   25   26   27   28   29   30
         DEPENDENT V'S :    31   32
         DEPENDENT F'S :     8    9   10   11   12

    NUMBER OF INDEPENDENT VARIABLES = 44
         INDEPENDENT F'S :   1    2    3    4    5    6    7
         INDEPENDENT E'S :   1    2    3    4    5    6    7    8    9   10
         INDEPENDENT E'S :  11   12   13   14   15   16   17   18   19   20
         INDEPENDENT E'S :  21   22   23   24   25   26   27   28   29   30
         INDEPENDENT E'S :  31   32
         INDEPENDENT D'S :   8    9   10   11   12

    NUMBER OF FREE PARAMETERS = 102
    NUMBER OF FIXED NONZERO PARAMETERS = 49

PARAMETER          CONDITION CODE
D10,D10            CONSTRAINED AT LOWER BOUND
```

The Bentler–Weeks representation summary of the hypothesized model is shown in Table 6.7. To assure full comprehension of the status of each variable in the model, it is helpful to check this decomposition of parameters for the model against its schematic presentation in Fig. 6.4. Review of Table 6.7 reveals the following:

- 37 dependent variables
  - ➢ 32 observed indicators (V1–V32)
  - ➢ 5 factors (F8–F12)
- 44 independent variables
  - ➢ 7 factors (F1–F7)
  - ➢ 32 error terms (E1–E32)
  - ➢ 5 disturbance terms (D8–D12)
- 102 estimated parameters

> ➤ 22 factor loadings (20 original, 2 additional)
> ➤ 44 variances (7 F's, 32 E's, 5 D's)
> ➤ 22 covariances (21 factor, 1 error)
> ➤ 14 structural regression paths
- 49 fixed parameters
> ➤ 32 error regression paths
> ➤ 5 disturbance regression paths
> ➤ 12 factor-loading regression paths

Of import also, is the Condition Code for parameter D10,D10, the disturbance variance for Factor 10 (Emotional Exhaustion). The program notes that this parameter has been constrained to lower bound, which means that it has been constrained to 0.0. Bentler (2005, p. 113) notes that "the constraint of a parameter at an upper or lower bound may be a cause for celebration or a reason for distress. If the bound is desired, the solution may be totally acceptable. If the bound is not desired, it implies a possible problem." In the present case, the disturbance variance for F10 is probably close to zero and, as a boundary parameter, can just as easily be a negative as a positive value. If the estimate is negative, EQS automatically constrains the value to zero because its variability cannot be computed accurately. Interpreted literally in the present case, this condition code implies that the combination of Role Conflict (F2), Work Overload (F3), and Classroom Climate (F4) was perfect in its prediction of Emotional Exhaustion (F10), thereby resulting in no residual variance. As shown in Table 6.8, whenever a condition code is identified, the program cautions about the appropriateness of the resulting parameter estimate. However, in the testing of full structural equation models, post hoc model-fitting often results in a solution in which the condition code disappears—which is the case in the present example.

Turning to the goodness-of-fit statistics in Table 6.8, notice first the substantial drop in χ^2 value between the ML uncorrected and the Satorra–Bentler scaled statistics, thereby providing evidence of some degree of non-normality in the data, as noted previously. Both the corrected CFI (i.e., *CFI) value of .944 and the *RMSEA value of .042 indicate that the hypothesized model sustained a very reasonable fit to the sample data. However, given that this model of burnout determinants was mapped solely from a review of the empirical literature, it is highly possible that other paths should be more appropriately added, whereas other paths already specified in the model may not be worthy of inclusion. Thus, the next step is to examine the LM Test statistics to determine what degree of modification, if any, might be considered. These statistics are presented in Table 6.9.

As noted earlier in this book EQS provides first, a set of ordered univariate LM Test statistics, together with both unstandardized and standardized expected parameter change statistics. Each univariate LM Test statistic is associated with an estimated value the parameter might assume if this fixed parameter is freely estimated rather than constrained. These values are followed by a set of multivariate

TABLE 6.8
Selected EQS Output for Initially Hypothesized Model: Goodness-of-Fit Statistics

```
*** WARNING *** TEST RESULTS MAY NOT BE APPROPRIATE DUE TO CONDITION CODE


            GOODNESS OF FIT SUMMARY FOR METHOD = ML

CHI-SQUARE =      1077.784 BASED ON      426 DEGREES OF FREEDOM
PROBABILITY VALUE FOR THE CHI-SQUARE STATISTIC IS         .00000

FIT INDICES
-----------
BENTLER-BONETT        NORMED FIT INDEX =        .911
BENTLER-BONETT NON-NORMED FIT INDEX =        .935
COMPARATIVE FIT INDEX (CFI)         =        .944
ROOT MEAN-SQUARE RESIDUAL (RMR)     =        .044
STANDARDIZED RMR                    =        .054
ROOT MEAN-SQUARE ERROR OF APPROXIMATION (RMSEA)    =        .046
90% CONFIDENCE INTERVAL OF RMSEA  (        .043,        .050)


          GOODNESS OF FIT SUMMARY FOR METHOD = ROBUST

SATORRA-BENTLER SCALED CHI-SQUARE =      963.3964 ON      426 DEGREES OF FREEDOM
PROBABILITY VALUE FOR THE CHI-SQUARE STATISTIC IS         .00000

FIT INDICES
-----------
BENTLER-BONETT        NORMED FIT INDEX =        .905
BENTLER-BONETT NON-NORMED FIT INDEX =        .935
COMPARATIVE FIT INDEX (CFI)         =        .944
ROOT MEAN-SQUARE ERROR OF APPROXIMATION (RMSEA)    =        .042
90% CONFIDENCE INTERVAL OF RMSEA  (        .039,        .046)
```

statistics. Decisions regarding which parameters to consider for addition to the model are based on the multivariate statistics because correlation among all variables has been taken into account. Examination of the column labeled Parameter shows that the variables suggested for addition to the model represent both structural paths (e.g., F11,F3) and correlated disturbance terms (D10,D8). The easiest way to identify the path being targeted as a misspecified parameter is to conceptualize the causal flow as going from the second factor in a pair of latent factors to the first factor in the pair. For example, the first parameter specified in the output is F11,F3; this parameter is interpreted as the structural path flowing from F3 (Work Overload) to F11 (Depersonalization). These results suggest that if this path were to be specified in the model, Work Overload would have a substantial impact on Depersonalization.

Given the substantive reasonableness of this new path, the sharp drop in the univariate increment from $\chi^2_{(1)} = 63.440$ to $\chi^2_{(2)} = 31.712$, and the substantial size of the expected parameter change statistic, this parameter certainly qualifies for inclusion in the model. Likewise, several other parameters representative of structural paths can be considered as logical candidates for inclusion and could all be included at this time. However, my preference, at this time, is to limit modification to the inclusion of only the first parameter. As with the CFA analyses conducted

TABLE 6.9
Selected EQS Output for Initially Hypothesized Model: Modification Indexes

LAGRANGE MULTIPLIER TEST (FOR ADDING PARAMETERS)

ORDERED UNIVARIATE TEST STATISTICS:

*** WARNING *** TEST RESULTS MAY NOT BE APPROPRIATE DUE TO CONDITION CODE

NO	CODE	PARAMETER	CHI-SQUARE	PROB.	HANCOCK 426 DF PROB.	PARAMETER CHANGE	STANDAR-DIZED CHANGE
1	2 16	F11,F3	63.440	.000	1.000	-3.277	-3.574
2	2 16	F11,F4	63.440	.000	1.000	-1.110	-3.525
3	2 10	D10,D8	31.688	.000	1.000	-.082	.000
4	2 22	F10,F8	31.414	.000	1.000	-1.141	-3.494
5	2 22	F8,F10	27.911	.000	1.000	-.167	-.510
6	2 22	F10,F11	24.033	.000	1.000	-.539	-.529
7	2 10	D11,D10	24.033	.000	1.000	-.337	.000
8	2 22	F9,F8	23.708	.000	1.000	-.309	-2.334
9	2 16	F8,F1	20.932	.000	1.000	.292	1.438
10	2 16	F9,F2	18.820	.000	1.000	.163	.493

STEP	PARAMETER	CUMULATIVE MULTIVARIATE STATISTICS CHI-SQUARE	D.F.	PROB.	UNIVARIATE INCREMENT CHI-SQUARE	PROB.	HANCOCK'S SEQUENTIAL D.F.	PROB.
1	F11,F3	63.440	1	.000	63.440	.000	426	1.000
2	D10,D8	95.152	2	.000	31.712	.000	425	1.000
3	F9,F8	120.344	3	.000	25.193	.000	424	1.000
4	F12,F5	136.719	4	.000	16.374	.000	423	1.000
5	F11,F12	147.255	5	.000	10.536	.001	422	1.000
6	F10,F6	156.239	6	.000	8.984	.003	421	1.000
7	F9,F2	165.073	7	.000	8.834	.003	420	1.000
8	F10,F11	170.974	8	.000	5.901	.015	419	1.000
9	F11,F6	176.041	9	.000	5.067	.024	418	1.000

previously, we now move into exploratory mode as we respecify and analyze models that vary from the one originally hypothesized and tested. This first respecified model is Model 2.

POST HOC ANALYSES: MODEL 2

The EQS Input File

Model respecification with the new parameter (F11,F3) included is shown in boldface in Table 6.10. Note that no start value is included because it is unnecessary.

The EQS Output File

Let's see now what difference the addition of this new path made to the model. In Table 6.11, note first that the condition code for the variance of D10 is still

TABLE 6.10

Selected EQS Input: Model 2

```
/TITLE
 FULL BURNOUT MODEL FOR SECONDARY TCHRS (GRP1); "BURNHS2.EQS"
 MODEL 2
 ADDED: F3 to F11 (Work —> DP)
     .
     .
     .
/EQUATIONS
     .
     .
     .
 F8  =  .363*F5 - .114*F6 -.044*F7 + 1.000 D8;
 F9  = -.262*F5 + 1.000 D9;
 F10 = -.128*F2 + .745*F3 -.898*F4 + 1.000 D10;
 F11 =  .549*F10 + .147*F2 + *F3 + 1.000 D11;
 F12 =  .512*F8 -.188*F9 + .019*F10 -.195*F11 -.041*F1 + 1.000 D12;
     .
     .
     .
/LMTEST
 SET=GFF, BFF, PDD;
/END
```

TABLE 6.11

Selected EQS Output for Model 2: Goodness-of-Fit Statistics

PARAMETER   **CONDITION CODE**
  D10,D10   CONSTRAINED AT LOWER BOUND

GOODNESS OF FIT SUMMARY FOR METHOD = ML

CHI-SQUARE =   1012.059 BASED ON   425 DEGREES OF FREEDOM
PROBABILITY VALUE FOR THE CHI-SQUARE STATISTIC IS   .00000

FIT INDICES

BENTLER-BONETT   NORMED FIT INDEX =   .917
BENTLER-BONETT NON-NORMED FIT INDEX =   .941
COMPARATIVE FIT INDEX (CFI)   =   .950
ROOT MEAN-SQUARE RESIDUAL (RMR)   =   .039
STANDARDIZED RMR   =   .049
ROOT MEAN-SQUARE ERROR OF APPROXIMATION (RMSEA)   =   .044
90% CONFIDENCE INTERVAL OF RMSEA (.040,   .047)

GOODNESS OF FIT SUMMARY FOR METHOD = ROBUST

SATORRA-BENTLER SCALED CHI-SQUARE = 903.1202 ON 425 DEGREES OF FREEDOM
PROBABILITY VALUE FOR THE CHI-SQUARE STATISTIC IS   .00000

FIT INDICES

BENTLER-BONETT   NORMED FIT INDEX =   .911
BENTLER-BONETT NON-NORMED FIT INDEX =   .942
COMPARATIVE FIT INDEX (CFI)   =   .951
ROOT MEAN-SQUARE ERROR OF APPROXIMATION (RMSEA)   =   .040
90% CONFIDENCE INTERVAL OF RMSEA (.036,   .043)

TABLE 6.12
Selected EQS Output for Model 2: Modification Indexes

MULTIVARIATE LAGRANGE MULTIPLIER TEST BY SIMULTANEOUS PROCESS IN STAGE 1
PARAMETER SETS (SUBMATRICES) ACTIVE AT THIS STAGE ARE:
  PDD GFF BFF

| | | CUMULATIVE MULTIVARIATE STATISTICS | | | UNIVARIATE INCREMENT | | HANCOCK'S SEQUENTIAL | |
STEP	PARAMETER	CHI-SQUARE	D.F.	PROB.	CHI-SQUARE	PROB.	D.F.	PROB.
1	D10,D8	38.225	1	.000	38.225	.000	425	1.000
2	F9,F8	63.285	2	.000	25.059	.000	424	1.000
3	D12,D9	80.017	3	.000	16.732	.000	423	1.000
4	F10,F6	89.151	4	.000	9.134	.003	422	1.000
5	F9,F2	98.219	5	.000	9.068	.003	421	1.000
6	F12,F3	105.312	6	.000	7.093	.008	420	1.000
7	F11,F6	109.563	7	.000	4.251	.039	419	1.000

there. Otherwise, the goodness-of-fit information reveals substantial improvement in overall fit as indicated by a *CFI value of .951 (from .944) and a *RMSEA value of .040 (from .042). In Table 6.12, there is a somewhat bewildering situation in which there are now two correlated disturbance terms noted, with the first one (D10,D8) showing the greatest potential improvement in model fit if this parameter is estimated. However, once again, I prefer to limit modification to only the structural path exhibiting the highest univariate incremental χ^2 value (F9,F8), a path leading from Self-esteem to External Locus of Control.

MODEL 3

The EQS Input File

Specification of this new structural path is shown in boldface in Table 6.13 and no start value has been included. To make it easier for you in keeping track of the changes made to this model, I have also included the /TITLE paragraph in which I have noted the most recent addition (F8 to F9) has been included.

The EQS Output File

Table 6.14 shows (a) evidence that the condition code is still maintained, and (b) that the inclusion of a path from Self-esteem to External Locus of Control resulted in a slight improvement to model fit (i.e., *CFI = .953; *RMSEA = .039). Review of the modification indexes in Table 6.15 shows the parameter D10,D8 still exhibiting the highest univariate incremental LM Test χ^2 value. Also shown, however, are five structural paths that represent reasonable additions to

TABLE 6.13
Selected EQS Input: Model 3

```
/TITLE
  FULL BURNOUT MODEL FOR SECONDARY TCHRS (GRP1); "BURNHS3.EQS"
  MODEL 3
  ADDED: F3 to F11 (Work -> DP)
  ADDED: F8 to F9 (SE -> XLOCUS)
    .
    .
    .
/EQUATIONS
    .
    .
    .
  F8 =  .363*F5 -.114*F6 -.044*F7 + 1.000 D8;
  F9 = -.262*F5 +  *F8 + 1.000 D9;
  F10 = -.128*F2 + .745*F3  -.898*F4 + 1.000 D10;
  F11 = .549*F10 + .147*F2 + *F3 + 1.000 D11;
  F12 = .512*F8 -.188*F9 + .019*F10 -.195*F11 -.041*F1 + 1.000 D12;
    .
    .
    .
/LMTEST
  SET=GFF, BFF, PDD;
/END
```

TABLE 6.14
Selected EQS Output for Model 3: Goodness-of-Fit Statistics

```
PARAMETER      CONDITION CODE
 D10,D10       CONSTRAINED AT LOWER BOUND

GOODNESS OF FIT SUMMARY FOR METHOD = ML

CHI-SQUARE =        988.239 BASED ON     424 DEGREES OF FREEDOM
PROBABILITY VALUE FOR THE CHI-SQUARE STATISTIC IS      .00000

FIT INDICES
-----------
BENTLER-BONETT      NORMED FIT INDEX =      .919
BENTLER-BONETT NON-NORMED FIT INDEX =      .943
COMPARATIVE FIT INDEX (CFI)          =     .952
ROOT MEAN-SQUARE RESIDUAL (RMR)      =     .038
STANDARDIZED RMR                     =     .046
ROOT MEAN-SQUARE ERROR OF APPROXIMATION (RMSEA)   =     .043
90% CONFIDENCE INTERVAL OF RMSEA   (      .040,      .047)

GOODNESS OF FIT SUMMARY FOR METHOD = ROBUST

SATORRA-BENTLER SCALED CHI-SQUARE =   882.3626 ON     424 DEGREES OF FREEDOM
PROBABILITY VALUE FOR THE CHI-SQUARE STATISTIC IS      .00000

FIT INDICES
-----------
BENTLER-BONETT      NORMED FIT INDEX =      .913
BENTLER-BONETT NON-NORMED FIT INDEX =      .944
COMPARATIVE FIT INDEX (CFI)          =     .953
ROOT MEAN-SQUARE ERROR OF APPROXIMATION (RMSEA)   =     .039
90% CONFIDENCE INTERVAL OF RMSEA   (      .035,      .043)
```

TABLE 6.15
Selected EQS Output for Model 3: Modification Indexes

MULTIVARIATE LAGRANGE MULTIPLIER TEST BY SIMULTANEOUS PROCESS IN STAGE   1
   PARAMETER SETS (SUBMATRICES) ACTIVE AT THIS STAGE ARE:
      PDD GFF BFF

| | | CUMULATIVE MULTIVARIATE STATISTICS | | | UNIVARIATE INCREMENT | | | |
STEP	PARAMETER	CHI-SQUARE	D.F.	PROB.	CHI-SQUARE	PROB.	HANCOCK'S SEQUENTIAL D.F.	PROB.
1	D10,D8	37.582	1	.000	37.582	.000	424	1.000
2	F12,F5	53.760	2	.000	16.178	.000	423	1.000
3	F9,F2	66.701	3	.000	12.941	.000	422	1.000
4	F10,F6	75.660	4	.000	8.959	.003	421	1.000
5	F12,F3	82.639	5	.000	6.978	.008	420	1.000
6	F11,F6	86.942	6	.000	4.303	.038	419	1.000

the model. Although cognizant of obtaining the most parsimonious model that concomitantly best represents the data and ever wary of overfitting a model, I nonetheless believe that each of these paths should be included because they all have substantive meaning. Indeed, research has shown that in an exploratory context, it is wise to overfit a model (i.e., add more parameters than may be needed) before considering which parameters to drop from the model (see, e.g., Bentler, 2005; and Green, Thompson, & Poirier, 1999).

MODEL 4

The EQS Input File

Table 6.16 shows the five additional paths specified for the model, again presented in boldface and without start values. The/TITLE paragraph was revised to include these new paths.

The EQS Output File

Reviewing the goodness-of-fit statistics in Table 6.17, note first that the D10 condition code is gone; this message was replaced by "no special problems were encountered during the minimization process." In the Robust statistics, the inclusion of these five parameters produced only a small increment in overall model fit (i.e., *CFI = .956; *RMSEA = .038).

In Table 6.18, the correlated disturbance term, D10,D8, still displays prominently as a parameter to be addressed. In many models, the covariance between two independent factors and the direct paths between them are identical and cannot be statistically differentiated (Bentler, pers. comm., November 2, 2004). For example,

TABLE 6.16
Selected EQS Input: Model 4

```
/TITLE
FULL BURNOUT MODEL FOR SECONDARY TCHRS (GRP1); "BURNHS4.EQS"
MODEL 4
ADDED: F3 to F11 (Work -> DP)
ADDED: F8 to F9 (SE -> XLOCUS)
ADDED: F5 to F12 (SSUP->PA; F2 to F9 (ROLEC->XLOCUS); F6 to F10 (PSUP->EE);
       F3 to F12 (WORK->PA); F6 to F11 (PSUP->DP)
   .
   .
/EQUATIONS
   .
   .
F8  =  .363*F5 -.114*F6 -.044*F7 + 1.000 D8;
F9  = -.262*F5 + *F8 + *F2 + 1.000 D9;
F10 = -.128*F2 + .745*F3 -.898*F4 + *F6 + 1.000 D10;
F11 = .549*F10 + .147*F2 + *F3 + *F6 + 1.000 D11;
F12 = .512*F8 -.188*F9 + .019*F10 -.195*F11 -.041*F1+ *F5 + *F3 + 1.000 D12;
   .
   .
/LMTEST
SET=GFF, BFF, PDD;
/END
```

F1 and F2: If these two factors are correlated, then an equivalent representation is F1->F2 (or F2->F1). However, if these two factors are dependent variables in a model, the same situation may or may not hold true. Conversely, Bentler further suggests that if their χ^2 values are identical, it is likely that equivalence of their covariance and direct path does hold true.

This information is important to the results presented in Table 6.18. Given the strength of the univariate incremental χ^2 statistic for D10,D8, it is evident that this parameter should be specified in the model. Although it appears to make little sense to include the correlation of D10,D8 in the model, it does make sense to include a structural path from F8 (self-esteem) to F10 (emotional exhaustion). Further support for this specification comes with a review of the expected parameter change statistic associated with each parameter. Indeed, the path F10,F8 is shown to have a particularly strong standardized change value (−3.685). Given that both of these factors are dependent variables in the model, I considered it important to check first on the equivalence of the fit indexes between two models according to Bentler's caveat: (a) Model A, in which D10,D8 was specified as the free parameter; and (b) Model B, in which, alternatively, a path from F8 to F10 was specified as the free parameter. In each case, the *CFI and *RMSEA were identical (.96 and .036, respectively) and the S-Bχ^2 statistic almost identical (808.13 versus 805.61). Based on these results, the model was respecified (i.e., Model 5) with an estimated path flowing from F8 to F10.

TABLE 6.17

Selected EQS Output for Model 4: Goodness-of-Fit Statistics

```
PARAMETER ESTIMATES APPEAR IN ORDER,
NO SPECIAL PROBLEMS WERE ENCOUNTERED DURING OPTIMIZATION.

        GOODNESS OF FIT SUMMARY FOR METHOD = ML

CHI-SQUARE =      935.518 BASED ON     419 DEGREES OF FREEDOM
PROBABILITY VALUE FOR THE CHI-SQUARE STATISTIC IS      .00000
FIT INDICES
-----------
BENTLER-BONETT       NORMED FIT INDEX =      .923
BENTLER-BONETT NON-NORMED FIT INDEX =      .948
COMPARATIVE FIT INDEX (CFI)         =      .956
ROOT MEAN-SQUARE RESIDUAL (RMR)     =      .033
STANDARDIZED RMR                    =      .041
ROOT MEAN-SQUARE ERROR OF APPROXIMATION (RMSEA)   =      .042
90% CONFIDENCE INTERVAL OF RMSEA  (      .038,     .045)

        GOODNESS OF FIT SUMMARY FOR METHOD = ROBUST

SATORRA-BENTLER SCALED CHI-SQUARE =    844.0545 ON   419 DEGREES OF FREEDOM
PROBABILITY VALUE FOR THE CHI-SQUARE STATISTIC IS      .00000
FIT INDICES
-----------
BENTLER-BONETT       NORMED FIT INDEX =      .917
BENTLER-BONETT NON-NORMED FIT INDEX =      .948
COMPARATIVE FIT INDEX (CFI)         =      .956
ROOT MEAN-SQUARE ERROR OF APPROXIMATION (RMSEA)   =      .038
90% CONFIDENCE INTERVAL OF RMSEA  (      .034,     .041)
```

TABLE 6.18

Selected EQS Output for Model 4: Modification Indexes

```
LAGRANGE MULTIPLIER TEST (FOR ADDING PARAMETERS)

ORDERED UNIVARIATE TEST STATISTICS:
```

NO	CODE	PARAMETER	CHI-SQUARE	PROB.	HANCOCK 419 DF PROB.	PARAMETER CHANGE	STANDAR-DIZED CHANGE
1	2 10	D10,D8	43.930	.000	1.000	-.095	-1.422
2	2 22	F10,F8	41.626	.000	1.000	-1.210	-3.685
3	2 22	F8,F11	25.169	.000	1.000	-.106	-.321
4	2 22	F8,F10	23.007	.000	1.000	-.200	-.610
5	2 10	D11,D8	17.885	.000	1.000	-.055	-.279

CUMULATIVE MULTIVARIATE STATISTICS   UNIVARIATE INCREMENT

STEP	PARAMETER	CHI-SQUARE	D.F.	PROB.	CHI-SQUARE	PROB.	HANCOCK'S SEQUENTIAL D.F.	PROB.
1	D10,D8	43.930	1	.000	43.930	.000	419	1.000
2	F9,F1	47.993	2	.000	4.063	.044	418	1.000

MODEL 5

The EQS Input File

Table 6.19 shows the partial input file for Model 5; in particular, the specification of a path leading from F8 to F10.

The EQS Output File

Goodness-of-fit statistics related to the estimation of Model 5 are shown in Table 6.20. As noted previously, this analysis resulted in excellent model fit that improved over that of Model 4 (*CFI = .960 versus .956; *RMSEA = .036 versus .038). Shown in Table 6.21 are the LM Test results for this model. Here we find yet another parameter to be considered for inclusion in the model, a path from Role Ambiguity to Depersonalization (F11,F1). Given that nonsignificant paths are identified and deleted before a final model is established, I considered it appropriate to test one more model in which this parameter was estimated.

TABLE 6.19
Selected EQS Input: Model 5

```
/TITLE
FULL BURNOUT MODEL FOR SECONDARY TCHRS (GRP1); "BURNHS5.EQS"
MODEL 5
ADDED: F3 to F11 (Work -> DP)
ADDED: F8 to F9 (SE -> XLOCUS)
ADDED: F5 to F12 (SSUP->PA; F2 to F9 (ROLEC->XLOCUS); F6 to F10 (PSUP->EE);
       F3 to F12 (WORK->PA); F6 to DP (PSUP->DP)
ADDED: F8 to F10 (SE -> EE)
    .
    .
    .
/EQUATIONS
    .
    .
    .
  F8  =   .363*F5 -.114*F6 -.044*F7 + 1.000 D8;
  F9  = -.262*F5 +  *F8 +  *F2 + 1.000 D9;
  F10 = -.128*F2 +  .745*F3  - .898*F4 +  *F6 +  *F8 + 1.000 D10;
  F11 =  .549*F10 +  .147*F2 +  *F3 +  *F6 + 1.000 D11;
  F12 =  .512*F8  - .188*F9 +  .019*F10 -  .195*F11 -  .041*F1 +  *F5 +  *F3 + 1.000 + D12;
    .
    .
/LMTEST
 SET=GFF, BFF, PDD;
/END
```

TABLE 6.20

Selected EQS Output for Model 5: Goodness-of-Fit Statistics

```
            GOODNESS OF FIT SUMMARY FOR METHOD = ML

CHI-SQUARE =        895.790 BASED ON      418 DEGREES OF FREEDOM
PROBABILITY VALUE FOR THE CHI-SQUARE STATISTIC IS       .00000

FIT INDICES
-----------
BENTLER-BONETT      NORMED FIT INDEX =       .926
BENTLER-BONETT NON-NORMED FIT INDEX =       .951
COMPARATIVE FIT INDEX (CFI)         =       .959
ROOT MEAN-SQUARE RESIDUAL (RMR)     =       .032
STANDARDIZED RMR                    =       .040
ROOT MEAN-SQUARE ERROR OF APPROXIMATION (RMSEA)   =         .040
90% CONFIDENCE INTERVAL OF RMSEA  (       .036,         .044)


            GOODNESS OF FIT SUMMARY FOR METHOD = ROBUST

SATORRA-BENTLER SCALED CHI-SQUARE =      808.1292 ON      418 DEGREES OF FREEDOM
PROBABILITY VALUE FOR THE CHI-SQUARE STATISTIC IS       .00000

FIT INDICES
-----------
BENTLER-BONETT      NORMED FIT INDEX =       .920
BENTLER-BONETT NON-NORMED FIT INDEX =       .952
COMPARATIVE FIT INDEX (CFI)         =       .960
ROOT MEAN-SQUARE ERROR OF APPROXIMATION (RMSEA)   =         .036
90% CONFIDENCE INTERVAL OF RMSEA  (       .032,         .040)
```

TABLE 6.21

Selected EQS Output for Model 5: Modification Indexes

```
MULTIVARIATE LAGRANGE MULTIPLIER TEST BY SIMULTANEOUS PROCESS IN STAGE 1
    PARAMETER SETS (SUBMATRICES) ACTIVE AT THIS STAGE ARE:
       PDD GFF BFF
```

		CUMULATIVE MULTIVARIATE STATISTICS			UNIVARIATE INCREMENT			
							HANCOCK'S SEQUENTIAL	
STEP	PARAMETER	CHI-SQUARE	D.F.	PROB.	CHI-SQUARE	PROB.	D.F.	PROB.
1	F11,F1	6.041	1	.014	6.041	.014	418	1.000

MODEL 6

The EQS Input File

Table 6.22 is the related EQS input file showing the specification of F1 leading to F11. The model changes are summarized in the /TITLE paragraph.

The EQS Output File

As shown in the goodness-of-fit summary in Table 6.23, incorporation of the path F11,F1 resulted in virtually no change in overall model fit from the previous model (i.e., Model 5). Thus, although the LM Test Statistics shown in Table 6.24 suggested another structural path to be incorporated into the model, this addition was not considered.

Thus far in this chapter, discussion related to model fit has considered only the addition of parameters to the model. However, another side to the question of fit—particularly as it pertains to a full causal model—is the extent to which certain initially hypothesized paths and possibly post hoc additional paths may be redundant to the model. One way to determine such redundancy is to examine the statistical significance of all structural parameter estimates. This information, as derived from the estimation of Model 6, is presented in Table 6.25.

Examining z-statistics associated with these structural estimates, we can determine five that are nonsignificant; these parameters are circled in Table 6.25 and represent structural paths flowing from F7 to F8, F1 to F11, F6 to F11, F10 to F12, and F1 to F12. The limiting factor in using these statistics as a basis for pinpointing redundant parameters, however, is that they represent univariate tests of significance. When sets of parameters are to be evaluated, a more appropriate approach is to implement a multivariate test of statistical significance. Indeed, the EQS program is unique in its provision of the Wald Test (WTest; Wald, 1943) for

TABLE 6.22
Selected EQS Input: Model 6

```
/TITLE
FULL BURNOUT MODEL FOR SECONDARY TCHRS (GRP1); "BURNHS6.EQS"
MODEL 6
ADDED:   F3 to F11 (Work -> DP)    ·
ADDED:   F8 to F9 (SE -> XLOCUS)
ADDED:   F5 to F12 (SSUP->PA; F2 to F9 (ROLEC->XLOCUS); F6 to F10 (PSUP->EE);
         F3 to F12 (WORK->PA); F6 to F11 (PSUP->DP)
ADDED:   F8 to F10 (SE -> EE)
ADDED:   F1 to F11 (ROLEA -> DP)
      ·
      ·
      ·
/EQUATIONS
      ·
      ·
      ·
F8 =   .363*F5 -.114*F6 -.044*F7 + 1.000 D8;
F9 = -.262*F5 + *F8 + *F2 + 1.000 D9;
F10 = -.128*F2 + .745*F3 -.898*F4 + *F6 + *F8 + 1.000 D10;
F11 = .549*F10 + .147*F2 + *F3 + *F6 + *F1 + 1.000 D11;
F12 = .512*F8 -.188*F9 + .019*F10 -.195*F11 -.041*F1 + *F5 + *F3 + 1.000 D12;
      ·
      ·
/LMTEST
SET=GFF, BFF, PDD;
/END
```

TABLE 6.23

Selected EQS Output for Model 6: Goodness-of-Fit Statistics

```
          GOODNESS OF FIT SUMMARY FOR METHOD = ML
CHI-SQUARE =      889.534 BASED ON     417 DEGREES OF FREEDOM
PROBABILITY VALUE FOR THE CHI-SQUARE STATISTIC IS      .00000

FIT INDICES
-----------
BENTLER-BONETT     NORMED FIT INDEX  =        .927
BENTLER-BONETT NON-NORMED FIT INDEX  =        .952
COMPARATIVE FIT INDEX (CFI)          =        .960
ROOT MEAN-SQUARE RESIDUAL (RMR)      =        .032
STANDARDIZED RMR                     =        .040
ROOT MEAN-SQUARE ERROR OF APPROXIMATION (RMSEA)   =      .040
90% CONFIDENCE INTERVAL OF RMSEA   (       .036,      .043)

          GOODNESS OF FIT SUMMARY FOR METHOD = ROBUST
SATORRA-BENTLER SCALED CHI-SQUARE =     802.7997 ON    417 DEGREES OF FREEDOM
PROBABILITY VALUE FOR THE CHI-SQUARE STATISTIC IS      .00000

FIT INDICES
-----------
BENTLER-BONETT     NORMED FIT INDEX  =        .921
BENTLER-BONETT NON-NORMED FIT INDEX  =        .952
COMPARATIVE FIT INDEX (CFI)          =        .960
ROOT MEAN-SQUARE ERROR OF APPROXIMATION (RMSEA)   =      .036
90% CONFIDENCE INTERVAL OF RMSEA   (       .032,      .040)
```

TABLE 6.24

Selected EQS Output for Model 6: Modification Indexes

```
MULTIVARIATE LAGRANGE MULTIPLIER TEST BY SIMULTANEOUS PROCESS IN STAGE 1
  PARAMETER SETS (SUBMATRICES) ACTIVE AT THIS STAGE ARE:
      PDD GFF BFF
```

		CUMULATIVE MULTIVARIATE STATISTICS			UNIVARIATE INCREMENT			HANCOCK'S SEQUENTIAL
STEP	PARAMETER	CHI-SQUARE	D.F.	PROB.	CHI-SQUARE	PROB.	D.F.	PROB.
1	F9,F3	3.870	1	.049	3.870	.049	417	1.000

this very purpose. Essentially, the WTest ascertains whether sets of parameters, specified as free in the model, can in fact be simultaneously set to zero without substantial loss in model fit. It does so by taking the least significant parameter (i.e., the one with the smallest z-statistic) and adding other parameters in such a way that the overall multivariate test yields a set of free parameters that with high probability can simultaneously be dropped from the model in future EQS runs without significant degradation in model fit (Bentler, 2005). In other words, this

TABLE 6.25
Selected EQS Output for Model 6: Structural Path Estimates

CONSTRUCT EQUATIONS WITH STANDARD ERRORS AND TEST STATISTICS
STATISTICS SIGNIFICANT AT THE 5% LEVEL ARE MARKED WITH @.
(ROBUST STATISTICS IN PARENTHESES)

```
SELF  =F8  =        .360*F5    -    .120*F6          -  .047*F7    +    1.000 D8
                    .060            .031                .034
                   5.984@         -3.827@             -1.374
              (    .068)     (    .035)          (    .042)
              (   5.310@     (   -3.405@         (   -1.120)

XLOC  =F9  =       -.269*F8    +    .131*F2    -       .081*F5    +    1.000 D9
                    .057            .037                .039
                  -4.672@          3.553@             -2.076@
              (    .072)     (    .036)          (    .040)
              (   -3.738@    (    3.641@         (   -2.033@

EE    =F10 =       -.828*F8    -   2.118*F2    +      2.223*F3    -     .929*F4
                    .133            .650                .548            .178
                  -6.247@         -3.259@              4.057@         -5.212@
              (    .168)     (    .687)          (    .569)     (     .187)
              (   -4.934@    (   -3.084@         (    3.907@     (    -4.957@

             -     .269*F6    +   1.000 D10
                    .108
                  -2.487@
              (    .126)
              (   -2.132@

DP    =F11 =        .996*F10   -    .452*F1    +      4.213*F2    -    3.548*F3
                    .177            .233               1.493            1.244
                   5.623@         -1.942               2.822@          -2.852@
              (    .194)     (    .241)          (   1.598)     (    1.307)
              (   5.124@     (   -1.874)         (   2.637@     (    -2.715@

             +     .276*F6    +   1.000 D11
                    .210
                   1.313
              (    .236)
              (   1.170)

PA    =F12 =        .465*F8    -    .174*F9    -       .017*F10   -     .159*F11
                    .102            .075                .049            .035
                   4.541@         -2.317@             -.345          -4.523@
              (    .132)     (    .074)          (    .051)     (     .041)
              (   3.521@     (   -2.360@         (   -.334)      (    -3.893@

             +     .043*F1    +    .165*F3    +       .268*F5    +    1.000 D12
                    .103            .064                .072
                    .411           2.596@              3.708@
              (    .118)     (    .067)          (    .078)
              (    .362)     (   2.476@          (   3.419@
```

TABLE 6.26

Selected EQS Output for Model 6: Wald Test Results

```
WALD TEST (FOR DROPPING PARAMETERS)
ROBUST INFORMATION MATRIX USED IN THIS WALD TEST
MULTIVARIATE WALD TEST BY SIMULTANEOUS PROCESS
```

		CUMULATIVE MULTIVARIATE STATISTICS			UNIVARIATE INCREMENT	
STEP	PARAMETER	CHI-SQUARE	D.F.	PROBABILITY	CHI-SQUARE	PROBABILITY
1	F12,F10	.111	1	.739	.111	.739
2	F12,F1	.186	2	.911	.074	.785
3	F11,F6	1.511	3	.680	1.325	.250
4	F8,F7	2.895	4	.576	1.385	.239
5	F11,F1	6.048	5	.302	3.152	.076

multivariate WTest operates in a stepwise manner that is analogous to stepwise backward regression. In contrast, the stepping procedure for the LM Test is forward. The value of this stepwise implementation in EQS is that it may determine that only a few parameters actually carry all the weight in the multivariate test (Bentler, 2005). Implementation of the WTest is simple and involves only the typing of a separate line, as follows: /WTEST. Essentially, this specification replaces the /LMTEST specification.

To test multivariately for redundant structural paths in the model, the /WTEST paragraph was added to the EQS input for Model 6 and the model was reestimated; for this run also, there was no specification of LM Test statistics. Results from this invocation of the WTest are presented in Table 6.26.

Interestingly, the WTest identified the same five parameters noted in Table 6.25 as being redundant to the model. Of the five nonsignificant parameters, three represent structural paths present in the originally hypothesized model (F7 ->F8; F10 ->F12; F1 ->F12) and two represent paths added during the post hoc model-fitting stage (F1 ->F11; F6 ->F11).

Revision of the model in accordance with these results led to deletion of structural paths describing the impact of: Role Ambiguity on Personal Accomplishment, Role Ambiguity on Depersonalization, Superior Support on Depersonalization, Peer Support on Self-esteem, and Emotional Exhaustion on Personal Accomplishment. These deletions resulted in the Role Ambiguity and Peer Support constructs being totally eliminated from the causal model. To obtain fit statistics and estimates for this final model of burnout for secondary school teachers, Model 6 was respecified with these five parameters deleted and labeled Model 7, which was then estimated. Goodness-of-fit statistics related to this final model of burnout are presented in Table 6.27.

Of import in reviewing these statistics is the fact that both the *CFI and the *RMSEA values remained unchanged (.960 and .036, respectively) from those for Model 6 in which these five structural paths were estimated. Although there was a

TABLE 6.27

Selected EQS Output for Final Model: Goodness-of-Fit Statistics

GOODNESS OF FIT SUMMARY FOR METHOD = ML

```
CHI-SQUARE =         901.634 BASED ON        422 DEGREES OF FREEDOM
PROBABILITY VALUE FOR THE CHI-SQUARE STATISTIC IS          .00000

FIT INDICES
-----------
BENTLER-BONETT     NORMED FIT INDEX =       .926
BENTLER-BONETT NON-NORMED FIT INDEX =       .952
COMPARATIVE FIT INDEX (CFI)         =       .959
ROOT MEAN-SQUARE RESIDUAL (RMR)     =       .032
STANDARDIZED RMR                    =       .040
ROOT MEAN-SQUARE ERROR OF APPROXIMATION (RMSEA)    =        .040
90% CONFIDENCE INTERVAL OF RMSEA   (        .036,         .043)
```

GOODNESS OF FIT SUMMARY FOR METHOD = ROBUST

```
SATORRA-BENTLER SCALED CHI-SQUARE =       812.6905 ON        422 DEGREES OF FREEDOM
PROBABILITY VALUE FOR THE CHI-SQUARE STATISTIC IS          .00000

FIT INDICES
-----------
BENTLER-BONETT     NORMED FIT INDEX =       .920
BENTLER-BONETT NON-NORMED FIT INDEX =       .952
COMPARATIVE FIT INDEX (CFI)         =       .960
ROOT MEAN-SQUARE ERROR OF APPROXIMATION (RMSEA)    =        .036
90% CONFIDENCE INTERVAL OF RMSEA   (        .032,         .040)
```

slight increase in the overall χ^2 statistic value from Model 6 (S-Bχ^2 = 802.80) to the Final Model (S-Bχ^2 = 812.69), such degradation is expected with the removal of five parameters from the model. Of substantial importance, however, is whether this S-Bχ^2 difference value is statistically nonsignificant, which it should be.

When analyses are based on the usual ML estimation with no correction for non-normality, a comparison of nested models[5] is simply a matter of computing the difference between the χ^2 values and related degrees of freedom for the two models. This difference value ($\Delta\chi^2$) is distributed as χ^2, with degrees of freedom equal to the difference in degrees of freedom (Δdf). However, when analyses are based on Robust (i.e., corrected) ML estimation, it is not possible to perform this straightforward computation of the difference test because the ΔS-Bχ^2 value is not χ^2-distributed. However, Satorra and Bentler (2001) have shown how the ΔS-Bχ^2 value can be corrected and therefore used in the same way as the $\Delta\chi^2$ to judge for statistical significance. Readers are now walked through the computations involved in making this correction to the ΔS-Bχ^2 value.

The nested models of interest here are Models 6 and 7, the final model in which five structural paths were deleted. In this instance, Model 7 is considered the

---

[5]Nested models are hierarchically related to one another in the sense that their parameter sets are subsets of one another. That is, particular parameters are freely estimated in one model but fixed to zero in a second model (Bentler & Chou, 1987; and Bollen, 1989a).

more restrictive model because it has fewer parameters to be estimated than does Model 6. Based on statistical convention, Model 6 represents the more general model and is given the label M_1; Model 7 is the more restrictive model and is labeled M_0. Steps in the computation process are as follows:

1. (Model 7) $k_0 = T_0/\overline{T}_0$, where $T_0 = \text{ML}\chi^2$ and $\overline{T}_0 = \text{S-B}\chi^2$

$$= \frac{901.634}{812.6905} = 1.109$$

2. (Model 6) $k_1 = T_1/\overline{T}_1$, where $T_1 = \text{ML}\chi^2$ and $\overline{T}_1 = \text{S-B}\chi^2$

$$= \frac{889.534}{802.7997} = 1.108$$

3. Compute from model comparisons:
   (a) usual difference test $(\Delta\chi^2; D) = T_0 - T_1$
   $$= 901.634 - 889.534 = 12.10$$
   (b) S-B scaling coefficient, with $d = d_0 - d_1$, where d = degrees of freedom and $k = (d_0k_0 - d_1k_1)/d$

   $$d = 422 - 417 = 5$$
   $$k = \frac{(422)(1.109) - (417)(1.108)}{5} = \frac{5.962}{5} = 1.1924$$

4. Compute $\Delta\text{S-B}\chi^2$ value

$$\overline{D} = D/k = \frac{12.10}{1.1924} = 10.148$$

As shown in these computations, the $\Delta\text{S-B}\chi^2$ value between Model 6 and the final model of burnout (Model 7) was nonsignificant. These findings, therefore, argue for the redundancy of the five deleted structural paths. Table 6.28 presents both the unstandardized and standardized estimates for all remaining structural paths in the final model of burnout for secondary school teachers; Fig. 6.10 is a schematic representation, in which solid lines represent the originally hypothesized paths and dotted lines represented the paths subsequently added as a result of post hoc model-fitting.

In summary, of 14 causal paths specified in the hypothesized model (see Fig. 6.4), 11 were found to be statistically significant for secondary school teachers. These paths reflected the impact of (a) role conflict, classroom climate, and work overload on emotional exhaustion; (b) decision-making on both self-esteem and external locus of control; (c) self-esteem, depersonalization, and external locus of control on perceived personal accomplishment; (d) role conflict and emotional exhaustion on depersonalisation; and (e) superior support on self-esteem. Seven paths, not specified a priori (Work Overload → Depersonalization; Work Overload → Personal Accomplishment; Role Conflict → External Locus of Control; Decision-making → Personal Accomplishment; Superior Support → Emotional

TABLE 6.28

Selected EQS Output for Final Model: Structural Path Coefficients

Unstandardized Solution

CONSTRUCT EQUATIONS WITH STANDARD ERRORS AND TEST STATISTICS
STATISTICS SIGNIFICANT AT THE 5% LEVEL ARE MARKED WITH @.
(ROBUST STATISTICS IN PARENTHESES)

```
SELF  =F8  =        .305*F5     -     .105*F6     +    1.000 D8
                    .040              .027
                    7.705@           -3.875@
               (    .043)       (     .030)
               (    7.116@      (    -3.441@


XLOC  =F9  =       -.268*F8     +     .129*F2     -     .084*F5    +   1.000 D9
                    .057              .036              .039
                   -4.690@            3.529@           -2.150@
               (    .072)       (     .036)       (     .040)
               (   -3.753@      (     3.621@      (    -2.078@


EE    =F10 =       -.801*F8     -    1.918*F2     +    2.137*F3    -   1.146*F4
                    .123              .562              .500             .212
                   -6.517@           -3.414@            4.275@          -5.405@
               (    .154)       (     .569)       (     .503)      (     .233)
               (   -5.202@      (    -3.370@      (     4.248@      (    -4.917@

                -   .120*F6     +    1.000 D10
                    .043
                   -2.796@
               (    .048)
               (   -2.518@


DP    =F11 =        .898*F10    +    2.552*F2     -    2.442*F3    +   1.000 D11
                    .127              .651              .634
                    7.067@            3.919@           -3.850@
               (    .140)       (     .670)       (     .648)
               (    6.411@      (     3.808@      (    -3.771@


PA    =F12 =        .467*F8     -     .166**F9    -     .166**F11  +    .175*F3
                    .094              .075              .031             .047
                    4.960@           -2.224@           -5.385@           3.718@
               (    .120)       (     .073)       (     .036)      (     .051)
               (    3.891@      (    -2.267@      (    -4.591@      (     3.457@

                +   .261*F5     +    1.000 D12
                    .059
                    4.428@
               (    .063)
               (    4.109@
```

Standardized Solution

```
SELF = F8  = .710*F5  -  .346*F6 +  .882 D8
XLOC = F9  = -.216*F8 +  .263*F2 -  .157*F5 + .852 D9
EE   = F10 = -.256*F8 - 1.564*F2 + 1.959*F3 - .352*F4 - .127*F6 + .544 D10
DP   = F11 = .893*F10 + 2.067*F2 - 2.224*F3 + .594 D11
PA   = F12 = .245*F8  -  .108*F9 -  .274*F11 +  .263*F3 + .318*F5 + .817 D12
```

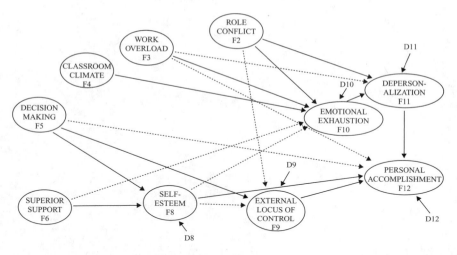

FIG. 6.10. Final model of teacher burnout. Solid lines represent originally hypothesized structural paths; broken lines represent structural paths added to the originally hypothesized model. *Note*: For simplicity, the measurement model is not included.

Exhaustion; Self-esteem → Emotional Exhaustion; Self-esteem → External Locus of Control), proved to be essential components of the causal structure; therefore, they were added to the model. Finally, three originally hypothesized paths (Role Ambiguity → Personal Accomplishment; Peer Support → Self-esteem; Emotional Exhaustion → Personal Accomplishment) were found to be not statistically significant and were therefore deleted from the model.

Overall, the conclusion from this study is that role conflict, work overload, classroom climate, participation in the decision-making process, and support of superiors are potent organizational determinants of burnout for high school teachers. The process appears to be tempered, however, by a general sense of self-worth and locus of control.

III

Multiple-Group Analyses

7

Application 5: Testing for the Factorial Invariance of a Measuring Instrument (First-Order CFA Model)

So far, previous applications have illustrated analyses based on single samples. In Part III, however, we focus on applications involving more than one sample in which the central concern is whether components of the measurement model and/or the structural model are invariant (i.e., equivalent) across particular groups.

In seeking evidence of multigroup invariance, researchers are typically interested in finding the answer to one of five questions. First, do the items composing a particular measuring instrument operate equivalently across different populations (e.g., gender, age, ability, culture)? In other words, is the measurement model group-invariant? Second, is the factorial structure of a single instrument or theoretical construct equivalent across populations as measured either by items of a single assessment measure or by subscale scores from multiple instruments? Typically, this approach exemplifies a construct-validity focus. In such instances, invariance of both the measurement and structural models is of interest. Third, are certain paths in a specified causal structure invariant across populations? Fourth, are the latent means of particular constructs in a model different across populations? *Finally*, does the factorial structure of a measuring instrument replicate across independent samples drawn from the same population? This last question, of course, addresses the issue of cross-validation.

Applications presented in this and the next three chapters provide specific examples of how each question can be answered using SEM based on EQS. The applications illustrated in chapters 7 and 8 are based on the analysis of covariance structures, whereas those in chapters 9 and 10 are based on the analysis of means and covariance structures; commonly used acronyms are the analyses of COVS and MACS, respectively. When analyses are based on COVS, only the variances and covariances of the observed variables are of interest; all single-group applications illustrated thus far have been based on the analysis of COVS. However, when analyses are based on MACS, the modeled data include both sample means and covariances. Details related to the MACS approach to invariance are addressed in chapter 9.

In the first multigroup application, hypotheses related to the invariance of a single measuring instrument are tested across two different panels of school teachers. Specifically, we test for equivalency of the factorial measurement (i.e., scale items) of the Maslach Burnout Inventory (MBI; Maslach & Jackson, 1986) and its underlying latent structure (i.e., relations among dimensions of burnout) across elementary and secondary school teachers. Purposes of the original study, from which this example is taken (Byrne, 1993), were (a) to test for the factorial validity of the MBI separately for each of three teacher groups;[1] (b) given findings of inadequate fit, to propose and test an alternative factorial structure; (c) to cross-validate this structure over independent samples within each teacher group; and (d) to test for the equivalence of item measurements and theoretical structure across the three teaching panels. Only analyses bearing on tests for invariance across calibration samples of elementary ($N = 580$) and secondary ($N = 692$) school teachers are central to this chapter. Before reviewing the model under scrutiny, however, an overview is provided of the general procedure involved in tests for invariance (or equivalence) across groups.

TESTING FOR MULTIGROUP INVARIANCE

Development of a procedure capable of testing for multigroup invariance derives from the seminal work of Jöreskog (1971b). Accordingly, Jöreskog recommended that all tests of invariance begin with a global test of the equality of covariance structures across the groups of interest. Expressed more formally, this initial step tests the null hypothesis (H_0), $\Sigma_1 = \Sigma_2 = \ldots \Sigma_G$, where Σ is the population variance–covariance matrix and G is the number of groups. Rejection of the null hypothesis argues for the nonequivalence of the groups and thus for the subsequent testing of increasingly restrictive hypotheses to identify the source of noninvariance. Conversely, if H_0 cannot be rejected, the groups are considered to have equivalent covariance structures and thus tests for invariance are not needed. Presented with such findings, Jöreskog recommended that group data be pooled and all subsequent investigative work be based on single-group analyses.

---

[1] Middle-school teachers composed the third group.

Although this omnibus test appears reasonable and fairly straightforward, it often leads to contradictory findings with respect to equivalencies across groups. For example, sometimes the null hypothesis is found to be tenable, yet subsequent tests of hypotheses related to the invariance of particular measurement or structural parameters must be rejected (see, e.g., Jöreskog, 1971b). Alternatively, the global null hypothesis may be rejected, yet tests for the invariance of measurement and structural invariance hold (see, e.g., Byrne, 1988a). Such inconsistencies in the global test for invariance stem from the fact that there is no baseline model for the test of invariant variance–covariance matrices, thereby making it substantially more restrictive than is the case for tests of invariance related to sets of model parameters. Indeed, any number of inequalities may possibly exist across the groups under study. Realistically then, testing for the equality of specific sets of model parameters appears to be the more informative and interesting approach to multigroup invariance.

In testing for equivalencies across groups, sets of parameters are put to the test in a logically ordered and increasingly restrictive fashion. Depending on the model and hypotheses to be tested, the following sets of parameters are most commonly of interest in answering questions related to multigroup invariance: (a) factor-loading paths, (b) factor covariances, and (c) structural regression paths. Historically, the Jöreskog tradition of invariance testing holds that the equality of these error variances and their covariances should also be tested. However, it is now widely accepted that to do so represents an overly restrictive test of the data. Indeed, Bentler (2005) contends that testing for the equality of error variances and covariances is probably of least interest and importance. Nonetheless, there may be particular instances where findings bearing on the equivalence or nonequivalence of these parameters can provide important information (e.g., scale items).

The Testing Strategy

Testing for factorial invariance encompasses a series of hierarchical steps that begin with the separate determination of a baseline model for each group. This model represents the one that best fits the data from the perspectives of both parsimony and substantive meaning. Addressing the somewhat tricky combination of model fit and model parsimony, it ideally represents one for which fit to the data and minimal parameter specification are optimal. Following completion of this preliminary task, tests for the equivalence of parameters are conducted across groups at each of several increasingly stringent levels. Jöreskog (1971b) argues that these tests should most appropriately begin with scrutiny of the measurement model. In particular, the pattern of factor loadings for each observed measure is tested for its equivalence across the groups. Once it is known which measures are group-invariant, these parameters are constrained equal while subsequent tests of the structural parameters are conducted. As each new set of parameters is tested, those known to be group-invariant are cumulatively constrained equal. Thus, the process of determining nonequivalence of measurement and structural parameters across groups involves the testing of a series of increasingly restrictive hypotheses.

TESTING FOR INVARIANCE ACROSS INDEPENDENT SAMPLES

The Hypothesized Model

The focus here is to test for the equivalence of the MBI across elementary and secondary school teachers. Details regarding the structure of this measuring instrument are discussed in chapter 4; thus, they will not be repeated here. Of key importance in testing for the invariance of the MBI across these two selected groups of teachers is its determined baseline model structure for each group, not the extent to which the instrument may have been validated for other populations. Once these models are established, they (if two different baseline models are ascertained) represent the hypothesized model under test.

Establishing Baseline Models

Because the estimation of baseline models involves no between-group constraints, the data can be analyzed separately for each group. However, in testing for invariance, equality constraints are imposed on particular parameters; therefore, the data for all groups must be analyzed simultaneously to obtain efficient estimates (Bentler, 2005; and Jöreskog & Sörbom, 1996). The pattern of fixed and free parameters nonetheless remains consistent with the baseline model specification for each group. However, measuring instruments are often group-specific in the way they operate; thus, it is possible that baseline models may not be completely identical across groups (Bentler, 2005; and Byrne, Shavelson, & Muthén, 1989). For example, it may be that the best-fitting model for one group includes an error covariance (see, e.g., Bentler, 2005) or a cross-loading[2] (see, e.g., Byrne, 1988b; and Reise, Widaman, & Pugh, 1993), whereas these parameters may not be specified for the other group. Presented with such findings, Byrne et al. (1989) showed that by implementing a condition of partial measurement invariance, multigroup analyses can still continue. As such, some but not all measurement parameters are constrained equal across groups in the testing for structural invariance or latent factor mean differences. A priori knowledge of such group differences, as illustrated in this chapter, is critical to the application of invariance-testing procedures.

---

[2]This is the loading of an observed variable on a factor other than the one on which it was designed to load (i.e., its targeted factor).

In testing for the validity of the three-factor structure of the MBI (see Fig. 4.1), findings were consistent in revealing goodness-of-fit statistics for this initial model that were less than optimal for both elementary teachers (S-B$\chi^2_{(206)}$ = 804.084; SRMR = .071; *CFI = .855; *RMSEA = .071; 90% C.I. .066, .076) and secondary teachers (S-B$\chi^2_{(206)}$ = 996.069; SRMR = .080; *CFI = .833; *RMSEA = .075; 90% C.I. .070, .079). Three exceptionally large error covariances and one cross-loading contributed identically to the misfit of the model for both teacher panels. The error covariances involved Items 1 and 2, Items 6 and 16, and Items 10 and 11; the cross-loading involved the loading of Item 12 on Factor 1 (Emotional Exhaustion) in addition to its targeted Factor 3 (Personal Accomplishment). Indeed, these findings replicate those reported in chapter 4 for male elementary school teachers. (For a discussion related to possible reasons for these misfitting parameters, see chap. 4.) To review the extent to which these four parameters erode fit of the originally hypothesized model to data for elementary and secondary school teachers we turn to Table 7.1, which is an abbreviated list of results from the LM Test that include the Ordered Univariate Test Statistics and the χ^2 Univariate Increments associated with the Cumulative Multivariate Statistics.

Review of both the parameter change statistics and the univariate increments of the multivariate statistics for elementary school teachers, clearly shows that all four parameters are contributing substantially to model misfit. The error covariance between Item 6 and Item 16 exhibit the most profound effect. The content of both items, focuses on the extent to which working with people all day is stressful.[3] These results, as they relate to secondary school teachers, exhibit precisely the same pattern, albeit the effect appears, to be even more pronounced than it was for elementary school teachers. However, there is one slight difference between the two groups of teachers regarding the impact of the four parameters on model misfit: Whereas the error covariance between Items 6 and 16 was found to be the most seriously misfitting parameter for elementary school teachers, the error covariance between Items 1 and 2 held this dubious honor for secondary school teachers. These items both focus on the extent to which teachers feel emotionally drained or used up from their work at the end of the day.

Given that both the cross-loading of Item 12 on Factor 1 and the error covariances can be substantively justified (for an elaboration, see chap. 4), they were subsequently specified as free parameters in the model for each teacher group and then the models were reestimated. Results from these analyses for both groups yielded model-fit statistics that were substantially and significantly improved

---

[3] Unfortunately I am unable to present the actual item context here as the publisher of the MBI refused copyright permission to do so. As a result, I am able only to describe the context of these and other items exhibiting poor loadings (Items 11, 9, 19).

TABLE 7.1
Selected EQS Output for Initally Hypothesized Model: Modification Indexes

Elementary Teachers

LAGRANGE MULTIPLIER TEST (FOR ADDING PARAMETERS)
ORDERED UNIVARIATE TEST STATISTICS:

NO	CODE	PARAMETER	CHI-SQUARE	PROB.	HANCOCK 206 DF PROB.	PARAMETER CHANGE	STANDAR-DIZED CHANGE
1	2 6	E16,E6	180.006	.000	.904	.895	.595
2	2 6	E2,E1	102.999	.000	1.000	.535	.494
3	2 12	V12,F1	81.163	.000	1.000	-.400	-.241
4	2 6	E11,E10	67.616	.000	1.000	.687	.828

	CUMULATIVE MULTIVARIATE STATISTICS				UNIVARIATE INCREMENT		HANCOCK'S SEQUENTIAL	
STEP	PARAMETER	CHI-SQUARE	D.F.	PROB.	CHI-SQUARE	PROB.	D.F.	PROB.
1	E16,E6	180.006	1	.000	180.006	.000	206	.904
2	E2,E1	277.423	2	.000	97.416	.000	205	1.000
3	V12,F1	358.585	3	.000	81.163	.000	204	1.000
4	E11,E10	426.201	4	.000	67.616	.000	203	1.000
5	E7,E4	466.869	5	.000	40.668	.000	202	1.000
6	E19,E18	501.328	6	.000	34.459	.000	201	1.000
7	V16,F2	533.006	7	.000	31.678	.000	200	1.000
8	V14,F3	556.432	8	.000	23.426	.000	199	1.000

Secondary Teachers

LAGRANGE MULTIPLIER TEST (FOR ADDING PARAMETERS)
ORDERED UNIVARIATE TEST STATISTICS:

NO	CODE	PARAMETER	CHI-SQUARE	PROB.	HANCOCK 206 DF PROB.	PARAMETER CHANGE	STANDAR-DIZED CHANGE
1	2 6	E2,E1	167.986	.000	.976	.618	.577
2	2 6	E11,E10	142.389	.000	1.000	1.219	1.509
3	2 6	E16,E6	130.671	.000	1.000	.692	.464
4	2 12	V12,F1	118.034	.000	1.000	-.467	-.291

	CUMULATIVE MULTIVARIATE STATISTICS				UNIVARIATE INCREMENT		HANCOCK'S SEQUENTIAL	
STEP	PARAMETER	CHI-SQUARE	D.F.	PROB.	CHI-SQUARE	PROB.	D.F.	PROB.
1	E2,E1	167.986	1	.000	167.986	.000	206	.976
2	E11,E10	310.374	2	.000	142.389	.000	205	1.000
3	E16,E6	435.076	3	.000	124.702	.000	204	1.000
4	V12,F1	553.110	4	.000	118.034	.000	203	1.000
5	V11,F1	609.593	5	.000	56.483	.000	202	1.000
6	E19,E9	652.274	6	.000	42.681	.000	201	1.000
7	E20,E2	685.208	7	.000	32.934	.000	200	1.000
8	V16,F2	715.198	8	.000	29.990	.000	199	1.000

from those for the initially hypothesized model (i.e., elementary: corrected ΔS-$B\chi^2_{(4)} = 197.159$; secondary: corrected ΔS-$B\chi^2_{(4)} = 268.560$). Additionally, all newly specified parameters were statistically significant. Model goodness-of-fit statistics were as follows.[4]

Elementary School Teachers: S-$B\chi^2_{(202)} = 471.180$; SRMR = .053; *CFI = .935; *RMSEA = .048, 90% C.I. .042, .054

Secondary School Teachers: S-$B\chi^2_{(202)} = 587.190$; SRMR = .059; *CFI = .918; *RMSEA = .053, 90% C.I. .048, .057

Let's turn now to Table 7.2 where an abbreviated list of the LM Test statistics associated with this modified model (Model 2) is presented. Review of these results for elementary school teachers shows that the two highest incremental χ^2 values represent error covariances (i.e., E7,E4 and E19,E18). Although, admittedly, the third parameter in this list represents a cross-loading that exhibits a fairly substantial parameter change value (i.e., .864), I consider it best to leave this model in place as the baseline model for this group. I make this decision based on the fact that (a) the model represents a fairly well-fitting model, and (b) the addition of more error covariances that are not distinctively different from one another runs counter to the criterion of parsimony.

In reviewing the results for secondary school teachers, however, there is more work to do in establishing an appropriate baseline model. This decision is based on two factors: (a) the model does not yet reflect a satisfactorily good fit to the data, and (b) in reviewing the multivariate LM Test statistics, there are perhaps two additional parameters (i.e., V11,F1 and E19,E9) that require scrutiny, as evidenced by both the large $\chi2$ values and the substantial drop between these values (71.235 and 48.570) and those for the remaining three parameters shown here (34.638, 29.330, and 26.730). The cross-loading of Item 11 (which expresses the concern that the job is hardening the teacher emotionally) onto Factor 1 (Emotional Exhaustion) appears to be reasonable. Likewise, a covariance between the error terms associated with Item 9 and Item 19 is meaningful in the sense that it reflects some degree of overlap in content. Item 19 measures the extent to which respondents believe they have accomplished many worthwhile things in the job; likewise, Item 9 measures the extent to which they believe they are positively influencing other peoples lives through their work. Consequently, both parameters were freely estimated and this new model (Model 3) was reestimated.[5] Results from the estimation of Model 3, for secondary school teachers, yielded goodness-of-fit statistics that represented a

---

[4]The decrease in the number of degrees of freedom from 206 to 202 represents the estimation of four additional parameters in the model, thereby using up 4 degrees of freedom.

[5]As a cautionary measure in adding these parameters to the model, each parameter was originally respecified separately (i.e., two separate models). Provided with no aberrant differences in the results, I therefore suggest the inclusion of both parameters in this newly specified model.

TABLE 7.2
Selected EQS Output for Model 2: Modification Indexes

Elementary Teachers

LAGRANGE MULTIPLIER TEST (FOR ADDING PARAMETERS)

ORDERED UNIVARIATE TEST STATISTICS:

NO	CODE		PARAMETER	CHI-SQUARE	PROB.	HANCOCK 206 DF PROB.	PARAMETER CHANGE	STANDAR-DIZED CHANGE
--	------		---------	------	-----	--------	---------	--------

ORDERED UNIVARIATE TEST STATISTICS:

NO	CODE		PARAMETER	CHI-SQUARE	PROB.	HANCOCK 206 DF PROB.	PARAMETER CHANGE	STANDAR-DIZED CHANGE
1	2	6	E7,E4	38.867	.000	1.000	.174	.284
2	2	6	E19,E18	38.659	.000	1.000	.267	.333
3	2	12	V14,F3	24.387	.000	1.000	.864	1.095
4	2	6	E12,E3	23.940	.000	1.000	-.251	-.227
5	2	6	E13,E12	20.444	.000	1.000	.231	.211

	CUMULATIVE MULTIVARIATE STATISTICS				UNIVARIATE INCREMENT			
					CHI-		HANCOCK'S SEQUENTIAL	
STEP	PARAMETER	CHI-SQUARE	D.F.	PROB.	SQUARE	PROB.	D.F.	PROB.
----	---------	----------	----	-----	------	-----	----	-----
1	E7,E4	38.867	1	.000	38.867	.000	202	1.000
2	E19,E18	73.644	2	.000	34.777	.000	201	1.000
3	V14,F3	98.031	3	.000	24.387	.000	200	1.000
4	E12,E3	121.544	4	.000	23.513	.000	199	1.000
5	E13,E12	136.775	5	.000	15.230	.000	198	1.000

Secondary Teachers

LAGRANGE MULTIPLIER TEST (FOR ADDING PARAMETERS)

ORDERED UNIVARIATE TEST STATISTICS:

NO	CODE		PARAMETER	CHI-SQUARE	PROB.	HANCOCK 206 DF PROB.	PARAMETER CHANGE	STANDAR-DIZED CHANGE
--	------		---------	------	-----	------	---------	------
1	2	12	V11,F1	71.235	.000	1.000	.470	.266
2	2	6	E19,E9	48.570	.000	1.000	.371	.380
3	2	6	E15,E11	38.034	.000	1.000	-.333	-.234
4	2	6	E15,E5	36.869	.000	1.000	.423	.323
5	2	6	E20,E16	29.335	.000	1.000	.229	.202

	CUMULATIVE MULTIVARIATE STATISTICS				UNIVARIATE INCREMENT			
					CHI-		HANCOCK'S SEQUENTIAL	
STEP	PARAMETER	CHI-SQUARE	D.F.	PROB.	SQUARE	PROB.	D.F.	PROB.
----	---------	----------	----	-----	------	-----	----	----
1	V11,F1	71.235	1	.000	71.235	.000	202	1.000
2	E19,E9	119.806	2	.000	48.570	.000	201	1.000
3	E18,E7	154.443	3	.000	34.638	.000	200	1.000
4	E20,E16	183.773	4	.000	29.330	.000	199	1.000
5	E15,E5	210.503	5	.000	26.730	.000	198	1.000

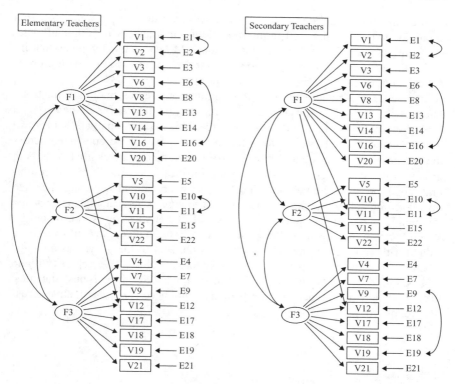

FIG. 7.1. Hypothesized multigroup model of factorial structure of the Maslach Burnout Inventory (Maslach & Jackson, 1986.

satisfactorily good fit to the data (S-B$\chi^2_{(200)}$ = 500.332; SRMR = .054; *CFI = .936; *RMSEA = .047, 90% C.I. .042, .052). This final model is determined to be the baseline model for secondary school teachers.

With these baseline models established, we are now ready to test hypotheses bearing on the equivalence of the MBI across elementary and secondary school teachers. The baseline models are shown in Fig. 7.1, which provides the foundation against which the series of increasingly stringent hypotheses related to MBI structure are tested.

Testing for Configural Invariance

This initial step in testing for invariance requires only that the same number of factors and factor-loading pattern be the same across groups. As such, no equality constraints are imposed on the parameters. That is, the same parameters estimated in the baseline model for each group separately are again estimated in this multigroup model. Goodness-of-fit related to this multigroup parameterization should be indicative of a well-fitting model. Of importance here is that although the factor structure is similar, it is not identical. More specifically, given that invariant latent factors have not been identified in the two groups, group differences on any parameters in the model cannot be tested.

In essence, the model being tested is a multigroup representation of the baseline models. Accordingly, it incorporates the baseline models for elementary and secondary school teachers within the same file. This multigroup model serves two important functions: First, it allows for invariance tests to be conducted across the two groups simultaneously. In other words, parameters are estimated for both groups at the same time. Second, in testing for invariance, the fit of this configural model provides the baseline value against which all subsequently specified invariance models are compared. In contrast to single-group analyses, however, this multigroup analysis yields only one set of fit statistics for overall model fit. When ML estimation is used, the χ^2 statistics are summative; thus, the overall χ^2 value for the multigroup model should equal the sum of the χ^2 values obtained when the baseline model is tested separately for each group of teachers (with no cross-group constraints imposed). If estimation is based on the robust statistics, the S-Bχ^2 statistic for each group separately is not necessarily summative across the groups.

The EQS Input File

To fully comprehend the specification of parameters representing the configural model, we turn Table 7.3 where the related multigroup input file is presented. In reviewing this file, you will see that it actually contains two sets of model parameters: The first part of the file specifies the model for elementary school teachers, whereas the second part specifies the model for secondary school teachers. Closer examination of each baseline model reveals the post hoc addition of parameters for each teacher group. Thus, for Group 1 (Elementary Teachers), note the cross-loading of V12 onto F1 in addition to the three error covariances (E2,E1; E16,E6; and E11,E10). For Group 2 (Secondary Teachers), there are the same four specifications but in addition, the cross-loading of V11 onto F1 and the error covariance between Items 19 and 9 (E19,E9). Basically, this initial multigroup file simply represents the input file for one group stacked on top of the input file for the other; however, there is one very critical piece of information that must be added to the /SPECIFICATION paragraph for the first group: the statement "GROUPS = 2;". This command tells the program how many groups are involved in the analysis. By default, if this information is not specified, the program assumes there is only one group and all action ceases when the analyses for Group 1 are completed.

TABLE 7.3

EQS Input File for Test for Invariance of MBI: The Configural Model

---

/TITLE

TESTING FOR INVARIANCE OF THE MBI FOR ELEMENTARY/SECONDARY TEACHERS "MBIINVelhs1"
GROUP 1: ELEMENTARY TEACHERS

/SPECIFICATIONS

DATA= ' C:\EQS61\files\books\data\mbielm1.ess ' ;
VARIABLES= 22; CASES= 580; GROUPS = 2;
METHODS=ML,ROBUST; MATRIX=RAW; FO= ' (22F1.0) ' ;

/LABELS

V1=MBI1; V2=MBI2; V3=MBI3; V4=MBI4; V5=MBI5; V6=MBI6; V7=MBI7; V8=MBI8;
V9=MBI9; V10=MBI10; V11=MBI11; V12=MBI12; V13=MBI13; V14=MBI14;
V15=MBI15; V16=MBI16; V17=MBI17; V18=MBI18; V19=MBI19; V20=MBI20;
V21=MBI21; V22=MBI22;
F1=EE;   F2=DP;   F3=PA;

/EQUATION

V1 = F1 + E1;
V2 = *F1 + E2;
V3 = *F1 + E3;
V6 = *F1 + E6;
V8 = *F1 + E8;
V13 = *F1 + E13;
V14 = *F1 + E14;
V16 = *F1 + E16;
V20 = *F1 + E20;
V5 = F2 + E5;
V10 = *F2 + E10;
V11 = *F2 + E11;
V15 = *F2 + E15;
V22 = *F2 + E22;
V4 = F3 + E4;
V7 = *F3 + E7;
V9 = *F3 + E9;
V12 = *F3 + *F1 + E12;
V17 = *F3 + E17;
V18 = *F3 + E18;
V19 = *F3 + E19;
V21 = *F3 + E21;

/VARIANCES

F1 to F3 = *;
E1 to E22 = *;

/COVARIANCES

F1 to F3 = *;
E2,E1 = *; E16,E6 = *; E11,E10 = *;

/PRINT

Fit = All;

/END

(Continued)

TABLE 7.3

(Continued)

/TITLE
TESTING FOR INVARIANCE OF THE MBI FOR ELEMENTARY/SECONDARY TEACHERS "MBIINVelhs1"
GROUP 2: SECONDARY TEACHERS
/SPECIFICATIONS
DATA=' C:\EQS61\files\books\data\mbisec1.ess ' ;
VARIABLES= 22; CASES= 692; DEL= 115;
METHODS=ML,ROBUST; MATRIX=RAW; FO=' (22F1.0)' ;
/LABELS
V1=MBI1; V2=MBI2; V3=MBI3; V4=MBI4; V5=MBI5; V6=MBI6; V7=MBI7; V8=MBI8;
V9=MBI9; V10=MBI10; V11=MBI11; V12=MBI12; V13=MBI13; V14=MBI14;
V15=MBI15; V16=MBI16; V17=MBI17; V18=MBI18; V19=MBI19; V20=MBI20;
V21=MBI21; V22=MBI22;
F1=EE;　F2=DP;　　F3=PA;
/EQUATION
　V1 = F1 + E1;
　V2 = *F1 + E2;
　V3 = *F1 + E3;
　V6 = *F1 + E6;
　V8 = *F1 + E8;
　V13 = *F1 + E13;
　V14 = *F1 + E14;
　V16 = *F1 + E16;
　V20 = *F1 + E20;
　V5 = F2 + E5;
　V10 = *F2 + E10;
　V11 = *F2 + *F1 + E11;
　V15 = *F2 + E15;
　V22 = *F2 + E22;
　V4 = F3 + E4;
　V7 = *F3 + E7;
　V9 = *F3 + E9;
　V12 = *F3 + *F1 + E12;
　V17 = *F3 + E17;
　V18 = *F3 + E18;
　V19 = *F3 + E19;
　V21 = *F3 + E21;
/VARIANCES
F1 to F3 = *;
E1 to E22 = *;
/COVARIANCES
F1 to F3 = *;
E2,E1 = *; E16,E6 = *; E11,E10 = *;
E19,E9 = *;
/PRINT
Fit = All;
/END

The EQS Output File

Results yielded from the testing of this configural model are shown in Table 7.4. As expected, goodness-of-fit statistics related to this model reveal a well-fitting multigroup model, with the S-B$\chi^2_{(402)}$ value of 971.991 closely (but not exactly) representing the sum of these values when the two baseline models were analyzed separately (i.e., Elementary: S-B$\chi^2_{(202)} = 471.180$; Secondary: S-B$\chi^2_{(200)} = 500.332$). Overall, the goodness-of-fit indexes suggest that the configural model fits the data well. Therefore, we can conclude that the structure of the MBI is optimally represented as a three-factor model, with the pattern of factor loadings specified in accordance with this initial multigroup model.

Testing for Measurement Invariance

The next step addresses the question of equality with respect to the measurement model. That is, only the invariance of factor loadings and measurement error variances–covariances are of interest. Typically, however, primary interest focuses on the factor loadings because tests for the equivalence of error variances–covariances are now widely considered excessively stringent. Nonetheless, from a psychometric perspective, when invariance hypotheses bear on a

TABLE 7.4
Selected EQS Output for the Configural Model: Goodness-of-Fit Statistics

GOODNESS OF FIT SUMMARY FOR METHOD = ML

```
CHI-SQUARE =       1221.325 BASED ON      402 DEGREES OF FREEDOM
PROBABILITY VALUE FOR THE CHI-SQUARE STATISTIC IS        .00000
```

FIT INDICES

```
BENTLER-BONETT     NORMED FIT INDEX   =     .899
BENTLER-BONETT NON-NORMED FIT INDEX   =     .919
COMPARATIVE FIT INDEX (CFI)           =     .929
ROOT MEAN-SQUARE RESIDUAL (RMR)       =     .111
STANDARDIZED RMR                      =     .053
ROOT MEAN-SQUARE ERROR OF APPROXIMATION (RMSEA)  =    .040
90% CONFIDENCE INTERVAL OF RMSEA  (        .037,        .043)
```

GOODNESS OF FIT SUMMARY FOR METHOD = ROBUST

```
SATORRA-BENTLER SCALED CHI-SQUARE =    971.9910 ON   402 DEGREES OF FREEDOM
PROBABILITY VALUE FOR THE CHI-SQUARE STATISTIC IS   .00000
```

FIT INDICES

```
BENTLER-BONETT     NORMED FIT INDEX   =     .896
BENTLER-BONETT NON-NORMED FIT INDEX   =     .926
COMPARATIVE FIT INDEX (CFI)           =     .936
ROOT MEAN-SQUARE ERROR OF APPROXIMATION (RMSEA)  =    .033
90% CONFIDENCE INTERVAL OF RMSEA  (        .031,      .036)
```

measuring instrument, it seems important to know whether additionally specified parameters—such as cross-loadings and error covariances—hold across groups (i.e., they are group-equivalent). These parameterizations speak for the quality of such items in the measurement of their related latent factors. In testing for invariance of the MBI measurement model across elementary and secondary school teachers, then, I include the one cross-loading (V12,F1) and three error covariances (E2,E1; E16,E6; E11,E10) found commonly specified for each group.

Testing for the equivalence of factor loadings entails specification of equality constraints for all freely estimated factor loadings that are similarly specified in both baseline models. The key conditions here require the factor loadings to be (a) freely estimated (as opposed to fixed at some value), and (b) consistently specified across groups. The first criterion addresses the issue of model identification and latent variable scaling (see chap. 2); the second addresses the issue of partial measurement invariance (addressed later in this chapter). For clarification of these points, the reader may review either the graphic representation of the model under study (see Fig. 7.1) or the EQS input file (see Table 7.3). The fixed parameters in the model for both groups are the factor loadings representing Item 1 (V1,F1), Item 5 (V1,F2), and Item 4 (V4,F3). Review of the input file shows that these parameters are not accompanied by an asterisk (*), indicating that they are fixed to a value of 1.0 (by default) by the program. On the issue of consistent specification, we note that whereas one cross-loading (*V11,F1) and one error covariance (*E19,E9) were specified for secondary school teachers, it was not so for elementary school teachers. Thus, in testing for factor-loading invariance, equality constraints are placed on all those that are freely estimated except the one that is unique to secondary school teachers. Likewise, in testing for the invariance of the error covariances, equality constraints are specified for all except the one involving Items 19 and 9 (E19,E9). The portion of the input file where these constraints are specified in shown in Table 7.5.

The EQS Input File

In testing for group invariance, equality constraints are specified in a paragraph labeled /CONSTRAINTS, which must be included in the file for the last group only. Thus, in the present case, this paragraph appears as a component of the specified model for secondary school teachers. Examination of the /CONSTRAINTS paragraph in Table 7.5 reveals that one equality specification is required for each parameter being constrained equal across groups, with the parameter relative to Group 1 being specified within the first parentheses and the parameter relative to Group 2 in the second parentheses. Note also that (a) all constrained parameters are estimable; and (b) given the same loading pattern for elementary and secondary school teachers, the cross-loading of Item 12 on the Emotional Exhaustion factor (V12,F1) is also tested for its equivalence across groups. Finally, unlike previous /LMTEST paragraphs observed thus far, the one shown in Table 7.5 involves no

TABLE 7.5
EQS Input for Test for Invariance of the Measurement Model: Equality Constraints

---

/TITLE
TESTING FOR INVARIANCE OF THE MBI FOR ELEMENTARY/SECONDARY TEACHERS "MBIINVelhs1"
GROUP2: SECONDARY TEACHERS
   .
   .
   .
   .
/PRINT
  Fit = All;
/CONSTRAINTS
  (1,V2,F1) = (2,V2,F1);
  (1,V3,F1) = (2,V3,F1);
  (1,V6,F1) = (2,V6,F1);
  (1,V8,F1) = (2,V8,F1);
  (1,V13,F1) = (2,V13,F1);
  (1,V14,F1) = (2,V14,F1);
  (1,V16,F1) = (2,V16,F1);
  (1,V20,F1) = (2,V20,F1);
  (1,V10,F2) = (2,V10,F2);
  (1,V15,F2) = (2,V15,F2);
  (1,V22,F2) = (2,V22,F2);
  (1,V7,F3) = (2,V7,F3);
  (1,V9,F3) = (2,V9,F3);
  (1,V12,F3) = (2,V12,F3);
  (1,V12,F1) = (2,V12,F1);
  (1,V17,F3) = (2,V17,F3);
  (1,V18,F3) = (2,V18,F3);
  (1,V19,F3) = (2,V19,F3);
  (1,V21,F3) = (2,V21,F3);
  (1,E2,E1) = (2,E2,E1);
  (1,E16,E6) = (2,E16,E6);
  (1,E11,E10) = (2,E11,E10);
/LMTEST
/END

SET command related to particular parameters. This omission exists because with multigroup invariance, the purpose of the LM Test is to test the null hypothesis that each specified constraint is true in the population.

The EQS Output File

Let's turn now to the results of this initial test for invariance, which are presented in Table 7.6. Shown first are the goodness-of-fit statistics describing the entire multigroup model. Conventionally, it is argued that invariance holds if goodness-of-fit related to this model is deemed adequate (Widaman & Reise, 1997) and if there is minimal difference in fit from that of the configural model. Likewise, these same criteria hold in the testing of all subsequent invariance models. Review of

TABLE 7.6

Selected EQS Output for Testing Invariance of Measurement Model: Goodness-of-Fit Statistics

```
GOODNESS OF FIT SUMMARY FOR METHOD = ML
CHI-SQUARE =        1268.803 BASED ON       424 DEGREES OF FREEDOM
PROBABILITY VALUE FOR THE CHI-SQUARE STATISTIC IS          .00000

FIT INDICES
-----------
BENTLER-BONETT        NORMED FIT INDEX =        .895
BENTLER-BONETT NON-NORMED FIT INDEX =        .921
COMPARATIVE FIT INDEX (CFI)          =        .927
ROOT MEAN-SQUARE RESIDUAL (RMR)      =        .118
STANDARDIZED RMR                     =        .058
ROOT MEAN-SQUARE ERROR OF APPROXIMATION (RMSEA)      =      .040
90% CONFIDENCE INTERVAL OF RMSEA   (          .037,        .042)


GOODNESS OF FIT SUMMARY FOR METHOD = ROBUST

SATORRA-BENTLER SCALED CHI-SQUARE =     1010.4789 ON   424 DEGREES OF FREEDOM
PROBABILITY VALUE FOR THE CHI-SQUARE STATISTIC IS     .00000

FIT INDICES
-----------
BENTLER-BONETT        NORMED FIT INDEX =        .892
BENTLER-BONETT NON-NORMED FIT INDEX =        .928
COMPARATIVE FIT INDEX (CFI)          =        .934
ROOT MEAN-SQUARE ERROR OF APPROXIMATION (RMSEA)      =      .033
90% CONFIDENCE INTERVAL OF RMSEA   (          .030,        .036)
```

the goodness-of-fit results reported in Table 7.6 show that despite the imposition of equality constraints on all appropriate factor loadings, as well as three error covariances, the multigroup model underwent some deterioration in model fit (corrected ΔS-B$\chi 2$ = 38.350, p < .01; Δ*CFI = .02). Overall, however, the multigroup model still exhibits a good fit to the data (*CFI = .934; *RMSEA = .033; 90% C.I. = .030, .036).

To determine which (if any) parameters were found not to be equivalent across elementary and secondary school teachers, we turn to Table 7.7. As shown here, the program first echoes the constraints specified and then presents the results. Although the program yields both univariate and multivariate tests of hypotheses, only the multivariate results are presented. Associated with each constraint is a cumulative multivariate LM Test χ^2 and an incremental univariate χ^2 value, along with their probability values. To locate parameters that are noninvariant across groups, we look for probability values associated with the incremental univariate χ^2 values that are <.05. Review of these values, as reported in Table 7.7, reveals three parameters that are not operating equivalently across elementary and secondary school teachers (i.e., Constraints 10, 22, and 11). A check of these specified constraints reveals two factor loadings (i.e., V15,F2 and V22,F2) and one commonly specified error covariance (i.e., E11,E10) to be noninvariant across the two teacher groups.

TABLE 7.7

Selected EQS Output for Testing Invariance of Measurement Model: LM Test Statistics

LAGRANGE MULTIPLIER TEST (FOR RELEASING CONSTRAINTS)

CONSTRAINTS TO BE RELEASED ARE:

CONSTRAINTS FROM GROUP 2

CONSTR:	1	(1,V2,F1)-(2,V2,F1)=0;
CONSTR:	2	(1,V3,F1)-(2,V3,F1)=0;
CONSTR:	3	(1,V6,F1)-(2,V6,F1)=0;
CONSTR:	4	(1,V8,F1)-(2,V8,F1)=0;
CONSTR:	5	(1,V13,F1)-(2,V13,F1)=0;
CONSTR:	6	(1,V14,F1)-(2,V14,F1)=0;
CONSTR:	7	(1,V16,F1)-(2,V16,F1)=0;
CONSTR:	8	(1,V20,F1)-(2,V20,F1)=0;
CONSTR:	9	(1,V10,F2)-(2,V10,F2)=0;
CONSTR:	10	(1,V15,F2)-(2,V15,F2)=0;
CONSTR:	11	(1,V22,F2)-(2,V22,F2)=0;
CONSTR:	12	(1,V7,F3)-(2,V7,F3)=0;
CONSTR:	13	(1,V9,F3)-(2,V9,F3)=0;
CONSTR:	14	(1,V12,F3)-(2,V12,F3)=0;
CONSTR:	15	(1,V12,F1)-(2,V12,F1)=0;
CONSTR:	16	(1,V17,F3)-(2,V17,F3)=0;
CONSTR:	17	(1,V18,F3)-(2,V18,F3)=0;
CONSTR:	18	(1,V19,F3)-(2,V19,F3)=0;
CONSTR:	19	(1,V21,F3)-(2,V21,F3)=0;
CONSTR:	20	(1,E2,E1)-(2,E2,E1)=0;
CONSTR:	21	(1,E16,E6)-(2,E16,E6)=0;
CONSTR:	22	(1,E11,E10)-(2,E11,E10)=0;

		CUMULATIVE MULTIVARIATE STATISTICS			UNIVARIATE INCREMENT	
STEP	PARAMETER	CHI-SQUARE	D.F.	PROBABILITY	CHI-SQUARE	PROBABILITY
1	CONSTR: 10	5.374	1	.020	5.374	.020
2	CONSTR: 22	12.330	2	.002	6.956	.008
3	CONSTR: 11	18.259	3	.000	5.929	.015
4	CONSTR: 16	21.928	4	.000	3.669	.055
5	CONSTR: 21	24.719	5	.000	2.792	.095
6	CONSTR: 12	26.350	6	.000	1.631	.202
7	CONSTR: 15	28.111	7	.000	1.761	.185
8	CONSTR: 5	30.703	8	.000	2.592	.107
9	CONSTR: 3	32.636	9	.000	1.934	.164
10	CONSTR: 9	33.889	10	.000	1.252	.263

It is interesting that all items found to be noninvariant are designed to measure the factor of Depersonalization. Thus, it appears that whereas the MBI may be a viable measure of the emotional exhaustion and personal accomplishment components of teacher burnout, item content designed to measure the depersonalization component is being differentially interpreted by elementary and secondary school teachers. Having determined evidence of noninvariance related to these three parameters, the question is: Can we still continue to test for invariance of the structural model (i.e., interfactor relations)? The answer to this question is "yes" if certain conditions can be met. To move ahead in testing for the invariance of the structural model, we invoke the use of partial measurement invariance. As such, all previously imposed equality constraints are retained except those found to be noninvariant; these parameters are allowed to be freely estimated in each group. However, the use of partial measurement invariance is contingent on the number of indicator variables used in measuring each latent construct. Given multiple indicators and at least one invariant measure (other than the one fixed to 1.00 for identification purposes), remaining noninvariant measures can be specified as unconstrained across groups; that is, they can be freely estimated (Byrne et al., 1989; and Muthén & Christoffersson, 1981). In the present case, there is no difficulty in meeting this requirement.

In testing for invariance related to the structural model, our interest focuses on the factor covariances. Although some researchers may also want to test for the equality of the factor variances, these parameters are typically of little interest. From a construct-validity perspective, we test only for the invariance of the factor covariances. The /CONSTRAINTS paragraph of this input file is discussed in the following subsection.

The EQS Input File

In reviewing this section of the input file in Table 7.8, there are two important points: (a) equality constraints related to the factor loadings for Item 15 (V15,F2) and Item 22 (V22,F2) are now absent, as is the constraint related to the error covariance between Items 11 and 10 (E11,E10); and (b) equality constraints are now specified for the three factor covariances (see the last three lines of the /CONSTRAINTS paragraph). Of importance here is that the equality of these structural parameters is tested while concomitantly maintaining the equality of specified measurement parameters across groups. Thus, it is easy to see why the invariance-testing criteria become increasingly stringent as a researcher progresses from tests of the measurement model to tests of the structural model.

The EQS Output File

Results related to this analysis are presented in Tables 7.9 and 7.10. Shown first in Table 7.9 are the goodness-of-fit statistics that reflect a model that still represents a good fit to the data and with negligible difference in fit from that of the configural model.[6] Indeed, comparison with the configural model yields a nonsignificant difference in S-Bχ^2 values (corrected ΔS-B$\chi^2_{(22)} = 23.224$, $p > .05$); likewise, the difference in *CFI values was minimal (Δ*CFI $= .01$). However, further insight into these results comes from the LM Test statistics shown in Table 7.10. Review of the univariate χ^2 incremental values reveals two with probabilities <.05. These probabilities are associated with Constraint 20, which represents, the factor covariance between Emotional Exhaustion and Depersonalization (F2,F1), and Constraint 10, which represents, the loading of Item 7 on the Personal Accomplishment

---

[6]Given that three previously specified parameters from Model 2 were not estimated but three newly specified parameters were, the degrees of freedom associated with Models 2 and 3 remain the same.

TABLE 7.8

Selected EQS Input for Testing Invariance of Structural Model: Equality Constraints

---

/TITLE

TESTING FOR INVARIANCE OF THE MBI FOR ELEMENTARY/SECONDARY TEACHERS "MBIINVelhs1"
GROUP 2: SECONDARY TEACHERS
.
.
.

/PRINT

Fit = All;

/CONSTRAINTS

(1,V2,F1) = (2,V2,F1);
(1,V3,F1) = (2,V3,F1);
(1,V6,F1) = (2,V6,F1);
(1,V8,F1) = (2,V8,F1);
(1,V13,F1) = (2,V13,F1);
(1,V14,F1) = (2,V14,F1);
(1,V16,F1) = (2,V16,F1);
(1,V20,F1) = (2,V20,F1);
(1,V10,F2) = (2,V10,F2);
(1,V7,F3) = (2,V7,F3);
(1,V9,F3) = (2,V9,F3);
(1,V12,F3) = (2,V12,F3);
(1,V12,F1) = (2,V12,F1);
(1,V17,F3) = (2,V17,F3);
(1,V18,F3) = (2,V18,F3);
(1,V19,F3) = (2,V19,F3);
(1,V21,F3) = (2,V21,F3);
(1,E2,E1) = (2,E2,E1);
(1,E16,E6) = (2,E16,E6);
(1,F1,F2) = (2,F1,F2);
(1,F1,F3) = (2,F1,F3);
(1,F2,F3) = (2,F2,F3);

/LMTEST

/END

(V7,F3). However, although these parameters have been pinpointed as not operating equivalently across elementary and secondary school teachers, the $\Delta S\text{-}B\chi^2$ test yielded a difference value that was not significant. Presented with these findings, it seems appropriate to adhere to results of the $\Delta S\text{-}B\chi^2$ test. As such, it is concluded that structural relations among the three factors of burnout, as measured by the modified MBI items determined in this study, are invariant across the two groups of teachers.

In this chapter, we tested for the invariance of MBI factorial structure across elementary and secondary school teachers based on the analysis of COVS. First, a baseline model for each teacher group was established separately; these analyses revealed the best-fitting model to include one cross-loading (i.e., V12,F1) and three error covariances (i.e., E2,E1; E16,E6; and E11,E10) for both teacher groups. For secondary teachers, however, this model also included an additional cross-loading (i.e., V11,F1) and one error covariance (i.e., E19,E9). Following the establishment

```
GOODNESS OF FIT SUMMARY FOR METHOD = ML

CHI-SQUARE =     1249.170  BASED  ON       424 DEGREES OF FREEDOM
PROBABILITY VALUE FOR THE CHI-SQUARE  STATISTIC  IS          .00000

FIT INDICES
-----------
BENTLER-BONETT      NORMED FIT INDEX =        .897
BENTLER-BONETT NON-NORMED FIT INDEX =        .923
COMPARATIVE FIT INDEX (CFI)         =        .929
ROOT MEAN-SQUARE RESIDUAL (RMR)     =        .127
STANDARDIZED RMR                    =        .060
ROOT MEAN-SQUARE ERROR OF APPROXIMATION (RMSEA)     =        .039
90% CONFIDENCE INTERVAL OF RMSEA (          .037,         .042)

GOODNESS OF FIT SUMMARY FOR METHOD = ROBUST

SATORRA-BENTLER SCALED CHI-SQUARE =      996.0734 ON 424 DEGREES OF FREEDOM
PROBABILITY VALUE FOR THE CHI-SQUARE STATISTIC  IS  .00000

FIT INDICES
-----------
BENTLER-BONETT      NORMED FIT INDEX =        .893
BENTLER-BONETT NON-NORMED FIT INDEX =        .930
COMPARATIVE FIT INDEX (CFI)         =        .935
ROOT MEAN-SQUARE ERROR OF APPROXIMATION (RMSEA)     =        .033
90% CONFIDENCE INTERVAL OF RMSEA (          .030,         .035)
```

of these baseline models and based on partial-measurement invariance, the equivalence of common parameters composing both the measurement (factor loadings and error covariances) and structural (factor covariances) models across groups was tested. Based on results from implementation of the LM Test, only two factor loadings (i.e., V15,F2 and V22,F2) and one error covariance (i.e., E11,E10) were determined to be noninvariant across elementary and secondary school teachers.

In the interest of completeness regarding the topic of multigroup invariance, there are two aspects of these analyses that require further elaboration. Although both issues are topics of considerable debate in the literature, they nonetheless need to be addressed: these are partial measurement and appropriate evaluative criteria in determining evidence of invariance.

OTHER CONSIDERATIONS IN TESTING FOR MULTIPLE-GROUP INVARIANCE

The Issue of Partial-Measurement Invariance

Perhaps the first paper to discuss the issue of partial-measurement invariance was that of Byrne et al., 1989, which addressed the difficulty commonly encountered in

TABLE 7.10

Selected EQS Output for Testing Invariance of Structural Model: LM Test Statistics

LAGRANGE MULTIPLIER TEST (FOR RELEASING CONSTRAINTS)

CONSTRAINTS TO BE RELEASED ARE:

CONSTRAINTS FROM GROUP   2

CONSTR:	1	$(1,V2,F1)-(2,V2,F1)=0;$
CONSTR:	2	$(1,V3,F1)-(2,V3,F1)=0;$
CONSTR:	3	$(1,V6,F1)-(2,V6,F1)=0;$
CONSTR:	4	$(1,V8,F1)-(2,V8,F1)=0;$
CONSTR:	5	$(1,V13,F1)-(2,V13,F1)=0;$
CONSTR:	6	$(1,V14,F1)-(2,V14,F1)=0;$
CONSTR:	7	$(1,V16,F1)-(2,V16,F1)=0;$
CONSTR:	8	$(1,V20,F1)-(2,V20,F1)=0;$
CONSTR:	9	$(1,V10,F2)-(2,V10,F2)=0;$
CONSTR:	10	$(1,V7,F3)-(2,V7,F3)=0;$
CONSTR:	11	$(1,V9,F3)-(2,V9,F3)=0;$
CONSTR:	12	$(1,V12,F3)-(2,V12,F3)=0;$
CONSTR:	13	$(1,V12,F1)-(2,V12,F1)=0;$
CONSTR:	14	$(1,V17,F3)-(2,V17,F3)=0;$
CONSTR:	15	$(1,V18,F3)-(2,V18,F3)=0;$
CONSTR:	16	$(1,V19,F3)-(2,V19,F3)=0;$
CONSTR:	17	$(1,V21,F3)-(2,V21,F3)=0;$
CONSTR:	18	$(1,E2,E1)-(2,E2,E1)=0;$
CONSTR:	19	$(1,E16,E6)-(2,E16,E6)=0;$
CONSTR:	20	$(1,F1,F2)-(2,F1,F2)=0;$
CONSTR:	21	$(1,F1,F3)-(2,F1,F3)=0;$
CONSTR:	22	$(1,F2,F3)-(2,F2,F3)=0;$

		CUMULATIVE MULTIVARIATE STATISTICS			UNIVARIATE INCREMENT	
STEP	PARAMETER	CHI-SQUARE	D.F.	PROBABILITY	CHI-SQUARE	PROBBILITY
1	CONSTR: 20	4.821	1	.028	4.821	.028
2	CONSTR: 10	9.735	2	.008	4.914	.027
3	CONSTR: 14	11.838	3	.008	2.103	.147
4	CONSTR: 19	13.520	4	.009	1.682	.195
5	CONSTR: 13	14.676	5	.012	1.156	.282
6	CONSTR: 5	16.417	6	.012	1.741	.187
7	CONSTR: 3	17.930	7	.012	1.512	.219
8	CONSTR: 9	19.361	8	.013	1.431	.232
9	CONSTR: 18	20.390	9	.016	1.029	.310
10	CONSTR: 11	21.007	10	.021	.617	.432

testing for multigroup invariance whereby certain parameters in the measurement model (typically, factor loadings) are found to be noninvariant across the groups of interest. At the time of writing that paper, researchers were generally under the impression that faced with such results, one should not continue to test for invariance of the structural model. Byrne and colleagues (1989) showed that as long as certain conditions were met (described previously), tests for invariance could continue by invoking the strategy of partial-measurement invariance.

More recently, however, the issue of partial-measurement invariance has been subject to some controversy in the technical literature (see, e.g., Marsh & Grayson, 1994; and Widaman & Reise, 1997). Review of the literature related to this topic reveals a modicum of experimental studies designed to test the impact of partial-measurement invariance on, for example, the power of the test when group sample sizes are widely disparate (Kaplan & George, 1995), the accuracy of selection in multiple populations (Millsap & Kwok, 2004), and the meaningful interpretation of latent mean differences across groups (Marsh & Grayson, 1994). Substantially more work needs to be done in this area of research before there is a comprehensive view of the extent to which implementation of partial-measurement invariance affects results yielded from tests for the equivalence of measuring instruments across groups.

The Issue of Appropriate Evaluative Criteria in Determining Evidence of Invariance

In reporting on evidence of invariance, it has become customary to report the difference in χ^2 values ($\Delta\chi^2$) derived from the comparison of χ^2 values associated with various models under test with the the baseline configural model. In this regard, Yuan and Bentler (2004a) recently reported that for virtually every SEM application, evidence in support of multigroup invariance has been based on the $\Delta\chi^2$ test. In chapter 6, it was explained that this computed value is possible because such models are nested (see chap. 3, footnote 9). It was also noted that although the same comparisons can be based on the S-Bχ^2 (ΔS-Bχ^2), a correction to the value is needed because this difference is not distributed as χ^2 (Bentler, 2005). The correction formula for computing this ΔS-Bχ^2 value was provided in chapter 6 and was used in computing these values in the present chapter as well as in all remaining chapters. If this difference value is statistically significant, it suggests that the constraints specified in the more restrictive model do not hold (i.e., the two models are not equivalent across groups). If, on the other hand, the $\Delta\chi^2$ value is statistically nonsignificant, this finding suggests that all specified equality constraints are tenable. Although Steiger, Shapiro, and Browne (1985) noted that, in theory, the $\Delta\chi^2$ test holds whether or not the baseline model is misspecified, Yuan and Bentler (2004a) reported findings that point to the unreliability of this test when the model is, in fact, misspecified. Given that in our present tests for invariance, we determined a very good fit of the baseline model to the data for both groups of teachers, I consider this baseline model to be well specified.

This evaluative strategy involving the $\Delta\chi^2$ (or ΔS-Bχ^2) represents the traditional approach to determining evidence of measurement invariance and follows from Jöreskog's (1971b) original technique in testing for multigroup equivalence. However, this traditional strategy was based on the LISREL program for which the only way to identify noninvariant parameters was to compare models in this manner. (For elaboration and illustration of the LISREL approach to invariance testing, see Byrne, 1998.) In contrast, this comparative approach is technically not necessary when analyses are based on EQS because the LM Test allows for immediate identification of equality constraints found to be noninvariant across groups. However, as revealed in this chapter, when there is minimal difference in fit between two nested models, it behooves the researcher to check the ΔS-Bχ^2 value.

Recently, however, researchers (e.g., Cheung & Rensvold, 2002; Marsh, Hey, & Roche, 1997; and Little, 1997) have argued that this $\Delta\chi^2$ value is as sensitive to sample size and non-normality as the χ^2 statistic itself, thereby rendering it an impractical and unrealistic criterion on which to base evidence of invariance. As a consequence, there is an increasing tendency to argue for evidence of invariance based on two alternative criteria: (a) the multigroup model exhibits an adequate fit to the data, and (b) the ΔCFI (or $*\Delta$CFI) values between models is negligible. Although Little (1997), basing his work on two earlier studies (McGaw & Jöreskog, 1971; and Tucker & Lewis, 1973), suggested that this difference should not exceed a value of .05, other researchers were less specific and based evidence for invariance merely on the fact that change in the CFI values between nested models is minimal. However, Cheung and Rensvold (2002) pointed out that the .05 criterion suggested by Little (1997) has neither strong theoretical nor empirical support. Thus, until their recent simulation research, use of the ΔCFI difference value has been of a purely heuristic nature. In contrast, Cheung and Rensvold (2002) examined the properties of 20 goodness-of-fit indexes within the context of invariance testing and recommended that the ΔCFI, ΔGamma hat, and/or ΔMcDonald's noncentrality values provide the best information for determining evidence of measurement invariance. With respect to the ΔCFI, they arbitrarily suggested that its difference value should not exceed .01. This recent approach to the determination of multigroup invariance takes a more practical approach to the process.

Table 7.11 reviews results from the tests for invariance of the MBI across elementary and secondary school teachers from both a traditional and a practical perspective. Presented in this table are goodness-of-fit statistics related to all models tested, along with the S-Bχ2 and *CFI difference values resulting from their comparisons with the configural model, the baseline against which all remaining models are compared in the process of determining evidence of invariance. Review of these results determines the extent of their consistency based on both traditional and practical evaluative criteria. Adhering to Cheung and Rensvold's (2002) recommended cutpoint of .01, results related to Model 2 (i.e., the measurement model) appear consistent across the two perspectives in detecting some evidence of noninvariance. To pinpoint which parameters are contributing to the inequality, the LM Test results need to be checked. With respect to Model 3 (i.e., the structural

TABLE 7.11

Tests for Invariance of MBI Factorial Structure: Summary of Goodness-of-Fit Statistics

Model	S-Bχ^2	df	*CFI	SRMR	*RMSEA	*RMSEA 90% CI	Model Comparison	Δ S-Bχ^{2a}	Δ df	Δ*CFI
Model 1 Configural No constraints	971.991	402	.936	.053	.033	.031, .036	------	------	---	------
Model 2 Measurement Model invariant (factor loadings; 1 cross-loading; 3 error covariances)	1010.479	424	.934	.063	.033	.030, .036	2 vs 1	38.350	22	.02
Model 3 Structural Model invariant (factor covariances; all *invariant* parameters from Model 2)	996.073	424	.935	.073	.033	.030, .035	3 vs 1	23.224	22	.01

[a]Corrected value (see chap. 6).

model), conclusions based on the difference tests are consistent; in this instance, however, results support the equivalence of interfactor covariances across the two groups of teachers. Although, in the present case, conclusions based on both the traditional and practical perspectives paralleled one another in the presentation of results, this is not always the case—in fact, it is usually not the case. Of importance in the present application, however, is the fact that if the evidence of invariance were limited to only the LM Test results, a quite different conclusion, would have been drawn regarding the equivalence of relations among the underpinning three factors of burnout across elementary and secondary school teachers.

The intent in presenting these two issues is to keep you abreast of the current literature regarding testing strategies associated with multigroup invariance. However, until such time that these issues are clearly resolved and documented with sound analytic findings, continued use of partial-measurement invariance and the traditional approach in determining evidence of multigroup invariance is suggested.

8

Application 6:
Testing for the Invariance
of a Causal Structure

In chapter 4, several problematic aspects of post hoc model-fitting in SEM were highlighted. Indeed, so common is this practice and so frequently is it conducted with little regard for the substantive meaningfulness of the respecified models that concerned researchers have provided various means by which such models can be tested more stringently (see, e.g., Anderson & Gerbing, 1988; Cudeck & Henly, 1991; MacCallum, 1995; and MacCallum et al., 1992, 1993). It was noted in chapter 4 that one approach to addressing problems associated with post hoc model-fitting is to apply some mode of cross-validation analysis; this is the focus of the present chapter. The application demonstrated herein is a follow-up to the analyses of chapter 6 in which the validity of a causal structure describing determinants of burnout for a calibration sample of secondary school teachers was tested. However, before a walk-through of this cross-validation procedure, it is important to review some of the related issues.

CROSS-VALIDATION IN SEM

Typically in applications of SEM, the researcher tests a hypothesized model and then, from an assessment of various goodness-of-fit criteria, concludes that a statistically better-fitting model could be attained by respecifying the model such that particular parameters previously constrained to zero are freely estimated (Breckler,

1990; MacCallum et al., 1992, 1993; and MacCallum, Roznowski, Mar, & Reith, 1994). Possibly as a consequence of considerable criticism of SEM procedures in the past (e.g., Biddle & Marlin, 1987; Breckler, 1990; and Cliff, 1983), most researchers who proceed with this respecification process are now generally familiar with the issues. In particular, they are cognizant of the exploratory nature of these follow-up procedures as well as the fact that additionally specified parameters in the model must be theoretically substantiated.

Indeed, the pros and cons of post hoc model-fitting have been rigorously debated in the literature. Although some have severely criticized the practice (e.g., Cliff, 1983; and Cudeck & Browne, 1983), others have argued that as long as researchers are fully cognizant of the exploratory nature of their analyses, the process can be substantively meaningful because both practical and statistical significance can be considered (Byrne et al., 1989; and Tanaka & Huba, 1984). However, Jöreskog (1993, p. 298) is clear in stating that "If the model is rejected by the data, the problem is to determine what is wrong with the model and how the model should be modified to fit the data better." The purists would argue that once a hypothesized model is rejected, it is the end of the story. More realistically, however, other researchers in this area recognize the obvious impracticality in the termination of all subsequent model analyses. Clearly, in the interest of future research, it behooves the investigator to probe deeper into the question of why the model is misfitting (Tanaka, 1993). As a consequence of the concerted efforts of statistical experts in addressing this issue, there are now several different approaches that can be used to increase the soundness of findings derived from these post hoc analyses.

Undoubtedly, post hoc model-fitting in the analysis of covariance structures is problematic. With multiple model specifications, there is a risk of capitalization on chance factors because model modification may be driven by characteristics of the particular sample on which the model was tested (e.g., sample size, sample heterogeneity) (MacCallum et al., 1992). As a consequence of this sequential testing procedure, there is increased risk of making either a Type I or Type II error and, at this point, there is no direct way to adjust for the probability of such error. Because hypothesized covariance structure models represent only approximations of reality and thus are not expected to fit real-world phenomena exactly (Cudeck & Browne, 1983; and MacCallum et al., 1992), most research applications are likely to require the specification of alternative models in the quest for one that fits the data well (Anderson & Gerbing, 1988; and MacCallum, 1986). Indeed, this aspect of covariance structure modeling represents a serious limitation; to date, several alternative strategies for model testing have been proposed (see, e.g., Anderson & Gerbing, 1988; Cudeck & Henly, 1991; MacCallum, 1995; and MacCallum et al., 1992, 1993).

One approach to addressing problems associated with post hoc model fitting is to employ a cross-validation strategy, whereby the final model derived from the post hoc analyses is tested on a second (or more) independent sample(s) from the same population. Barring the availability of separate data samples, albeit a sufficiently large sample, the researcher may want to randomly split the data into two (or more) parts, thereby making it possible to cross-validate the findings (Cudeck & Browne, 1983). As such, Sample A serves as the calibration sample on which the initially hypothesized model is tested as well as any post hoc analyses conducted in the process of attaining a well-fitting model. Once this final model is determined, the validity of its structure can then be tested based on Sample B (the validation sample). In other words, the final best-fitting model for the calibration sample becomes the hypothesized model under test for the validation sample.

There are several ways to test the similarity of model structure (e.g., MacCallum et al., 1994). For example, Cudeck and Browne (1983) suggested the computation of a Cross-Validation Index (CVI) that measures the distance between the restricted (i.e., model-imposed) variance–covariance matrix for the calibration sample and the unrestricted variance–covariance matrix for the validation sample. Because the estimated predictive validity of the model is gauged by the smallness of the CVI value, evaluation is facilitated by their comparison based on a series of alternative models. It is important to note, however, the CVI estimate reflects overall discrepancy between "the actual population covariance matrix, Σ, and the estimated population covariance matrix reconstructed from the parameter estimates obtained from fitting the model to the sample" (MacCallum et al., 1994, p. 4). More specifically, this global index of discrepancy represents combined effects arising from the discrepancy of approximation (e.g., nonlinear influences among variables) and the discrepancy of estimation (e.g., representative sample; sample size). (For more discussion of these discrepancy aspects, see Browne & Cudeck, 1989; Cudeck & Henly, 1991; and MacCallum et al., 1994.)

In this chapter, we examine another approach to cross-validation. Specifically, we use an invariance-testing strategy to test for the replicability of both the measurement and structural models across groups. Although there are numerous approaches to cross-validation in SEM depending on the focus of the study (Anderson & Gerbing, 1988; Browne & Cudeck, 1989; and Cudeck & Browne, 1983), the application described herein is straightforward in addressing the question of whether a model that has been respecified in one sample replicates over a second independent sample from the same population. (For another approach in addition to the one demonstrated here, see Byrne & Baron, 1994.)

TESTING FOR INVARIANCE ACROSS CALIBRATION/VALIDATION SAMPLES

The present example comes from the same study briefly described in chapter 6 (Byrne, 1994c). The intent of this original study was to (a) validate a causal structure involving the impact of organizational and personality factors on three facets of burnout for elementary, intermediate, and secondary school teachers; (b) cross-validate this model across a second independent sample within each teaching panel; and (c) test for the invariance of common structural paths across teaching panels. In chapter 6, we tested for the validity of this causal structure for the "calibration" sample of secondary school teachers ($n = 716$); following several respecifications of the model, a final best-fitting model was determined that was deemed valid from the perspective of substantive meaningfulness. (For an in-depth examination of invariance-testing procedures within and between the three teacher groups, see Byrne, 1994b.) The task in this chapter is to cross-validate this final model of burnout structure across a second independent group of high school teachers, which we'll call the "validation group" ($n = 714$).

Although the present example of cross-validation is based on a full structural equation model, the practice is in no way limited to such applications. Indeed, cross-validation is equally as important for CFA models, and examples of such applications are found in various disciplines: for those relevant to psychology, see Byrne, Stewart, & Lee, 2004; to education, see Benson and Bandalos (1992); and to medicine, see Francis, Fletcher, and Rourke (1988).

THE HYPOTHESIZED MODEL

The originally hypothesized model (shown in chap. 6) was tested and modified based on data from the calibration sample (Sample A) of high school teachers. The final best-fitting model for this sample yielded the following goodness-of-fit statistics: S-B$\chi^2_{(422)} = 812.691$; SRMR $= .040$; *CFI $= .960$; *RMSEA $= .036$ with 90% C.I. $= .032, .040$; it is graphically described in Fig. 8.1. The task now is to determine if this final model replicates over Sample B, the validation group of high school teachers.

THE EQS INPUT FILE

In chapter 7, we tested for the equivalence of a measuring instrument across two different panels of school teachers: elementary and secondary. We first established a baseline model of best fit for each group separately, prior to testing for invariance across groups. However, in cross-validating either a CFA or full structural equation model across groups, the only baseline model determined is for the calibration group. In the present case, this baseline model represents the final best-fitting

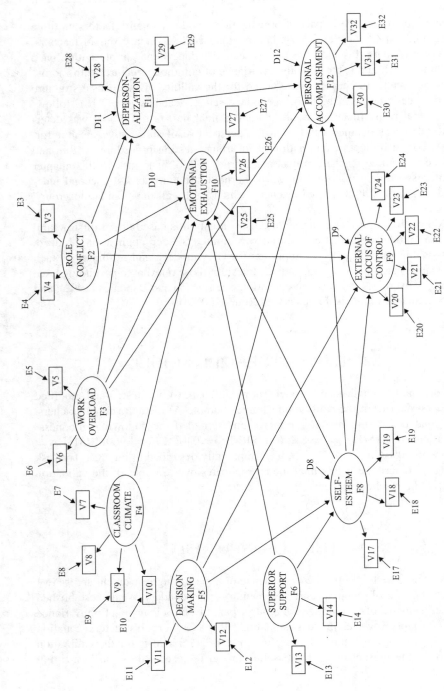

FIG. 8.1. Hypothesized multigroup model of causal structure reflecting determinants of teacher burnout.

254

model as determined from the analyses presented in chapter 6 and as shown in Fig. 8.1.[1] The rationale here is that the focus in testing across the calibration and validation groups is to determine the extent to which this final model replicates across a second independent sample from the same population.

Consistent with this conceptual rationale, model specification for the validation group should be identical to that for the calibration group. Although space constraints only permit the presentation of EQS input for the calibration group, the exact same specifications are made for the validation group, including two cross-loadings, one error covariance, and all specified start values. This partial file is shown in Table 8.1.

In Table 8.1, we turn first to the /TITLE and /SPECIFICATIONS paragraphs pertinent to Group 1, the calibration group. There is only one major difference in the /SPECIFICATIONS paragraph from the one presented for the same sample of high school teachers in Table 6.1: the statement "Groups = 2." As explained in chapter 7, this statement tells the program that analyses are to be based on two groups. In the same two paragraphs for Group 2, the validation group, observe three (albeit expected) differences in model specification: sample size, data filename, and absence of deleted cases. As noted in Table 8.1, other than these specification differences, the /LABELS, /EQUATIONS, /VARIANCES, and /COVARIANCES paragraphs for the validation group remain identical to those for the calibration group.

In the /CONSTRAINTS paragraph, all factor and cross-loadings, all structural paths, and one error covariance are constrained equal across the two groups. Although the specification of an equality constraint pertinent to the error covariance might be perceived as somewhat excessive (which it is), it is of interest and important to determine if this systematic error holds across the calibration/validation samples. Indeed, the present set of equality constraints represents a very rigorous although necessary test of multigroup invariance. Some researchers might contend that in the case of a full causal model only the structural paths are of interest; however, I maintains that to ensure meaningful and credible interpretation of findings bearing on equality of the structural paths, it is important to know that the measurement parameters (specifically the factor loadings) are operating in the same way for both groups under study.

---

[1] With reference to the measurement model, the two cross-loadings (i.e., V12→F6 and V30→F10) and one error covariance (i.e., E26, E25) are not included here in the interest of clarity.

TABLE 8.1
EQS Input for Test of Invariant Causal Structure Across Calibration and Validation
Samples of Secondary School Teachers

/TITLE
 CROSS-VALIDATION OF FINAL BURNOUT MODEL FOR SECONDARY TCHRS "CVBURNHSF"
 GROUP 1: CALIBRATION GROUP
/SPECIFICATIONS
 CASE=716; VAR=32; ME=ML,ROBUST; MA=RAW; FO='(19F4.2/13F4.2)'; Groups=2;
 DATA='C:\EQS61\Files\Books\Data\secind1.ess'; DEL=440,77;
/LABELS
 V1=ROLEA1; V2=ROLEA2; V3=ROLEC1; V4=ROLEC2; V5=WORK1; V6=WORK2; V7=CLIMATE1;
 V8=CLIMATE2; V9=CLIMATE3; V10=CLIMATE4; V11=DEC1; V12=DEC2; V13=SSUP1; V14=SSUP2;
 V15=PSUP1; V16=PSUP2; V17=SELF1; V18=SELF2; V19=SELF3; V20=XLOC1; V21=XLOC2;
 V22=XLOC3; V23=XLOC4; V24=XLOC5; V25=EE1; V26=EE2; V27=EE3; V28=DP1; V29=DP2;
 V30=PA1; V31=PA2; V32=PA3; F1=ROLEA; F2=ROLEC; F3=WORK; F4=CLIMATE; F5=DEC; F6=SSUP;
 F7=PSUP; F8=SELF; F9=XLOC; F10=EE; F11=DP; F12=PA;
/EQUATIONS
 V1 = 1.000 F1 + 1.000 E1 ;
 V2 = 1.308*F1 + 1.000 E2 ;
 V3 = 1.000 F2 + 1.000 E3 ;
 V4 = 1.253*F2 + 1.000 E4 ;
 V5 = 1.000 F3 + 1.000 E5 ;
 V6 = .708*F3 + 1.000 E6 ;
 V7 = 1.000 F4 + 1.000 E7 ;
 V8 = 1.664*F4 + 1.000 E8 ;
 V9 = .987*F4 + 1.000 E9 ;
 V10 = 1.385*F4 + 1.000 E10 ;
 V11 = 1.000 F5 + 1.000 E11 ;
 V12 = .242*F5   + .898*F6 + 1.000 E12 ;
 V13 = 1.000 F6 + 1.000 E13 ;
 V14 = 1.101*F6 + 1.000 E14 ;
 V15 = 1.000 F7 + 1.000 E15 ;
 V16 = 1.060*F7 + 1.000 E16 ;
 V17 = 1.000 F8 + 1.000 E17 ;
 V18 = 1.263* F8 + 1.000 E18 ;
 V19 = 1.417*F8 + 1.000 E19 ;
 V20 = 1.000 F9 + 1.000 E20 ;
 V21 = .911*F9 + 1.000 E21 ;
 V22 = 1.060*F9 + 1.000 E22 ;
 V23 = .957*F9 + 1.000 E23 ;
 V24 = 1.246*F9 + 1.000 E24 ;
 V25 = 1.000 F10 + 1.000 E25 ;
 V26 = 1.052*F10 + 1.000 E26 ;
 V27 = 1.219*F10 + 1.000 E27 ;
 V28 = 1.000 F11 + 1.000 E28 ;
 V29 = .920*F11 + 1.000 E29 ;
 V30 = -.171*F10 + 1.000 F12 + 1.000 E30 ;
 V31 = 1.234*F12 + 1.000 E31 ;
 V32 = 1.179*F12 + 1.000 E32 ;
 F8 = .363*F5   -.114*F6 + 1.000 D8 ;
 F9 = -.262*F5 + *F8 + *F2 + 1.000 D9 ;
 F10 = -.128*F2 + .745*F3   -.898*F4 + *F6 + *F8 + 1.000 D10 ;
 F11 = .549*F10 + .147*F2 + *F3 + 1.000 D11 ;
 F12 = .512*F8   -.188*F9 -.195*F11 + *F5 + *F3 + 1.000 D12 ;
/VARIANCES
 F1= .388* ; F2= .676* ; F3= .897* ; F4= .097* ; F5= .566* ; F6= 1.146* ; F7= .622* ;
 E1= .446* ; E2= .321* ; E3= .612* ; E4= .543* ; E5= .561* ; E6= .690* ; E7= .182* ; E8= .138* ;
 E9= .146* ; E10= .323* ; E11= .501* ; E12= .541* ; E13= .452* ; E14= .171* ; E15= .330* ; E16= .154*;
 E17= .072* ; E18= .070* ; E19= .075* ; E20= .211* ; E21= .275* ; E22= .128* ; E23= .235* ; E24= .171* ;
 E25= .688* ; E26= .426* ; E27= .212* ; E28= .246* ; E29= .671* ; E30= .301* ; E31= .308* ; E32= .382* ;
 D8= .077* ; D9= .127* ; D10= .493* ; D11= .628* ; D12= .270* ;

(Continued)

TABLE 8.1
(Continued)

/COVARIANCES

F2,F1 = 389* ; F3,F1 = .408* ; F3,F2 = .720* ; F4,F1 = -.038* ; F4,F2 = -.075* ; F4,F3 = -.062* ; F5,F1 = -.382* ;
F5,F2 = -.493* ; F5,F3 = -.550* ; F5,F4 = .092* ; F6,F1 = -.358* ; F6,F2 = -.497* ; F6,F3 = -.484* ; F6,F4 = .100* ;
F6,F5 = .636* ; F7,F1 = -.227* ; F7,F2 = -.255* ; F7,F3 = -.286* ; F7,F4 = .049* ; F7,F5 = .417* ; F7,F6 = .391* ;
E26,E25 = .259* ;

/PRINT

 FIT=ALL;

/END

/TITTLE

 GROUP 2: VALIDATION GROUP

/SPECIFICATIONS

 CASE=714; VAR=32; ME=ML,ROBUST; MA=RAW; FO='(19F4.2/13F4.2)';
 DATA='C:\EQS61\Files\Books\Data\secind2l.ess';

/LABELS
/EQUATIONS
/VARIANCES   }   Same as for Calibration group
/COVARIANCES
/CONSTRAINTS

 (1,V2,F1) = (2,V2,F1);
 (1,V4,F2) = (2,V4,F2);
 (1,V6,F3) = (2,V6,F3);
 (1,V8,F4) = (2,V8,F4);
 (1,V9,F4) = (2,V9,F4);
 (1,V10,F4) = (2,V10,F4);
 (1,V12,F5) = (2,V12,F5);
 (1,V12,F6) = (2,V12,F6);
 (1,V14,F6) = (2,V14,F6);
 (1,V16,F7) = (2,V16,F7);
 (1,V18,F8) = (2,V18,F8);
 (1,V19,F8) = (2,V19,F8);
 (1,V21,F9) = (2,V21,F9);
 (1,V22,F9) = (2,V22,F9);
 (1,V23,F9) = (2,V23,F9);
 (1,V24,F9) = (2,V24,F9);
 (1,V26,F10) = (2,V26,F10);
 (1,V27,F10) = (2,V27,F10);
 (1,V29,F11) = (2,V29,F11);
 (1,V30,F10) = (2,V30,F10);
 (1,V31,F12) = (2,V31,F12);
 (1,V32,F12) = (2,V32,F12);
 (1,F8,F5) = (2,F8,F5);
 (1,F8,F6) = (2,F8,F6);
 (1,F9,F5) = (2,F9,F5);
 (1,F9,F8) = (2,F9,F8);
 (1,F9,F2) = (2,F9,F2);
 (1,F10,F2) = (2,F10,F2);
 (1,F10,F3) = (2,F10,F3);
 (1,F10,F4) = (2,F10,F4);
 (1,F10,F6) = (2,F10,F6);
 (1,F10,F8) = (2,F10,F8);
 (1,F11,F10) = (2,F11,F10);
 (1,F11,F2) = (2,F11,F2);
 (1,F11,F3) = (2,F11,F3);
 (1,F12,F8) = (2,F12,F8);
 (1,F12,F9) = (2,F12,F9);
 (1,F12,F11) = (2,F12,F11);
 (1,F12,F5) = (2,F12,F5);
 (1,F12,F3) = (2,F12,F3);
 (1,E26,E25) = (2,E26,E25);

/LMTEST
/END

THE EQS OUTPUT FILE

Let's turn now to Table 8.2 where the goodness-of-fit results related to the test for multigroup invariance are presented. Somewhat surprisingly (given the rigor of the constraints), these findings reveal a remarkably well-fitting multigroup model (S-B$\chi^2_{(885)}$ = 1623.682; SRMR = .043; *CFI = .961; *RMSEA = .024 with 90% C.I. = .022, .026). Indeed, these results speak well for the general equivalence of the model specifications across calibration and validation samples.

We turn next to Table 8.3 where results from the LM Test of equality constraints are displayed. As explained in chapter 7, in determining evidence of noninvariance based on the LM Test of equality constraints, we look for univariate incremental χ^2 values with probability values < .05. In reviewing these values here, we find two such cases. The one with the smaller probability (Constraint 31; F10, F6) identifies the structural path flowing from Superior Support to Emotional Exhaustion (SSUP → EE); the second (Constraint 4; V8, F4) pinpoints the factor loading of Climate2 onto Factor 4 (Classroom Climate) as being noninvariant across the calibration and validation samples of high school teachers.

In summary, based on these findings we can conclude that with the exception of one structural path flowing from Superior Support to Emotional Exhaustion (SSUP → EE) and the factor loading of V8 (Climate2) onto Factor 4 (Classroom Climate), the hypothesized causal pattern of organizational and personality factor determinants of burnout shown in Fig. 8.1 are equivalent across two independent samples of high school teachers. That the analyses did not yield completely invariant parameters across groups is somewhat disappointing. Nonetheless, given the rigor of the equality constraints imposed, these findings speak well for the cross-validation of this causal structure as it relates to high school teachers.

TABLE 8.2

Selected EQS Output for Test of Invariant Causal Structure: Goodness-of-Fit Statistics

```
GOODNESS OF FIT SUMMARY FOR METHOD = ML

CHI-SQUARE =      1807.331 BASED ON     885 DEGREES OF FREEDOM
PROBABILITY VALUE FOR THE CHI-SQUARE STATISTIC IS          .00000

FIT INDICES
-----------
BENTLER-BONETT      NORMED FIT INDEX =       .924
BENTLER-BONETT NON-NORMED FIT INDEX =       .955
COMPARATIVE FIT INDEX (CFI)         =       .960
ROOT MEAN-SQUARE RESIDUAL (RMR)     =       .037
STANDARDIZED RMR                    =       .043
ROOT MEAN-SQUARE ERROR OF APPROXIMATION (RMSEA)    =     .027
90% CONFIDENCE INTERVAL OF RMSEA   (      .025,        .029)

GOODNESS OF FIT SUMMARY FOR METHOD = ROBUST

SATORRA-BENTLER SCALED CHI-SQUARE =    1623.6828 ON       885 DEGREES OF FREEDOM
PROBABILITY VALUE FOR THE CHI-SQUARE STATISTIC IS          .00000

FIT INDICES
-----------
BENTLER-BONETT      NORMED FIT INDEX =       .919
BENTLER-BONETT NON-NORMED FIT INDEX =       .957
COMPARATIVE FIT INDEX (CFI)         =       .961
ROOT MEAN-SQUARE ERROR OF APPROXIMATION (RMSEA)    =     .024
90% CONFIDENCE INTERVAL OF RMSEA   (      .022,        .026)
```

TABLE 8.3

Selected EQS Output for Test of Invariant Causal Structure: LM Test Results

```
LAGRANGE MULTIPLIER TEST (FOR RELEASING CONSTRAINTS)

CONSTRAINTS TO BE RELEASED ARE:

      CONSTRAINTS FROM GROUP 2
         CONSTR:    1    (1,V2,F1)-(2,V2,F1)=0;
         CONSTR:    2    (1,V4,F2)-(2,V4,F2)=0;
         CONSTR:    3    (1,V6,F3)-(2,V6,F3)=0;
         CONSTR:    4    (1,V8,F4)-(2,V8,F4)=0;
         CONSTR:    5    (1,V9,F4)-(2,V9,F4)=0;
         CONSTR:    6    (1,V10,F4)-(2,V10,F4)=0;
         CONSTR:    7    (1,V12,F5)-(2,V12,F5)=0;
         CONSTR:    8    (1,V12,F6)-(2,V12,F6)=0;
         CONSTR:    9    (1,V14,F6)-(2,V14,F6)=0;
         CONSTR:   10    (1,V16,F7)-(2,V16,F7)=0;
         CONSTR:   11    (1,V18,F8)-(2,V18,F8)=0;
         CONSTR:   12    (1,V19,F8)-(2,V19,F8)=0;
         CONSTR:   13    (1,V21,F9)-(2,V21,F9)=0;
         CONSTR:   14    (1,V22,F9)-(2,V22,F9)=0;
         CONSTR:   15    (1,V23,F9)-(2,V23,F9)=0;
         CONSTR:   16    (1,V24,F9)-(2,V24,F9)=0;
         CONSTR:   17    (1,V26,F10)-(2,V26,F10)=0;
         CONSTR:   18    (1,V27,F10)-(2,V27,F10)=0;
         CONSTR:   19    (1,V29,F11)-(2,V29,F11)=0;
```

(Continued)

TABLE 8.3
(Continued)

LAGRANGE MULTIPLIER TEST (FOR RELEASING CONSTRAINTS)

CONSTRAINTS TO BE RELEASED ARE:

CONSTRAINTS FROM GROUP 2

CONSTR:	20	(1,V30,F10)-(2,V30,F10)=0;
CONSTR:	21	(1,V31,F12)-(2,V31,F12)=0;
CONSTR:	22	(1,V32,F12)-(2,V32,F12)=0;
CONSTR:	23	(1,F8,F5)-(2,F8,F5)=0;
CONSTR:	24	(1,F8,F6)-(2,F8,F6)=0;
CONSTR:	25	(1,F9,F5)-(2,F9,F5)=0;
CONSTR:	26	(1,F9,F8)-(2,F9,F8)=0;
CONSTR:	27	(1,F9,F2)-(2,F9,F2)=0;
CONSTR:	28	(1,F10,F2)-(2,F10,F2)=0;
CONSTR:	29	(1,F10,F3)-(2,F10,F3)=0;
CONSTR:	30	(1,F10,F4)-(2,F10,F4)=0;
CONSTR:	31	(1,F10,F6)-(2,F10,F6)=0;
CONSTR:	32	(1,F10,F8)-(2,F10,F8)=0;
CONSTR:	33	(1,F11,F10)-(2,F11,F10)=0;
CONSTR:	34	(1,F11,F2)-(2,F11,F2)=0;
CONSTR:	35	(1,F11,F3)-(2,F11,F3)=0;
CONSTR:	36	(1,F12,F8)-(2,F12,F8)=0;
CONSTR:	37	(1,F12,F9)-(2,F12,F9)=0;
CONSTR:	38	(1,F12,F11)-(2,F12,F11)=0;
CONSTR:	39	(1,F12,F5)-(2,F12,F5)=0;
CONSTR:	40	(1,F12,F3)-(2,F12,F3)=0;
CONSTR:	41	(1,E26,E25)-(2,E26,E25)=0;

		CUMULATIVE MULTIVARIATE STATISTICS			UNIVARIATE INCREMENT	
STEP	PARAMETER	CHI-SQUARE	D.F.	PROBABILITY	CHI-SQUARE	PROBABILITY
1	CONSTR: 31	6.539	1	.011	6.539	.011
2	CONSTR: 4	11.279	2	.004	4.740	.029
3	CONSTR: 18	14.852	3	.002	3.574	.059
4	CONSTR: 39	18.529	4	.001	3.676	.055
5	CONSTR: 7	21.725	5	.001	3.196	.074
6	CONSTR: 30	24.251	6	.000	2.527	.112
7	CONSTR: 11	26.139	7	.000	1.888	.169
8	CONSTR: 35	28.051	8	.000	1.912	.167
9	CONSTR: 14	29.902	9	.000	1.851	.174
10	CONSTR: 16	33.172	10	.000	3.269	.071
11	CONSTR: 27	34.493	11	.000	1.321	.250
12	CONSTR: 13	36.429	12	.000	1.937	.164

9

Application 7: Testing for Latent Mean Differences Based on a First-Order CFA Model

In the years since the printing of my first EQS book in 1994, there has been a steady albeit moderate increase in reported findings from tests for multigroup equivalence. Review of the SEM literature, however, reveals that most tests for invariance have been based on the analysis of covariance structures COVS, as exemplified in chapters 7 and 8. Despite Sörbom's (1974) introduction of the mean and covariance structures (MACS) strategy in testing for latent mean differences 30 years ago, few studies have been designed to test for latent mean differences across groups based on real (as opposed to simulated) data (see, e.g., Aiken, Stein, & Bentler, 1994; Byrne, 1988b; Cooke et al., 2001; Little, 1997; Marsh & Grayson, 1994; Reise et al., 1993; and Widaman & Reise, 1997). This chapter introduces you to basic concepts associated with the analysis of latent mean structures and walks you through an application that tests for the invariance of latent means across two different cultural groups. Specifically, we test for differences in the latent means of four nonacademic self-concepts (SCs)—Physical SC (Appearance), Physical SC (Ability), Social SC (Peers), and Social SC (Parents)—across Australian and Nigerian adolescents; these constructs comprise the four nonacademic SC components of the Self-Description Questionnaire I (SDQ-I; Marsh, 1992). The present application is taken from a study by Byrne and Watkins (2003) but extends this previous work in two ways: (a) analyses are based on MACS rather than only on COVS, and (b) analyses address the issue of missing data with respect to the Nigerian sample (data were complete for the Australian sample).

BASIC CONCEPTS UNDERLYING TESTS
OF LATENT MEAN STRUCTURES

In the usual univariate or multivariate analyses involving multigroup comparisons, researchers are typically interested in testing whether the observed means representing the various groups are statistically significantly different from each other. Because these values are directly calculable from the raw data, they are considered to be observed values. In contrast, the means of latent variables (i.e., latent constructs) are unobservable; that is, they are not directly observed. Rather, these latent constructs derive their structure indirectly from their indicator variables, which in turn are directly observed and, hence, measurable. Testing for the invariance of mean structures conveys the notion that we intend to test for the equivalence of means related to each underlying construct or factor. Another way of saying this is that we intend to test for differences in the latent means (of factors for each group).

For all examples considered thus far, the analyses were based on covariance structures. In other words, only parameters representing regression coefficients, variances, and covariances have been of interest. Accordingly, the covariance structure of the observed variables constitutes the crucial parametric information; thus, a hypothesized model can be estimated and tested via the sample covariance matrix. One limitation of this level of invariance is that whereas the unit of measurement for the underlying factors (i.e., the factor loading) is identical across groups, the origin of the scales (i.e., the intercepts) is not. As a consequence, comparison of latent factor means is not possible, thereby leading Meredith (1993) to categorize this level of invariance as "weak" factorial invariance. This limitation, notwithstanding, evidence of invariant factor loadings nonetheless permits researchers to move on in testing further for the equivalence of factor variances, factor covariances, and pattern of these factorial relations, a focus of substantial interest to researchers more concerned with construct validity issues than in testing for latent mean differences. These subsequent tests continue to be based on the analysis of COVS.

In the analysis of COVS, it is implicitly assumed that all observed variables are measured as deviations from their means; in other words, *their* means are equal to zero. As a consequence, the intercept terms generally associated with regression equations are not relevant to the analyses. However, when the observed means take on nonzero values, the intercept parameter must be considered, thereby necessitating a reparameterization of the hypothesized model. Such is the case when one is interested in testing for the invariance of latent mean structures. An example taken from the EQS manual (Bentler, 2005) should help to clarify both the concept and the term "mean structures". First consider the following regression equation:

$$y = \alpha + \beta x + \varepsilon$$

where α is an intercept parameter. Although the intercept can assist in defining the mean of y, it does not generally equal the mean. Considering expectations of both sides of this equation and assuming that the mean of ε is zero, the above expression yields:

$$\mu_y = \alpha + \beta\mu_x$$

where μ_y is the mean of y and μ_x is the mean of x. As such, y and its mean can now be expressed in terms of the model parameters α, β, and μ_x. It is this decomposition of the mean of y, the dependent variable, that leads to the term *mean structures*. More specifically, it serves to characterize a model in which the means of the dependent variables can be expressed or "structured" in terms of structural coefficients and the means of the independent variables. The previous equation illustrates how incorporating a mean structure into a model necessarily includes the new parameters α and μ_x, the intercept and observed mean (of x), respectively. Thus, models with structured means merely extend the basic concepts associated with the analysis of covariance structures.

In each previous application involving the analysis of COVS, variances of dependent variables were never parameters in the model. The same dictum holds true in the analysis of mean structures; dependent variable means cannot be parameters in the model. However, as will become clear in the next sub-section, the intercepts of dependent variables actually do become parameters in the model—but only because they operate as the regression coefficients of a "constant" variable that EQS creates to carry out the analyses of mean structures. It functions as an independent variable within the context of the Bentler–Weeks schema. In summary, any model involving mean structures may include the following parameters:

- regression coefficients
- variances and covariances of the independent variables
- intercepts of the dependent variables
- means of the independent variables

MODELING MEAN STRUCTURES IN EQS

Basic Parameterization

It may be obvious that to accommodate two additional parameters in the model and yet retain the restriction that means and variances of dependent variables cannot be parameterized, the model must be restructured in some way. This is exactly what does take place for EQS to complete the analyses. Achievement of this task entails the utilization of two unique tricks: (a) creation of a constant variable that

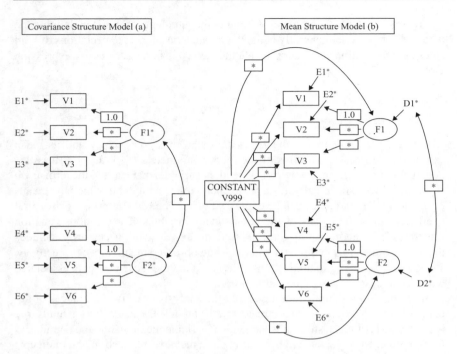

FIG. 9.1.   Sample models of covariance and mean structures.

EQS designates V999,[1] and (b) reconceptualization of the independent variables as dependent variables, in the Bentler–Weeks sense. A simple CFA model presented in Fig. 9.1 illustrates these points and conceptualizes how the covariance structure model transforms into a mean structure model.

The same set of variables and factors are parameterized in two different configurations: in (a) as a covariance structure model and in (b) as a mean structure model. In the covariance structure model, there are three measured variables each regressed on two factors; the factors are hypothesized to be correlated. Consistent with EQS notation, the asterisks (*) represent parameters to be estimated; the first of each set of congeneric measures is fixed to 1.00 for purposes of model identification and latent variable scaling. In terms of the Bentler–Weeks conceptualization, this model has eight independent variables (i.e., two F's and six E's) and six dependent variables (six V's). Typically variances can be estimated for only the independent variables. Finally, with 21 elements in the sample covariance matrix $(6[6 + 1]/2)$ and 13 estimable parameters, this model is overidentified with eight overidentifying restrictions.

---

[1]The rationale is that relative to the measured variables in the input file, the constant is always considered last.

Turning next to the mean structure model in Fig. 9.1 (b), we see a schematic representation that is vastly different from its covariance structure counterpart in (a). Let's now examine these differences more closely. First, you will see the inclusion in the model of a constant that EQS labels V999. The important aspect of this variable is that although it is an independent variable, in the Bentler–Weeks sense, it has no variance, no covariance with other variables in the model, and always remains fixed at a value of 1.0.

Second, note that the six observed variables and the two factors are regressed onto the constant. Each coefficient associated with these regression one-way arrows represents an intercept, which in turn expresses a mean value. Regression of the two factors onto the constant yields intercepts that represent the latent factor means; regression of the measured variables onto the constant represent the observed variable intercepts. Whenever there are no indirect effects of the constant on the measured variables, each intercept value represents a direct effect and should equal the observed mean.[2] On the other hand, if there are indirect effects in the model, as in Fig. 9.1 (b), the expected mean of a measured variable is represented by a total effect (i.e., direct effect + indirect effect). A brief example clarifies these points. Suppose the intercept for Factor 1 (V999 → F1) were fixed to zero. The expected mean value of V2 would then be determined solely by the direct effect of the constant (V999) on V2; this value would therefore equal the observed mean. By contrast, the expected mean value of V5 would be determined by both the direct effect of V999 on V5 and the indirect effect of V999 → F2 on V5, with these values in combination representing a total effect. Based on the tracing rule used in path analysis, the indirect effect on V5 would equal the product of paths V999 → F2 and F2 → V5. The decomposition of effects can be obtained as an option within the /PRINT paragraph of EQS.

As a consequence of regression onto the constant V999, the two factors are now dependent variables and, as such, cannot have variances and covariances. Instead, the residual of a variable that is a dependent variable by sole virtue of its regression onto the constant manifests the variance and covariance information for that variable. Thus, as shown in Fig. 9.1 (b), variances associated with D1 and D2 are estimated as well as the covariance between them.

Bentler (2005) has noted that in analyzing structured means models, there must always be fewer intercepts than there are measured variables. The intent of this requirement is to guard against possible underidentification related to the structured-means portion of the model. To fully comprehend this advice, let's reexamine Fig. 9.1 (b) more closely: It is actually composed of both a covariance structure as depicted in Fig. 9.1 (a) and a mean structure. Consider these two structures in terms of sample data. From all previous examples, we know that data for the covariance structure derive from the sample variance–covariance matrix. As noted

---

[2]Direct effects represent the impact of one variable on another, with no mediation by any other variable; indirect effects operate through at least one intervening variable (Bollen, 1989a).

previously, this portion of the model was overidentified with eight restrictions that provide degrees of freedom (df) in the model-testing process.

But what about the mean structure portion of the model in terms of model identification? It was discussed previously that to analyze a structured-means model, the user must input the observed mean value for each measured variable; these provide the data and are fundamental in determining the status of model identification. Thus, if the number of intercepts being estimated exceeds the amount of information coming into the structured means portion of the model as per the observed mean values, the model is underidentified. Indeed, the model in Fig. 9.1 (b) exemplifies this situation. There are six measured variables and, consequently, six pieces of information (i.e., six observed mean values) from which to estimate the means-related parameters. However, as indicated by the asterisks, the number of intercepts to be estimated is eight (i.e., six variable intercepts and two factor intercepts), thereby rendering the model underidentified. Thus, to estimate a mean structure as in Fig 9.1(b), two or more intercept restrictions must be imposed. The factor intercepts can be fixed to zero, yielding a just-identified mean structure that would yield identical covariance parameter results, as in Fig. 9.1(a) At the other extreme, all the V999 → V paths could be fixed to zero, in which case the means of the V's are explained solely by the means of the F's. In multisample models, as we shall see shortly, this type of situation can be resolved with the imposition of equality constraints across groups.

Multigroup Parameterization

As with previous examples of multigroup invariance, applications based on structured-means models involve testing simultaneously across two or more groups. However, in testing for invariance based on the analysis of MACS, the multigroup specification is unique in two important ways. First, because the two (or more) groups under study are tested simultaneously, evaluation of the identification criterion is considered across groups. As a consequence, although the structured-means model may not be identified in one group, it can become so when analyzed across groups. This outcome occurs as a function of specified equality constraints across groups.

Second, the multigroup model demands the specification of an additional constraint to satisfy the need for factor identification. The reason for this added constraint derives from the fact that when the intercepts of the measured variables are constrained equal across groups (as they typically should be), the latent factor intercepts have an arbitrary origin. A standard way of addressing this situation is to constrain the latent factor intercepts of one group to zero (Bentler, 2005). This group then operates as a reference group against which latent means for the other group(s) are compared. Consequently, latent factor means are interpretable only in a relative sense. Statistical significance associated with the differences between the latent mean(s) for the reference group (i.e., fixed at 0.0) and those freely estimated for the other group(s) can be determined on the basis of the z-statistic.

TESTING FOR LATENT MEAN DIFFERENCES OF A FIRST-ORDER CFA MODEL

The Strategy

The approach to testing for differences in latent factor means follows the same pattern as the one outlined and applied in chapter 7. That is, we first establish a well-fitting baseline model for each group separately. This step is followed by a hierarchically ordered series of analyses that test for the invariance of particular sets of parameters across groups. The primary difference in the tests for invariance in chapter 7 (based on the analysis of COVS) and those based on the analysis of MACS illustrated in this chapter (and in chap. 10) is the additional tests for the equivalence of intercepts and latent factor means across groups. The difference between the present chapter and chapter 10, however, lies with the levels of invariance testing involved. We turn now to the hypothesized model under study and the related tests for invariance of a first-order CFA structure.

THE HYPOTHESIZED MODEL

The application to be examined in this chapter bears on the equivalency of latent mean structures related to four nonacademic SC dimensions—Physical SC (appearance), Physical SC (ability), Social SC (peers), and Social SC (parents)—across Australian and Nigerian adolescents. These constructs comprise the four nonacademic SC components of the SDQ-I (Marsh, 1992). Although the data for Australian adolescents are complete ($n = 497$), those for Nigerian ($n = 463$) adolescents are incomplete. Provided with evidence of substantial multivariate kurtosis, as indicated by Mardia's normalized estimate of 80.70 for the Australians, and Yuan, Lambert, and Fouladi's (2004) normalized estimate of 71.20 for the Nigerians,[3] all analyses were based on the Robust statistics. The originally hypothesized model tested separately for each group is presented schematically in Fig. 9.2.

---

[3] When data are incomplete, there are typically many different patterns of missingness; thus, methods designed for one complete data set cannot be used. The Yuan, Lambert, and Fouladi (2004) coefficient is an extension of the Mardia (1970, 1974) test of multivariate kurtosis that can be used effectively with missing data. Essentially, it aggregates information across the missing data patterns to yield one overall summary statistic. Whenever a model is tested with missing data, EQS automatically computes and reports this coefficient along with its normalized estimate.

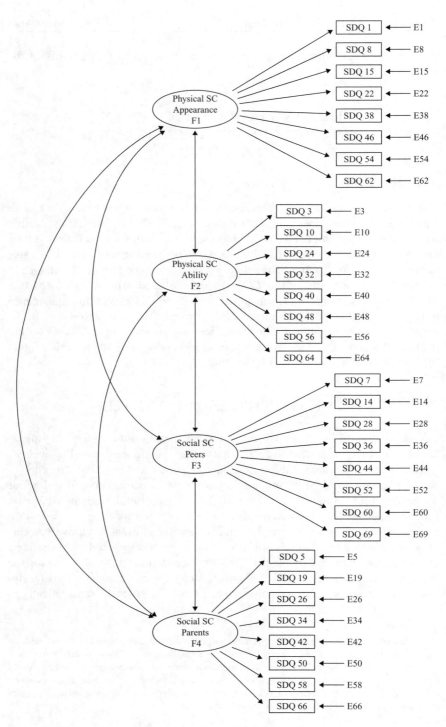

FIG. 9.2. Hypothesized model of factorial structure for the Self-Description Questionnaire-I (SDQ-I; Marsh, 1992; non-academic subscales).

Testing for Baseline Models

Australian Adolescents.

Initial testing of the hypothesized model for this group yielded only a marginally good fit to the data (S-B$\chi^2_{(458)}$ = 1059.29; SRMR = .07; *CFI = .90; *RMSEA = .05; 90% C.I. = .047, .055). Review of the LM Test statistics revealed one cross-loading (F3 → SDQ38) and two error covariances (SDQ40/SDQ24; SDQ26/SDQ19) to be markedly misspecified. Of the three parameters, the cross-loading exhibited the largest standardized parameter change statistic, whereas the error covariance between Items 40 and 24 exhibited the largest univariate incremental χ^2 statistic. These SDQ items are as follows:

- Item 19: I like my parents.
- Item 26: My parents like me.
- Item 24: I enjoy sports and games.
- Item 40: I am good at sports.
- Item 38: Other kids think I am good-looking.

Given that the cross-loading of Item 38 on Factor 3 (Social [Peers]) seemed reasonable, this parameter was added to the model first. Based on a comparison of *CFI values, this respecification resulted in a trivial improvement in model fit (S-B$\chi^2_{(457)}$ = 1003.701; SRMR = .063; *CFI = .905; *RMSEA = .049; 90% C.I. = .045, .053). Analogously, because the overlap of content between Items 19 and 26 was obvious and that between Items 24 and 40 seemed highly possible, the model was subsequently respecified and reestimated with these two error covariances included. This reparameterization resulted in a further slight improvement in model fit (S-B$\chi^2_{(455)}$ = 903.88; SRMR = .06; *CFI = .91; *RMSEA = .05; 90% C.I. = .045, .053). Although review of the LM Test statistics suggested the addition of a second cross-loading to the model (F1 → SDQ32), this parameter was not incorporated for two reasons: (a) considerations of parsimony, and (b) the questionable meaningfulness of this cross-loading across males and females. The content of this item reads as "I have good muscles." This content was considered possibly gender-specific, thereby arguing against its model specification. Thus, the baseline model considered the most appropriate and of reasonably good model fit for the Australian data consisted of the one cross-loading and two error covariances noted previously.

Nigerian Adolescents

Given the incomplete nature of SDQ-I responses for these adolescents, it was necessary that missingness be addressed in the analyses of these data. Although many approaches can be taken in dealing with missing data, the one considered most efficient and is therefore the most highly recommended is that of ML estimation (see, e.g., Arbuckle, 1996; Enders & Bandalos, 2001; Gold & Bentler,

TABLE 9.1
EQS Input: Test of Hypothesized Model for Nigerian Adolescents

---

/SPECIFICATIONS
```
DATA='C:\EQS61\files\books\data\nigerom.ess';
VARIABLES= 79; CASES=465;
METHODS=ML,ROBUST; MATRIX=RAW; ANALYSIS=MOMENT;
MISSING=ML; SE=FISHER;
```

2000; and Schafer & Graham, 2002). Nonetheless, Bentler (2005) notes that when the amount of missing data is extremely small, there may be some conditions in which some of the more commonly used methods, such as listwise and pairwise deletion, hot deck, and mean imputation, may suffer only marginal loss of accuracy and efficiency compared with the ML method pairwise. (For an abbreviated review of the issues, advantages and disadvantages of various approaches to handling missing data, see Byrne, 2001; for a more extensive and comprehensive treatment of these topics, see Arbuckle, 1996, and Schafer & Graham, 2002; for a comparison of missing data methods, see Enders & Bandalos, 2001; and for a review of ML methods, see Enders, 2001.) In testing for the validity of the hypothesized model for Nigerian adolescents, analyses were based on the ML estimation approach to missing data. The /SPECIFICATIONS paragraph of the related input file is shown in Table 9.1.

Review of this command paragraph shows three specifications that have not appeared in previous input files. The first is ANALYSIS=MOMENT. When analyses are based on MACS, the data to be modeled include both sample means and sample covariances. This information is typically contained in the moment matrix, although the format by which it is contained varies differently among SEM programs. For example, whereas LISREL organizes these in a moment matrix that combines means and covariances as cross-products of sample data, EQS analyzes means and covariances separately. In EQS, this is done by adding a "constant" variable to the input, with the recognition that a coefficient for regressing any variable on a constant is an intercept of that variable. For independent variables, the intercept is that variable's model-based mean; for other variables, the total effect of the constant on that variable is the variable's model-based mean (Bentler, 2005). The statistical theory assumes that the sample means and covariances are being analyzed in all groups; that is, the variables have not been standardized.

The second specification to note is MISSING=ML.[4] EQS uses the expectation maximization (EM) type of ML estimation procedure. Based on the work of Jamshidian and Bentler (1999), this approach provides optimal results when the data are multivariate normal; when this condition does not hold (i.e., data are non-normally distributed), a correction to the test statistics and standard errors

---

[4]MISSING=COMPLETE is equivalent to listwise deletion of missing data. It is the default condition for EQS and, therefore, has not been used in previous application input files.

must be made. Yuan and Bentler (2000) provided these corrections such that the Yuan–Bentler scaled statistic (Y-Bχ^2) is analogous to the S-Bχ^2 when data are both incomplete and non-normally distributed. Consistent with computation of the S-Bχ^2, the Y-Bχ^2 requires the specification of ME=ML, ROBUST, which is shown in Table 9.1.

The final specification of note is that of SE=FISHER, which indicates that the Fisher information matrix is used to compute the standard errors. This is the sensible standard error option if sample size is not too small; otherwise, the SE=OBSERVED option would be chosen.

Let's return now, to findings related to testing of the hypothesized model for Nigerian adolescents. In contrast to the Australian group, these results revealed a fairly well-fitting model (Y-B$\chi^2_{(458)}$ = 729.88; SRMR = .05; *CFI = .93; *RMSEA = .04; 90% C.I. = .031, .041). Review of the LM Test statistics revealed one parameter that could be regarded as misspecified: an error covariance between Items 26 and 19. This covariance replicates the same finding for Australian adolescents. Consequently, the model was subsequently respecified and reestimated with this parameter freely estimated. The respecification led to a slight improvement in model fit, thereby resulting in a fairly good fit to the data (Y-B$\chi^2_{(457)}$ = 699.54; SRMR = .05; *CFI = .94; *RMSEA = .03; 90% C.I. = .029, .039). Given no further clear evidence of badly specified parameters, this model was deemed the most appropriate baseline model for Nigerian adolescents.

With an established baseline model for both groups of adolescents, we now proceed in testing for the validity of the multigroup model in which both baseline models are tested simultaneously to determine evidence of invariance. This multigroup model is shown in Fig. 9.3.

Testing Validity of the Configural Model

As discussed in chapter 7, the model under test in this step of the invariance-testing process is a multigroup model in which no parameter constraints are imposed. The configural model simply incorporates the baseline models for both groups and allows for their simultaneous analyses. However, there is an important difference between the testing of the configural model in this chapter compared with the one in chapter 7 that arises solely as a result of the structure of the data. In this chapter, the Nigerian data comprise incomplete scores; consequently, this missingness must be considered in all analyses. In the current version of the program (EQS6.1), this requisite demands that analyses be based on mean as well as covariance structures. Conversely if the data for both groups had been based on complete data, tests for invariance related to both the configural and measurement models would have followed the same strategy illustrated in chapter 7. Because it is likely to be easier for you to follow specifications in the input file of the configural model if you can visualize the parameters in the related path diagram, I present this baseline model in Fig. 9.4. However, due to space restrictions, only the baseline model

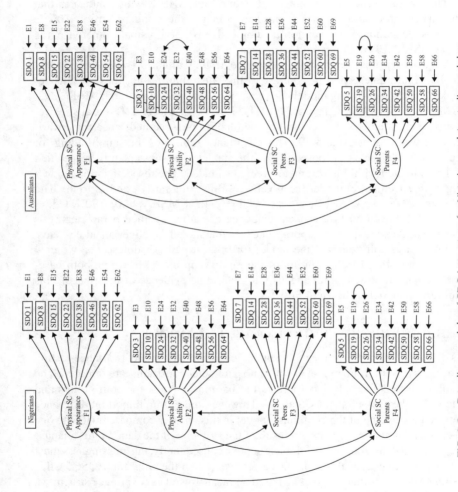

FIG. 9.3. Baseline models of SDQ-I structure for Nigerian and Australian adolescents.

272

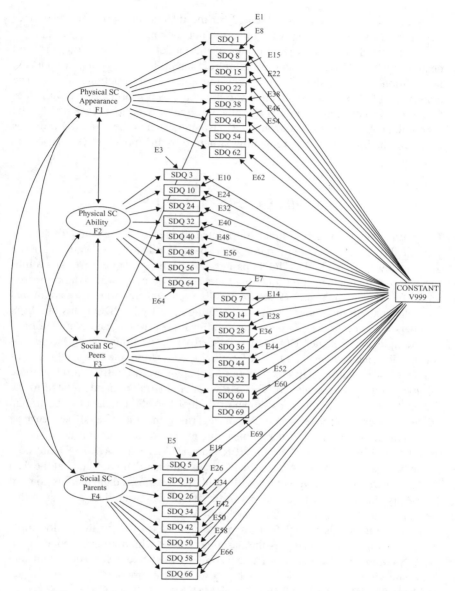

FIG. 9.4. Mean structure model of SDQ-I structure showing only observed variable intercepts.

for Australian adolescents is presented; in the interest of clarity, the two error covariances specified for the Australians are not shown.

The rectangle located at right center of the model is labeled "Constant" and designated "V999." Because intercepts are coefficients for regression on a constant, its addition to the model allows for the introduction of structured means. The constant (in EQS) is an independent variable that has no variance or covariances with other variables in the model and always remains fixed to a value of 1.0. The regression paths radiating out from the Constant to each of the observed variables represent the intercepts. The remaining structure of this model, of course will be familiar to you.

THE EQS INPUT FILE

Let's turn now, then, to the input file related to the configural model which is presented in Table 9.2. Again, to conserve space, duplicate specifications are not shown. However, the /EQUATIONS paragraph is included for both groups to eliminate any confusion in the presentation of subsequent output in which the numbered variables (V's) are presented. Because the Nigerian data comprise three additional variables that are incorporated into the data file prior to the SDQ items, the EQS numbers assigned to the V's necessarily differ for Australian and Nigerian files; for example, whereas the SDQ1 item is labeled V1 for Australians, it is labeled V4 for the Nigerians. Other than this differential specification, the key specifications here and for all subsequent analyses in this chapter are (a) notification that there are two groups to be analyzed (GROUPS=2), and (b) commands related to the fact that data are incomplete, as shown in Table 9.1. Although data for Australian adolescents are complete, specifications regarding method of analyses must be consistent across the groups in a multisample model. As a result, it is necessary to specify METHODS=ML, SE=FISHER, and ANALYSIS=MOMENT anyway. Nonetheless, as you will see later, the program automatically detects that the data for the Australians are complete. Finally, with the use of raw data, there is no need to specify the observed mean values in the input file; if the data are not in this form, this input is required in the analysis of MACS.

Evaluation of this model focuses on its goodness-of-fit to the multisample data, with this value serving as the baseline against which all subsequent models are compared. Results from the testing of this model for Australian and Nigerian adolescents revealed a modestly well-fitting model (i.e., Y-B$\chi^2_{(912)}$ = 1644.55; SRMR = .068; *CFI = .92; *RMSEA = .03; 90% C.I. = .027, .031). Because one of the groups has incomplete data, the overall robust statistic is based on the Yuan–Bentler scaled value. The 912 df represent the summed df associated with the final baseline model for Australian (455 df) and Nigerian (457 df) adolescents.

/TITLE
Testing for Invariance of SDQ Nonacademic SCs "sdqinvan1"
GROUP1: Australian Adolescents
CONFIGURAL MODEL
/SPECIFICATIONS
DATA='C:\EQS61\files\books\data\ausdata.ess';
VARIABLES=77; CASES=497; GROUPS=2;
METHODS=ML,ROBUST; MATRIX=RAW;
MISSING=ML; SE=FISHER; ANALYSIS=MOMENT;
/LABELS
V1=SDQ1; V2=SDQ2; V3=SDQ3; V4=SDQ4; V5=SDQ5; V6=SDQ6; V7=SDQ7; V8=SDQ8; V9=SDQ9;
V10=SDQ10; V11=SDQ11; V12=SDQ12; V13=SDQ13; V14=SDQ14; V15=SDQ15; V16=SDQ16; V17=SDQ17;
V18=SDQ18; V19=SDQ19; V20=SDQ20; V21=SDQ21; V22=SDQ22; V23=SDQ23; V24=SDQ24; V25=SDQ25;
V26=SDQ26; V27=SDQ27; V28=SDQ28; V29=SDQ29; V30=SDQ30; V31=SDQ31; V32=SDQ32; V33=SDQ33;
V34=SDQ34; V35=SDQ35; V36=SDQ36; V37=SDQ37; V38=SDQ38; V39=SDQ39; V40=SDQ40; V41=SDQ41;
V42=SDQ42; V43=SDQ43; V44=SDQ44; V45=SDQ45; V46=SDQ46; V47=SDQ47; V48=SDQ48; V49=SDQ49;
V50=SDQ50; V51=SDQ51; V52=SDQ52; V53=SDQ53; V54=SDQ54; V55=SDQ55; V56=SDQ56; V57=SDQ57;
V58=SDQ58; V59=SDQ59; V60=SDQ60; V61=SDQ61; V62=SDQ62; V63=SDQ63; V64=SDQ64; V65=SDQ65;
V66=SDQ66; V67=SDQ67; V68=SDQ68; V69=SDQ69; V70=SDQ70; V71=SDQ71; V72=SDQ72; V73=SDQ73;
V74=SDQ74; V75=SDQ75; V76=SDQ76; V77=GEN;
/EQUATIONS
V1 = *V999+F1+E1;
V8 = *V999+*F1+E8;
V15 = *V999+*F1+E15;
V22 = *V999+*F1+E22;
V38 = *V999+*F1+*F3+ E38;
V46 = *V999+*F1+E46;
V54 = *V999+*F1+E54;
V62 = *V999+*F1+E62;
V3 = *V999+F2+E3;
V10 = *V999+*F2+E10;
V24 = *V999+*F2+E24;
V32 = *V999+*F2+E32;
V40 = *V999+*F2+E40;
V48 = *V999+*F2+E48;
V56 = *V999+*F2+E56;
V64 = *V999+*F2+E64;
V7 = *V999+F3+E7;
V14 = *V999+*F3+E14;
V28 = *V999+*F3+E28;
V36 = *V999+*F3+E36;
V44 = *V999+*F3+E44;
V52 = *V999+*F3+E52;
V60 = *V999+*F3+E60;
V69 = *V999+*F3+E69;
V5 = *V999+F4+E5;
V19 = *V999+*F4+E19;
V26 = *V999+*F4+E26;
V34 = *V999+*F4+E34;
V42 = *V999+*F4+E42;
V50 = *V999+*F4+E50;
V58 = *V999+*F4+E58;
V66 = *V999+*F4+E66;
/VARIANCES
E1 =*; E3 =*; E5 =*; E7 =*; E8 =*; E10 =*; E14 =*; E15 =*; E19 =*; E22 =*; E24 =*; E26 =*; E28 =*; E32 =*;
E34 =*; E36 =*; E38 =*; E40 =*; E42 =*; E44 =*; E46 =*; E48 =*; E50 =*; E52 =*; E54 =*; E56 =*; E58 =*;
E60 =*; E62 =*; E64 =*; E66 =*; E69 =*;
F1 to F4 = *;
/COVARIANCES
F1 to F4 = *;
E40,E24 = *; E26,E19 = *;
/END

(Continued)

TABLE 9.2

(Continued)

/TITLE
GROUP2: NIGERIAN ADOLESCENTS
/SPECIFICATIONS
DATA='C:\EQS61\files\books\data\nigerom.ess';
VARIABLES= 79; CASES=465;
METHODS=ML,ROBUST; MATRIX=RAW;
MISSING=ML; SE=FISHER; ANALYSIS=MOMENT;
/LABELS
V1=ID; V2=SEX; V3=AGE; V4=SDQ1; V5=SDQ2; V6=SDQ3; V7=SDQ4; V8=SDQ5; V9=SDQ6; V10=SDQ7;
V11=SDQ8; V12=SDQ9; V13=SDQ10; V14=SDQ11; V15=SDQ12; V16=SDQ13; V17=SDQ14; V18=SDQ15;
V19=SDQ16; V20=SDQ17; V21=SDQ18; V22=SDQ19; V23=SDQ20; V24=SDQ21; V25=SDQ22; V26=SDQ23;
V27=SDQ24; V28=SDQ25; V29=SDQ26; V30=SDQ27; V31=SDQ28; V32=SDQ29; V33=SDQ30; V34=SDQ31;
V35=SDQ32; V36=SDQ33; V37=SDQ34; V38=SDQ35; V39=SDQ36; V40=SDQ37; V41=SDQ38; V42=SDQ39;
V43=SDQ40; V44=SDQ41; V45=SDQ42; V46=SDQ43; V47=SDQ44; V48=SDQ45; V49=SDQ46; V50=SDQ47;
V51=SDQ48; V52=SDQ49; V53=SDQ50; V54=SDQ51; V55=SDQ52; V56=SDQ53; V57=SDQ54; V58=SDQ55;
V59=SDQ56; V60=SDQ57; V61=SDQ58; V62=SDQ59; V63=SDQ60; V64=SDQ61; V65=SDQ62; V66=SDQ63;
V67=SDQ64; V68=SDQ65; V69=SDQ66; V70=SDQ67; V71=SDQ68; V72=SDQ69; V73=SDQ70; V74=SDQ71;
V75=SDQ72; V76=SDQ73; V77=SDQ74;V78=SDQ75; V79=SDQ76;
/EQUATIONS
V4 = *V999+F1+E4;
V11 = *V999+*F1+E11;
V18 = *V999+*F1+E18;
V25 = *V999+*F1+E25;
V41 = *V999+*F1+E41;
V49 = *V999+*F1+E49;
V57 = *V999+*F1+E57;
V65 = *V999+*F1+E65;
V6 = *V999+F2+E6;
V13 = *V999+*F2+E13;
V27 = *V999+*F2+E27;
V35 = *V999+*F2+E35;
V43 = *V999+*F2+E43;
V51 = *V999+*F2+E51;
V59 = *V999+*F2+E59;
V67 = *V999+*F2+E67;
V10 = *V999+F3+E10;
V17 = *V999+*F3+E17;
V31 = *V999+*F3+E31;
V39 = *V999+*F3+E39;
V47 = *V999+*F3+E47;
V55 = *V999+*F3+E55;
V63 = *V999+*F3+E63;
V72 = *V999+*F3+E72;
V8 = *V999+F4+E8;
V22 = *V999+*F4+E22;
V29 = *V999+*F4+E29;
V37 = *V999+*F4+E37;
V45 = *V999+*F4+E45;
V53 = *V999+*F4+E53;
V61 = *V999+*F4+E61;
V69 = *V999+*F4+E69;
/VARIANCES
 .
 .
 .
/COVARIANCES
F1 to F4 = *;
E29,E22 = *;
/PRINT
Fit = all;
/END

THE EQS OUTPUT FILE

In addition to the goodness-of-fit statistics, EQS provides a tremendous amount of helpful and important information related to missing data, some of which is introduced here. Although this material was presented in the separate model output for the Nigerians, it was not, of course in the output for the Australians. However, in the multigroup configural model, specification related to missing data must be the same across the two groups regardless of the fact that the data are complete for the Australians. The related output is presented in Table 9.3 for the Australians and in Table 9.4 for the Nigerians.

In the EQS output for the Australians, we see that there were no cases with missing data; therefore, data from all 497 cases were used in the analysis. The output for the Nigerians is a totally different picture. Here we note first a warning that, of the 465 cases in the data set, two were skipped because all variables were missing. Thus, the sample size is now 463 rather than 465.

Next we are advised that, of the 463 cases, there are 93 with missing data, thereby resulting in 48 different patterns of missing data. The program presents a summary of these various data patterns. Let's examine a few of these entries. Following the column headings, we determine that in the first row, there are 370 (79.91%) cases with no missing data. In the second row, there is one case with 13 missing scores on Variables 4 and 13 through 24 inclusive. In the third row, there are two cases with missing data on 12 variables (V13–V24) inclusive. In the fourth row, there is one case with missing data on four variables (V21–V24) inclusive, and so on. In reviewing these missing data patterns, it is evident that both the amount and type of data available across all cases vary immensely. Following this missing data pattern summary, EQS prints a pair-wise-present covariance matrix showing the sample sizes for each pair of cases. Also provided in the output are three sets of estimates of means and covariance matrices: (a) ML estimates of means

TABLE 9.3

Selected EQS Output: Missing Data Specification for Australian Adolescents

---

MULTIPLE POPULATION ANALYSIS, INFORMATION IN GROUP 1

MAXIMUM LIKELIHOOD SOLUTION (NORMAL DISTRIBUTION THEORY)

```
NUMBER OF CASES USED                 =   497
NUMBER OF CASES WITH POSITIVE WEIGHT =   497
NUMBER OF CASES WITH MISSING DATA    =     0
NUMBER OF MISSING PATTERNS IN THE DATA =   1
```

IN THE SUMMARY OF MISSING PATTERNS, M REPRESENTS A MISSING VALUE

```
                              VARIABLES
    #        #        %        1          2          3
 MISSING   CASES    CASES   12345678901234567890123456789012
 -------   -----    -----
       0     497   100.00
```

TABLE 9.4

Selected EQS Output: Missing Data Specification for Nigerian Adolescents

---

`*** WARNING *** THESE CASES ARE SKIPPED BECAUSE ALL VARIABLES ARE MISSING--`
     `265   272`

MULTIPLE POPULATION ANALYSIS, INFORMATION IN GROUP 2

MAXIMUM LIKELIHOOD SOLUTION (NORMAL DISTRIBUTION THEORY)

```
NUMBER OF CASES USED                    =   463
NUMBER OF CASES WITH POSITIVE WEIGHT    =   463
NUMBER OF CASES WITH MISSING DATA       =    93
NUMBER OF MISSING PATTERNS IN THE DATA  =    48
```

IN THE SUMMARY OF MISSING PATTERNS, M REPRESENTS A MISSING VALUE

```
                                    VARIABLES
    #        #        %              1         2         3
MISSING    CASES    CASES   123456789012345678901234567890 12
-------    -----    -----
      0      370    79.91
     13        1     .22    M           MMMMMMMMMMM
     12        2     .43                MMMMMMMMMMM
      4        1     .22                    MMMM
      1        3     .65                    M
      2        1     .22                    M       M
      1        2     .43                         M
      1        3     .65                          M
      1        2     .43                   M
      3        1     .22                   M       M       M
      1        2     .43                       M
      1        3     .65                          M
      2        1     .22                         MM
      1        1     .22                           M
      1        1     .22                             M
      2        1     .22                M             M
      1        4     .86                M
      3        1     .22                MM        M
      4       10    2.16               MMM        M
      5        1     .22               MMM        M       M
      6        1     .22    M          MMM        M       M
      2        6    1.30                  M        M
      3        1     .22               M  M        M
      1        3     .65                M
      2        1     .22                M              M
      1        2     .43                              M
      1        2     .43                    M
      1        3     .65                       M
      1        1     .22                        M
      1        2     .43    M
      2        1     .22    M        M
      1        1     .22                   M
      1        1     .22                             M
      2        1     .22                M             M
      1        1     .22                M
```

TABLE 9.4

(Continued)

```
   #        #        %             1         2         3
MISSING   CASES    CASES   12345678901234567890123456789012
-------   -----    -----
   1        1       .22         M
   1        2       .43                   M
   1        2       .43      M
   2        1       .22      M M
   1        3       .65                              M
   2        1       .22         M                    M
   2        1       .22                              M     M
   1        1       .22      M
   1        1       .22                    M
   1        1       .22                 M
   4        1       .22            M     M  M                M
   8        9      1.94                            MMMMMMMM
   6        1       .22      MMMM   M              M
```

TABLE 9.5

Selected EQS Output: GLS Tests of Missingness for Nigerian Adolescents

GLS TEST OF HOMOGENEITY OF MEANS

```
CHI-SQUARE =      1796.254 BASED ON     1388 DEGREES OF FREEDOM
PROBABILITY VALUE FOR THE CHI-SQUARE STATISTIC IS      .00000
```

GLS TEST OF HOMOGENEITY OF COVARIANCE MATRICES

```
CHI-SQUARE =     18983.662 BASED ON     8821 DEGREES OF FREEDOM
PROBABILITY VALUE FOR THE CHI-SQUARE STATISTIC IS      .00000
```

GLS COMBINED TEST OF HOMOGENEITY OF MEANS/COVARIANCES

```
CHI-SQUARE =     20779.916 BASED ON    10209 DEGREES OF FREEDOM
PROBABILITY VALUE FOR THE CHI-SQUARE STATISTIC IS      .00000
```

and covariance matrix based on the saturated (unstructured) model, (b) imputed estimates of means and sample covariance matrix based on the saturated model, and (c) imputed means and sample covariance matrix based on the structured model. The residual matrix used to evaluate fit is computed as (b)-(c). Readers are referred (to the manual [Bentler, 2005] for more details related to these matrices).

In addition to this output, EQS also provides information related to the extent to which the various patterns of data can be considered as samples from a single population with one mean (μ) and one covariance matrix (Σ). This information derives from three GLS tests of homogeneity: means, covariance matrices, and means and covariances combined (Kim & Bentler, 2002). These results are shown in Table 9.5.

In a cursory overview of these reported findings, you might be somewhat astounded at the large number of df. However, given that these tests (particularly the combined test reported here) reflect the many means and covariances from numerous patterns of data but with relatively few estimated common means and covariances, the df are exceedingly large. Probability values >0.05 provide support that the various patterns of missing data represent samples from a single population. Review of results from the three tests clearly show that the various patterns of data for Nigerian adolescents differ among themselves in terms of means and covariances, as evidenced by the probability values of 0.0 associated with each. Thus, technically, some of the missing data patterns provide different estimates of μ and Σ. However, given that the bulk of the data comprises 80% of the cases and the many patterns have few cases, the results of these tests are not discussed further. EQS currently provides no suggestions on which patterns might be deviant, and Bentler (2005) suggests that there are times that this test can be ignored.

Testing for Invariance of Factor Loadings

As illustrated in chapter 7, in testing for the invariance of factor loadings across groups, equality constraints were imposed on all factor loadings except (a) those that were fixed to 1.00 for identification and scaling,[5] and (b) the cross-loading specific to Australian adolescents. This test yielded a marginally acceptable fit to the multisample data (i.e., Y-B$\chi^2_{(940)}$ = 1810.03; SRMR = 0.07; *CFI = 0.91; *RMSEA = 0.03; 90% C.I. = 0.029, 0.033). However, these results are not surprising given the size of the model and the fact that the baseline model for Australian adolescents fit the data less well than for the Nigerian adolescents.

THE EQS OUTPUT FILE

Results arising from this test for invariant factor loadings are shown in Table 9.6. Review of the LM Test statistics related to this model reveals four univariate incremental χ^2 values with probabilities less than 0.05. A check of these parameters against the list of constraints to be released shows that they represent two items (24 and 40) measuring Factor 2 (Physical SC, ability) and two items (19 and 26) measuring Factor 4 (Social SC, Parents). These same items were cited previously with respect to their error covariances relative to the baseline models. Nonetheless, their content is repeated as follows:

- Item 24: I enjoy sports and games.
- Item 40: I am good at sports.
- Item 19: I like my parents.
- Item 26: My parents like me.

---

[5] Actually, EQS prompts the user with an error message if equality constraints on these fixed parameters are imposed.

TABLE 9.6
Selected EQS Output: Test for Invariant Factor Loadings - LM Test Statistics

LAGRANGE MULTIPLIER TEST (FOR RELEASING CONSTRAINTS)

CONSTRAINTS TO BE RELEASED ARE:

CONSTRAINTS FROM GROUP 2

CONSTR:	1	(1,V8,F1)-(2,V11,F1)=0;
CONSTR:	2	(1,V15,F1)-(2,V18,F1)=0;
CONSTR:	3	(1,V22,F1)-(2,V25,F1)=0;
CONSTR:	4	(1,V38,F1)-(2,V41,F1)=0;
CONSTR:	5	(1,V46,F1)-(2,V49,F1)=0;
CONSTR:	6	(1,V54,F1)-(2,V57,F1)=0;
CONSTR:	7	(1,V62,F1)-(2,V65,F1)=0;
CONSTR:	8	(1,V10,F2)-(2,V13,F2)=0;
CONSTR:	9	(1,V24,F2)-(2,V27,F2)=0;
CONSTR:	10	(1,V32,F2)-(2,V35,F2)=0;
CONSTR:	11	(1,V40,F2)-(2,V43,F2)=0;
CONSTR:	12	(1,V48,F2)-(2,V51,F2)=0;
CONSTR:	13	(1,V56,F2)-(2,V59,F2)=0;
CONSTR:	14	(1,V64,F2)-(2,V67,F2)=0;
CONSTR:	15	(1,V14,F3)-(2,V17,F3)=0;
CONSTR:	16	(1,V28,F3)-(2,V31,F3)=0;
CONSTR:	17	(1,V36,F3)-(2,V39,F3)=0;
CONSTR:	18	(1,V44,F3)-(2,V47,F3)=0;
CONSTR:	19	(1,V52,F3)-(2,V55,F3)=0;
CONSTR:	20	(1,V60,F3)-(2,V63,F3)=0;
CONSTR:	21	(1,V69,F3)-(2,V72,F3)=0;
CONSTR:	22	(1,V19,F4)-(2,V22,F4)=0;
CONSTR:	23	(1,V26,F4)-(2,V29,F4)=0;
CONSTR:	24	(1,V34,F4)-(2,V37,F4)=0;
CONSTR:	25	(1,V42,F4)-(2,V45,F4)=0;
CONSTR:	26	(1,V50,F4)-(2,V53,F4)=0;
CONSTR:	27	(1,V58,F4)-(2,V61,F4)=0;
CONSTR:	28	(1,V66,F4)-(2,V69,F4)=0;

		CUMULATIVE MULTIVARIATE STATISTICS			UNIVARIATE INCREMENT	
STEP	PARAMETER	CHI-SQUARE	D.F.	PROBABILITY	CHI-SQUARE	PROBABILITY
1	CONSTR: 9	18.163	1	.000	18.163	.000
2	CONSTR: 11	28.415	2	.000	10.252	.001
3	CONSTR: 23	34.953	3	.000	6.538	.011
4	CONSTR: 22	44.684	4	.000	9.730	.002
5	CONSTR: 19	48.570	5	.000	3.886	.049
6	CONSTR: 7	51.831	6	.000	3.261	.071
7	CONSTR: 4	54.606	7	.000	2.774	.096
8	CONSTR: 20	57.245	8	.000	2.639	.104
9	CONSTR: 13	59.272	9	.000	2.028	.154
10	CONSTR: 24	60.738	10	.000	1.465	.226

From a substantive perspective, the challenging question to be answered (if it is even possible) is: What is it about the content of these items that cause them to be differentially valid across the two cultural groups? Although space limitations prevent a full exploration of possible reasons, an elaboration of the topic as it relates to the current data for both cultural groups is presented in Byrne and Watkins (2003) and Byrne (2003).

Testing Invariance of Common Error Covariance

As discussed in chapter 7, testing for the invariance of error variance is considered extremely stringent and unnecessary (see, e.g., Widaman & Reise, 1997). Nonetheless, given that the error covariance between Items 26 and 19 is an important parameter in the baseline models for both Australian and Nigerian adolescents, I consider it important from a psychometric perspective to test for its invariance across the two groups. Before testing for this equivalency, however, the issue of the four noninvariant factor loadings needs to be addressed; accordingly, these constraints are released, thereby allowing the parameters to be freely estimated.

Results related to the testing of this model yielded a slightly better fit to the data than was the case for the last model (i.e., Y-B$\chi^2_{(937)}$ = 1728.78; SRMR = .06; *CFI = .92; *RMSEA = .03; 90% C.I. = .027, .032). The drop from 940 df to 937 df is accounted for by the estimation of the four freely estimated factor loadings, which is offset by the added equality constraint placed on one error covariance, thus leading to a reduction of 3 df.

EQS output showing LM Test statistics is presented in Table 9.7. As you will readily see, the error covariance under test was found to be invariant across the two groups; given the previous findings of noninvariant factor loadings related to Items 19 and 26, this result is somewhat surprising. However, this analysis revealed two additional factor loadings to be noninvariant across groups: Item 62 measuring Factor 1 (Physical SC, Appearance) and Item 52 measuring Factor 3 (Social SC, Peers). The content of these items is as follows:

- Item 62: I have nice features like nose, and eyes, and hair.
- Item 52: I have more friends than most other kids.

Testing for Invariance of Intercepts

Thus far in this chapter, all analyses have been based on the analysis of COVS. As discussed previously, researchers interested in testing for the invariance of the factor covariances—a focus of substantial interest in construct validity work—would continue their investigation within the framework of COVS. However, when interest focuses on differences in latent factor means, the next step in the process necessarily involves testing for the invariance of the intercepts. These tests must

TABLE 9.7

Selected EQS Output: Test for Invariant Common Error Covariance - LM Test Statistics

LAGRANGE MULTIPLIER TEST (FOR RELEASING CONSTRAINTS)

CONSTRAINTS TO BE RELEASED ARE:

CONSTRAINTS FROM GROUP 2

CONSTR:	1	(1,V8,F1)-(2,V11,F1)=0;
CONSTR:	2	(1,V15,F1)-(2,V18,F1)=0;
CONSTR:	3	(1,V22,F1)-(2,V25,F1)=0;
CONSTR:	4	(1,V38,F1)-(2,V41,F1)=0;
CONSTR:	5	(1,V46,F1)-(2,V49,F1)=0;
CONSTR:	6	(1,V54,F1)-(2,V57,F1)=0;
CONSTR:	7	(1,V62,F1)-(2,V65,F1)=0;
CONSTR:	8	(1,V10,F2)-(2,V13,F2)=0;
CONSTR:	9	(1,V32,F2)-(2,V35,F2)=0;
CONSTR:	10	(1,V48,F2)-(2,V51,F2)=0;
CONSTR:	11	(1,V56,F2)-(2,V59,F2)=0;
CONSTR:	12	(1,V64,F2)-(2,V67,F2)=0;
CONSTR:	13	(1,V14,F3)-(2,V17,F3)=0;
CONSTR:	14	(1,V28,F3)-(2,V31,F3)=0;
CONSTR:	15	(1,V36,F3)-(2,V39,F3)=0;
CONSTR:	16	(1,V44,F3)-(2,V47,F3)=0;
CONSTR:	17	(1,V52,F3)-(2,V55,F3)=0;
CONSTR:	18	(1,V60,F3)-(2,V63,F3)=0;
CONSTR:	19	(1,V69,F3)-(2,V72,F3)=0;
CONSTR:	20	(1,V34,F4)-(2,V37,F4)=0;
CONSTR:	21	(1,V42,F4)-(2,V45,F4)=0;
CONSTR:	22	(1,V50,F4)-(2,V53,F4)=0;
CONSTR:	23	(1,V58,F4)-(2,V61,F4)=0;
CONSTR:	24	(1,V66,F4)-(2,V69,F4)=0;
CONSTR:	25	(1,E26,E19)-(2,E29,E22)=0;

		CUMULATIVE MULTIVARIATE STATISTICS				UNIVARIATE INCREMENT	
STEP	PARAMETER	CHI-SQUARE	D.F.	PROBABILITY		CHI-SQUARE	PROBABILITY
1	CONSTR: 17	7.633	1	.006		7.633	.006
2	CONSTR: 7	13.612	2	.001		5.979	.014
3	CONSTR: 11	17.447	3	.001		3.835	.050
4	CONSTR: 18	20.544	4	.000		3.098	.078
5	CONSTR: 4	23.672	5	.000		3.128	.077
6	CONSTR: 22	26.107	6	.000		2.435	.119
7	CONSTR: 1	28.211	7	.000		2.103	.147
8	CONSTR: 15	30.429	8	.000		2.218	.136
9	CONSTR: 24	31.986	9	.000		1.557	.212
10	CONSTR: 12	33.514	10	.000		1.529	.216

be based on the analysis of MACS. Meredith (1993) argued that only tests based on the analysis of MACS allow for "strong" tests for invariance; those based on the analysis of COVS are only capable of testing for "weak" forms of invariance. At first blush, Meredith's categorization of invariance tests as "weak" versus "strong" would appear to cast a rather negative shadow over such tests based only on the analysis of COVS, with the implication that the latter are in some way less worthy than those based on the analysis of MACS. Realistically, this perceived implication does not hold because the analysis of only COVS may be the most appropriate approach to take in addressing the issues and interests of a particular study.

Testing for the invariance of intercepts across groups entailed equality constraints being placed on all invariant factor loadings, the common error covariance (E26,E19), and all observed variable intercepts—regardless of whether the factor loading for a variable is fixed to 1.0 for model identification and latent variable scaling or freely estimated due to its noninvariance across groups. It may be helpful to review the modeling of these parameters as shown in Fig. 9.4.

Results from this test yielded a modestly well-fitting model (i.e., Y-B$\chi^2_{(967)}$ = 2483.21; SRMR = .11; *CFI = .92; *RMSEA = .04; 90% C.I. = .038, .042). Review of the LM Test statistics, however, revealed 25 of the 32 intercepts to be noninvariant; these results are shown in Table 9.8.

The question is: How does a researcher interpret and make sense of these noninvariant intercepts? Chan (2000) presented one useful approach to the interpretation of noninvariant findings by weaving together application based on the analysis of MACS with interpretation based on Item Response Theory (IRT) analysis. (For an application based on this approach, see Byrne and Stewart [in press]). In testing for the invariance of a measuring instrument within the framework of MACS based on CFA modeling, interest focuses on the extent to which the factor loadings and intercepts are equivalent across groups. In testing for such equality based on IRT modeling, analyses seek to identify differential item functioning (DIF), with interest focusing on two characteristics (termed *parameters* in IRT lexicon) associated with each item: the level of item difficulty and the level of item discrimination—both of which describe the link between a test item and its underlying latent factor (Widaman & Reise, 1997). Within the framework of MACS, Chan (2000) and Ferrando (1996) (see also Widaman & Reise, 1997) show that the item intercept corresponds to the item difficulty parameter, whereas the item factor loading is analogous to the item discrimination parameter. Interpreted within the CFA framework, the higher an intercept value (or item difficulty level), the more attractive the item is in the sense that its average response level reflects its stronger endorsement. In contrast, the higher a factor-loading value (or item discrimination level), the more concrete (i.e., less ambiguous) an item is perceived to be (Chan, 2000; and Ferrando, 1996).

Presented with evidence of noninvariance related to factor loadings and intercepts, Cooke, Kosson, and Michie (2001) contended that of the two, noninvariant factor loadings are by far the more serious. They further argue that group differences in intercepts need not preclude the usefulness of these items in measuring their underlying constructs. As a result, we now move on to test for differences in the latent factor means, forcing the intercepts to be identical across groups.

LAGRANGE MULTIPLIER TEST (FOR RELEASING CONSTRAINTS)

CONSTRAINTS TO BE RELEASED ARE:
      CONSTRAINTS FROM GROUP 2

CONSTR:	1	(1,V8,F1)-(2,V11,F1)=0;
CONSTR:	2	(1,V15,F1)-(2,V18,F1)=0;
CONSTR:	3	(1,V22,F1)-(2,V25,F1)=0;
CONSTR:	4	(1,V38,F1)-(2,V41,F1)=0;
CONSTR:	5	(1,V46,F1)-(2,V49,F1)=0;
CONSTR:	6	(1,V54,F1)-(2,V57,F1)=0;
CONSTR:	7	(1,V10,F2)-(2,V13,F2)=0;
CONSTR:	8	(1,V32,F2)-(2,V35,F2)=0;
CONSTR:	9	(1,V48,F2)-(2,V51,F2)=0;
CONSTR:	10	(1,V56,F2)-(2,V59,F2)=0;
CONSTR:	11	(1,V64,F2)-(2,V67,F2)=0;
CONSTR:	12	(1,V14,F3)-(2,V17,F3)=0;
CONSTR:	13	(1,V28,F3)-(2,V31,F3)=0;
CONSTR:	14	(1,V36,F3)-(2,V39,F3)=0;
CONSTR:	15	(1,V44,F3)-(2,V47,F3)=0;
CONSTR:	16	(1,V60,F3)-(2,V63,F3)=0;
CONSTR:	17	(1,V69,F3)-(2,V72,F3)=0;
CONSTR:	18	(1,V34,F4)-(2,V37,F4)=0;
CONSTR:	19	(1,V42,F4)-(2,V45,F4)=0;
CONSTR:	20	(1,V50,F4)-(2,V53,F4)=0;
CONSTR:	21	(1,V58,F4)-(2,V61,F4)=0;
CONSTR:	22	(1,V66,F4)-(2,V69,F4)=0;
CONSTR:	23	(1,E26,E19)-(2,E29,E22)=0;
CONSTR:	24	(1,V1,V999)-(2,V4,V999)=0;
CONSTR:	25	(1,V8,V999)-(2,V11,V999)=0;
CONSTR:	26	(1,V15,V999)-(2,V18,V999)=0;
CONSTR:	27	(1,V22,V999)-(2,V25,V999)=0;
CONSTR:	28	(1,V38,V999)-(2,V41,V999)=0;
CONSTR:	29	(1,V46,V999)-(2,V49,V999)=0;
CONSTR:	30	(1,V54,V999)-(2,V57,V999)=0;
CONSTR:	31	(1,V62,V999)-(2,V65,V999)=0;
CONSTR:	32	(1,V3,V999)-(2,V6,V999)=0;
CONSTR:	33	(1,V10,V999)-(2,V13,V999)=0;
CONSTR:	34	(1,V24,V999)-(2,V27,V999)=0;
CONSTR:	35	(1,V32,V999)-(2,V35,V999)=0;
CONSTR:	36	(1,V40,V999)-(2,V43,V999)=0;
CONSTR:	37	(1,V48,V999)-(2,V51,V999)=0;
CONSTR:	38	(1,V56,V999)-(2,V59,V999)=0;
CONSTR:	39	(1,V64,V999)-(2,V67,V999)=0;
CONSTR:	40	(1,V7,V999)-(2,V10,V999)=0;
CONSTR:	41	(1,V14,V999)-(2,V17,V999)=0;
CONSTR:	42	(1,V28,V999)-(2,V31,V999)=0;
CONSTR:	43	(1,V36,V999)-(2,V39,V999)=0;
CONSTR:	44	(1,V44,V999)-(2,V47,V999)=0;
CONSTR:	45	(1,V52,V999)-(2,V55,V999)=0;
CONSTR:	46	(1,V60,V999)-(2,V63,V999)=0;
CONSTR:	47	(1,V69,V999)-(2,V72,V999)=0;
CONSTR:	48	(1,V5,V999)-(2,V8,V999)=0;
CONSTR:	49	(1,V19,V999)-(2,V22,V999)=0;
CONSTR:	50	(1,V26,V999)-(2,V29,V999)=0;
CONSTR:	51	(1,V34,V999)-(2,V37,V999)=0;
CONSTR:	52	(1,V42,V999)-(2,V45,V999)=0;
CONSTR:	53	(1,V50,V999)-(2,V53,V999)=0;
CONSTR:	54	(1,V58,V999)-(2,V61,V999)=0;
CONSTR:	55	(1,V66,V999)-(2,V69,V999)=0;

(Continued)

TABLE 9.8

(Continued)

		CUMULATIVE MULTIVARIATE STATISTICS			UNIVARIATE INCREMENT	
STEP	PARAMETER	CHI-SQUARE	D.F.	PROBABILITY	CHI-SQUARE	PROBABILITY
1	CONSTR: 40	70.621	1	.000	70.621	.000
2	CONSTR: 35	121.755	2	.000	51.134	.000
3	CONSTR: 33	153.070	3	.000	31.315	.000
4	CONSTR: 39	185.873	4	.000	32.803	.000
5	CONSTR: 34	202.710	5	.000	16.837	.000
6	CONSTR: 43	218.708	6	.000	15.998	.000
7	CONSTR: 46	234.300	7	.000	15.592	.000
8	CONSTR: 24	245.381	8	.000	11.082	.001
9	CONSTR: 29	257.586	9	.000	12.204	.000
10	CONSTR: 26	269.816	10	.000	12.230	.000
11	CONSTR: 27	282.710	11	.000	12.895	.000
12	CONSTR: 28	300.923	12	.000	18.212	.000
13	CONSTR: 25	315.878	13	.000	14.955	.000
14	CONSTR: 31	343.879	14	.000	28.001	.000
15	CONSTR: 30	376.739	15	.000	32.860	.000
16	CONSTR: 36	388.656	16	.000	11.918	.001
17	CONSTR: 37	400.649	17	.000	11.993	.001
18	CONSTR: 44	410.047	18	.000	9.398	.002
19	CONSTR: 45	417.974	19	.000	7.928	.005
20	CONSTR: 47	425.674	20	.000	7.699	.006
21	CONSTR: 41	436.185	21	.000	10.511	.001
22	CONSTR: 53	442.955	22	.000	6.771	.009
23	CONSTR: 52	449.414	23	.000	6.459	.011
24	CONSTR: 51	455.743	24	.000	6.329	.012
25	CONSTR: 1	458.960	25	.000	3.217	.073
26	CONSTR: 42	461.493	26	.000	2.533	.112
27	CONSTR: 49	464.118	27	.000	2.626	.105
28	CONSTR: 50	469.093	28	.000	4.974	.026
29	CONSTR: 11	471.238	29	.000	2.145	.143
30	CONSTR: 9	474.105	30	.000	2.867	.090

Testing the Invariance of Latent Factor Means

Previously in this chapter (see Fig. 9.1), we reviewed a simple CFA model, presented first as a COVS structure and then as a MACS structure. Analogously, in Fig. 9.5, the MACS model as it relates to the cross-cultural application is presented. However, for reasons of clarity and simplicity, I present only the baseline model for the Australian group. Also included in the model shown in Fig. 9.5 is a variety of symbols associated with particular parameters, which I hope will be helpful to you in visualizing the test for latent factor mean differences.

Before explaining the symbols in this model, however, we briefly review three major changes that occur in the transition from a COVS model to a MACS model to test for latent mean differences. First, given that latent factor means are represented

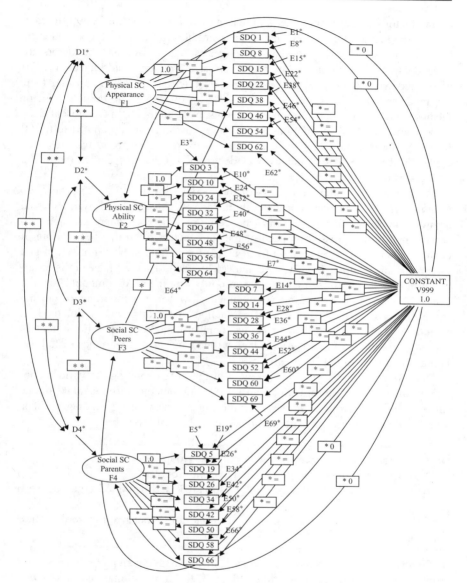

FIG. 9.5. Mean structure model representing test for latent factor mean differences.

by the factor intercepts (i.e., the path leading from the Constant [V999] to each factor), the factors thus become dependent variables in the model; consequently, their variances and covariances are no longer estimable. Because the factors are dependent variables in the model, they each have a related disturbance term (D) associated with them, and these residuals operate as proxies in carrying their variances and covariances. Second, in testing for differences in the latent factor means, the factor intercepts for one group must be fixed to 0.0. In the present case, these intercepts were specified as free for the Australian group and fixed to 0.0 for the Nigerian group; the latter then served as the reference group against which evidence of statistical significance was determined. Finally, specification of the LM Test is not included in the input file.

We now examine the parameters of the model shown in Fig. 9.5. There are four factors (F1–F4), each correlated with the other as indicated by the curved arrows connecting their related disturbance terms (D1–D4). There are eight observed measures regressed on each of the four factors, with the first loading of each congeneric set of measures fixed at 1.0 for purposes of identification and latent variable scaling. Finally, associated with each observed measure is an error term (E). To minimize the graphics in portraying the MACS model shown in Fig. 9.5, the error covariances are not included. However, it is important to note that these parameters were, of course, still maintained in the original baseline models, with the error covariance between Items 26 and 19 and between Items 40 and 24 estimated for the Australian group, albeit with the one error covariance (E26,E19) being constrained equal across groups.

The explanation of symbols presented in Fig. 9.5. depicting the various constraints in the model is meant only as an aid to a simultaneous portrayal of the model representing each group of adolescents; it is not a conventional path diagram. The symbols denoting these constraints are explained as follows:

>   * A parameter to be freely estimated in one group.
>   ** A parameter to be freely estimated in each group.
> *= A parameter that although freely estimated is constrained equal across groups.
> *0 A parameter to be freely estimated in one group but fixed to zero in the other group.

So now, let's once again review Fig. 9.5, this time taking all paths and assigned symbols into account. Interpretation of the model can be summarized as follows:

- As indicated by the assigned * *'s, the variances of the D's are freely estimated in each group, as are the covariances among them.
- To minimize clutter in the diagram, the variances of the E's are assigned *'s. However, they are freely estimated in each group.
- As indicated by the assigned *, the cross-loading of Item 38 (SDQ 38) on F3 is freely estimated only for the Australian group.

- As indicated by the assigned * =, all factor loadings are constrained equal across groups except for those factor loadings fixed to 1.00.
- As indicated by the assigned * =, all intercepts for the observed measures are constrained equal across groups.
- As indicated by the assigned * 0, the four factor intercepts are freely estimated in one group (Australians) and constrained equal to zero in the other group (Nigerians); the latter is therefore regarded as the "reference" group.
- As noted previously, variance associated with the constant (V999) is not estimated; the constant remains fixed to 1.00.

Before turning to the EQS input file related to this model, it is worthwhile to review two important points with respect to MACS models. First, the number of estimated intercepts must be less than the number of measured variables. In a multigroup model, this is controlled by the imposition of equality constraints across the groups. In the present case, review of the structured-means portion of the model in Fig. 9.5 reveals 64 measured variables (32 for each group). Relatedly, there are 64 observed variable intercepts; of these, 32 are freely estimated for the Australian group and 32 are constrained equal across the Nigerian group. In addition, there are four intercept parameters for factors being estimated. Thus, these model parameters are overidentified, with 28 df.

Second, in the present application, we are primarily interested in the comparison of latent mean values and, thus, in values representing the factor intercepts only. Nonetheless, a brief explanation of effects related to the observed variable intercepts is helpful. When there are no indirect effects, the variable intercepts should equal the actual observed means if the model is plausible. Relatedly, because the factor intercepts are fixed to zero for the Nigerian group (the reference group), there are consequently no indirect effects; thus, the expected means should approximate the observed sample means for that group. For the Australian group, expected means for the measured variables derive from the indirect effect of the constant via the related factor and its loading plus the direct effect of the constant on the variable itself.

THE EQS INPUT FILE

Table 9.9 shows selected portions of the input file used in testing for differences in the latent factor means. Given that this input basically replicates the one for testing the configural model shown in Table 9.2, only the portions of the file relevant to the present analysis are included.

In the /EQUATIONS paragraph for Group 1, Australian adolescents, there are four entries for the factor intercepts; these represent the latent factor means and are therefore estimated for the Australian group. Under the /VARIANCES paragraph, only variances related to the disturbance terms (D1–D4) are shown. In the /COVARIANCES paragraph, the specification of their covariances, along with

TABLE 9.9

Selected EQS Input: Test for Latent Mean Differences

```
/TITLE
Testing for Invariance of SDQ Nonacademic SCs "sdqinvan5"
GROUP1: Australian Adolescents
TESTING FOR LATENT MEAN DIFFERENCES
  - ALL INTERCEPTS INVARIANT
  - 6 NONINVARIANT FACTOR LOADINGS RELEASED
  - 1 ERROR CORR (E26,E19) INVARIANT
/SPECIFICATIONS
    .
    .
    .
/LABELS
    .
    .
    .
/EQUATIONS
V1 = *V999+F1+E1;
    .
    .
    .
F1 = *V999+D1;
F2 = *V999+D2;
F3 = *V999+D3;
F4 = *V999+D4;
/VARIANCES
    .
    .
    .
D1 to D4 = *;
/COVARIANCES
D1 to D4 = *;
E40,E24 = *;  E26,E19 = *;
/END
/TITLE
GROUP2: NIGERIAN ADOLESCENTS
/SPECIFICATIONS
    .
    .
    .
/LABELS
    .
    .
    .
/EQUATIONS
V4 = *V999+F1+E4;
    .
    .
    .
F1 = 0.0 V999+D1;
F2 = 0.0 V999+D2;
F3 = 0.0 V999+D3;
F4 = 0.0 V999+D4;
/VARIANCES
    .
    .
    .
D1 to D4 = *;
/COVARIANCES
D1 to D4 = *;
E29,E22 = *;
/PRINT
Fit = all;
/CONSTRAINTS
    .
    .
    .
/END
```

---

the two error covariances specific to this group, are shown. The main point to be made with specifications related to the Nigerian group lies within the /EQUATIONS paragraph, where we see the factor intercepts are fixed to zero. Of course, the constraints specified for this model are consistent with those specified for the configural model (see Table 9.2).

THE EQS OUTPUT FILE

To answer the primary question of whether the latent factor means for the two cultural groups are significantly different, interest focuses on the construct equations. Given that the Nigerian group was designated as the reference group—thus, their factor means were fixed to zero—we concentrate solely on estimates as they relate to the Australian group. These equations are presented in Table 9.10. The key parameters in answering this question are the factor intercepts as they represent the latent mean values. Because analyses were based on the robust statistics, these estimates are interpreted in terms of the robust standard errors and the resulting z-statistics. Accordingly, these results indicate that whereas the means of Factor 1 (Physical SC, Appearance) and Factor 3 (Social SC, Peers) for Australian

TABLE 9.10
Selected EQS Output: Group 1 Latent Mean Estimates

CONSTRUCT EQUATIONS WITH STANDARD ERRORS AND TEST STATISTICS
STATISTICS SIGNIFICANT AT THE 5% LEVEL ARE MARKED WITH @.
(ROBUST STATISTICS IN PARENTHESES)

```
     F1   =F1   =    -1.136*V999   +   1.000 D1
                         .060
                      -18.868@
                    (    .058)
                    ( -19.714@
     F2   =F2   =      .040*V999    +   1.000 D2
                         .062
                         .648
                    (    .059)
                    (    .673)
     F3   =F3   =     -.275*V999    +   1.000 D3
                         .036
                       -7.693@
                    (    .034)
                    (  -8.088@
     F4   =F4   =     -.076*V999    +   1.000 D4
                         .044
                       -1.730
                    (    .042)
                    (  -1.811)
```

adolescents were significantly different from those for Nigerian adolescents, the means for Factor 2 (Physical SC, Ability) and Factor 4 (Social SC, Parents) were not. More specifically, in light of the negative signs associated with these statistically significant values, the findings convey the notion that Physical SC as it relates to appearance, and Social SC as it relates to the peer group for Australian adolescents, appear to be less positive on average than is the case for Nigerian adolescents. That is, Australian youth report being more negative about their appearance and social self-concepts than Nigerian youth. Such a mean difference effect cannot be found when only covariances are analyzed.

The interesting question now, of course, is why these results should be what they are. Most appropriately, interpretation must be made within the context of theory and empirical research. However, when data are based on two vastly different cultural groups, such as this case, the task can be particularly challenging. Clearly, knowledge of the societal norms, values, and identities associated with each culture is an important requisite in any speculative interpretation of these findings, a task that is not undertaken herein.

10

Application 8:
Testing for Latent Mean
Differences Based on a
Second-Order CFA Model

As in chapter 9, analyses in this chapter are based on mean and covariance structures (MACS). However, whereas the previous application was based on a first-order CFA model, the work in the present chapter focuses on a higher order CFA model. Building on the work of chapter 9, we test for latent mean differences in both the lower and higher order factors of an assessment measure. In reality, however, the work of this chapter addresses an impossible situation and provides alternative approaches to how a researcher might deal with the situation. Essentially, the major interest of this chapter is to obtain a mean structure for a second-order multiple-group model. However, such models are generally not identified (Lubke, Dolan, & Kelderman, 2001). To obtain any meaningful results, additional specialized constraints have to be added to ordinary mean structure models. Although there is no truly satisfactory solution, the discussion of the issues and an illustration of several approaches on how such constraints might be considered and implemented may be fruitful.

This application is taken from a study by Byrne and Stewart (in press) in which we tested (a) for equivalence of the Beck Depression Inventory II (BDI-II; Beck, Steer, & Brown, 1996) across Hong Kong ($n = 1460$) and American ($n = 451$) nonclinical adolescents, and (b) for latent mean differences in the related underlying constructs. In this chapter, we focus on the latter and test for the extent to which the latent mean scores on three lower order factors (Negative Attitude, Performance Difficulty, Somatic Elements) and one higher order factor (General

Depression) of the BDI-II are equivalent across these two cultural groups. (For more details regarding these samples, see Byrne & Stewart, in press).

TESTING FOR LATENT MEAN DIFFERENCES OF A SECOND-ORDER MODEL

The Strategy

In chapter 9, we tested first for the establishment of a baseline model for each group under study. Once these models were determined, we next combined their specifications into one file and tested for the multigroup fit of these baseline models (termed the *configural model*). These initial tests were then followed by three additional ones that tested for the invariance of factor loadings, observed variable intercepts, and latent factor means. When analyses are based on higher order CFA models, however, the latter three tests for invariance must be conducted for each level of the factor structure (i.e., first- and second-order levels).

THE HYPOTHESIZED MODEL

In chapter 5, we tested for the validity of the BDI (Beck, Ward, Mendelson, Mock, & Erbaugh, 1961) for female adolescent high school students. In this chapter, the work involves the BDI-II, the second edition of this original measure of depression.[1] Essentially, the BDI-II was designed to parallel refinements in the definition of depression and to address recommendations that the instrument be made more compatible with criteria set forth in the diagnostic and statistical manual of mental disorders (DSM-IV; American Psychiatric Association, 1994; Dozois, Dobson, & Ahnberg, 1998). Although the BDI and BDI-II are consistent in being comprised of 21 items based on a four-point scale, several changes were implemented in the latter.[2] First, several items were reworded in the interest of clarity. Second, content designed to tap sleep and appetite changes was modified to reflect both increases and decreases in this behavior. Third, four new items assessing agitation, worthlessness, concentration difficulty, and loss of energy were added, and four old items assessing body image, work difficulty, weight loss, and hypochondria

---

[1]In chapter 5, analyses were based on covariance structures and were able to take the ordinality of the variables into account. However, at the time of writing this book, EQS was not yet capable of basing analyses on categorical data when analyses are based on MACS.

[2]In the present data, Item 21 was not included. This item is designed to tap changes in sexual interest and was considered objectionable by several Hong Kong school principals the item was therefore deleted from the Chinese version of the inventory.

were deleted. Finally, two items were relocated to a different area of the inventory (Beck et al., 1996).

As in chapter 5, the postulated structure of the BDI-II is based on the early work of Byrne and colleagues (for a comprehensive list of studies, see chap. 5).[3] Accordingly, it is argued that scores from the BDI-II are most adequately represented by a hierarchical four-factor structure comprising three first-order factors (Negative Attitude, Performance Difficulty, Somatic Elements) and one higher order factor (General Depression). This hypothesized model is presented schematically in Fig. 10.1.[4] Review of this model, may prompt a query about the rationale in the selection of factor loadings fixed to 1.0 for purposes of model identification and scaling. Although the first of each congeneric set of loadings is typically constrained to 1.00, this specification does not necessarily have to be the case. Indeed, it has been argued that because this loading sets the scale of its underlying latent variable, the strongest factor loading of any set should be the one that is fixed to 1.0. In the present case, exploratory factor analyses revealed the loadings for these items to be similarly the highest across the two groups.

Testing for Baseline Models

Given that the BDI-II is a clinical measure designed to tap aspects of depression, it is not surprising that scores based on this instrument for community samples are typically found to be at least moderately kurtotic. Consistent with past research, analysis of these data revealed substantial multivariate kurtosis, as indicated by Mardia's normalized estimate of 87.15 for Hong Kong adolescents and 75.89 for American adolescents. Consequently, all analyses were based on the robust statistics.

Hong Kong Adolescents

Scores for these adolescents were based on a Chinese version of the BDI-II (Chinese Behavioural Sciences Society, 2000). Cross-validated findings based on three independent groups of Hong Kong adolescents showed the structure displayed in Fig. 10.1 to fit the data extremely well (Byrne, Stewart, & Lee, 2004). As expected, testing of the hypothesized model for the full sample of Hong Kong adolescents yielded an excellent fit to the data (i.e., S-B$\chi^2_{(168)}$ = 491.13; SRMR = .04; *CFI = .95; *RMSEA = .04; 90% C.I. = .033, .040). Given that a review of the LM Test statistics revealed no cause for concern regarding

---

[3]This postulated structure includes the one equality constraint between D1 and D2. This restriction addresses the issue of statistical identification at the higher order level of the model, given only three first-order factors (see chap. 5 for elaboration on this point).

[4]Within each rectangle representing the observed variable, the numeral represents the BDI item number. As such, readers may query why the E labeling does not match these item numbers. The reason is that the first BDI item score entered the data as V5, as shown in the /LABELS paragraph in Table 10.1.

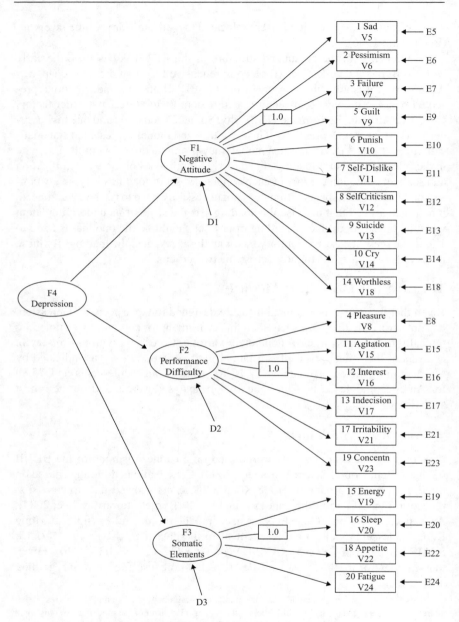

FIG. 10.1. Hypothesized model of second-order factorial structure for the BDI-II (Beck, Steer, & Brown, 1996).

TABLE 10.1

Selected EQS Input: Testing Validity of Configural Model

```
/TITLE
Testing for Invariance of BDI-II across HK and US Adolescents "HKUSInv0"
HK Adolescents (GROUP 1)
No Constraints Imposed
/SPECIFICATIONS
CASE=1460; VAR=44; ME=ML, ROBUST; MA=RAW; Groups=2; FO='(8X,20F1.0,20X)';
DATA='C:\EQS61\Files\Books\Data\BDIHK2C.ess';
/LABELS
V1=Cultural; V2=Linkvar; V3=Gender; V4=Age; V5=1SAD; V6=2PESSM; V7=3FAIL;
V8=4PLEASUR; V9=5GUILT; V10=6PUNISH;  V11=7SELFD;  V12=8SELFCR; 13=9SUICIDE;
V14=10CRY;  V15=11AGITN; V16=12INTRST;  V17=13INDEC; V18=14WORTH; 19=15ENERGY;
V20=16SLEEP; V21=17IRRIT; V22=18APPET;  V23=19CONCN; V24=20FATIG;  V25=H1_2;
V26=H2_2;   V27=H3_2;   V28=H4_2;  V29=H5_2;  V30=H6_2;  V31=H7_2;  V32=H8_2;
V33=H9_2;   V34=H10_2;  V35=H11_2; V36=H12_2; V37=H13_2;  V38=H14_2; V39=H15_2;
V40=H16_2;  V41=H17_2;  V42=H18_2; V43=H19;  V44=H20_2;

F1=NEGATT;   F2=PERFDIFF;   F3=SOMELEM;   F4=DEPRESS;
/EQUATIONS
    V5 =  *F1 + E5;
    V6 =  *F1 + E6;
    V7 =   F1 + E7;
    V9 =  *F1 + E9;
   V10 =  *F1 + E10;
   V11 =  *F1 + E11;
   V12 =  *F1 + E12;
   V13 =  *F1 + E13;
   V14 =  *F1 + E14;
   V18 =  *F1 + E18;
          V8 =  *F2 + E8;
         V15 = *F2 + E15;
         V16 =  F2 + E16  ;
         V17 = *F2 + E17  ;
         V21 = *F2 + E21  ;
         V23 = *F2 + E23  ;
                V19 = *F3 + E19  ;
                V20 =  F3 + E20  ;
                V22 = *F3 + E22  ;
                V24 = *F3 + E24  ;
   F1= *F4 + D1;
   F2= *F4 + D2;
   F3= *F4 + D3;
/VARIANCES
   F4=  1.0;
   D1=  *;
   D2=  *;
   D3=  *;
   E5 to E24 = *;
/END
```

(Continued)

TABLE 10.1

(Continued)

```
/TITLE
 US Adolescents - Group 2
/SPECIFICATIONS
 CASE=451; VAR=44; ME=ML,ROBUST; MA=RAW; FO='(8X,20F1.0,20X)';
 DATA='C:\EQS61\Files\Books\Data\BDIUS2C.ess';
                    ALL INTERVENING SPECIFICATIONS THE SAME AS ABOVE
/CONSTRAINTS
     (D2,D2) = (D1,D1)
/PRINT
 FIT = ALL;
/LMTEST
 SET=PEE,GVF;
/END
```

misspecified parameters, the baseline model for Hong Kong adolescents remained consistent with the hypothesized model.

American Adolescents

Scores for these adolescents were based on the English version of the BDI-II. Testing for the validity of the instrument again yielded an excellent fit to the data for these adolescents, with no reason for respecification of the model (i.e., S-B$\chi^2_{(168)}$ = 234.89; SRMR = .04; *CFI = .97; *RMSEA = .03; 90% C.I. = .020, .038). Thus, the baseline model for American adolescents is also consistent with the hypothesized model.

Testing for Validity of the Configural Model

The EQS input file for this hypothesized model is presented in Table 10.1. However, because the baseline models for both Hong Kong and American adolescents are identical, only an abbreviated version is presented here. Testing for the validity of this configural model yielded an excellent fit to the multisample data (i.e., S-B$\chi^2_{(336)}$ = 707.494; SRMR = .036; *CFI = .950; *RMSEA = .024, 90% C.I. = .022, .027). It is perhaps worth noting that the 336 df represent the sum of the number associated with each separately tested baseline model (i.e., 168).

TESTING FOR INVARIANCE

In the two previous CFA multisample applications tested thus far, we followed the traditional method for determining evidence of noninvariance across groups. However, as discussed in chapter 7, there has been a recent calling among researchers for a more practical approach to this evaluative task (see, e.g., Cheung

& Rensvold, 2002; Little, 1997; Marsh, Hey, & Roche, 1997; and Tomarken & Waller, 2005). Increasingly, these calls have argued for evidence of invariance based on two alternative criteria: (a) the multigroup model exhibits an adequate fit to the data, and (b) the ΔCFI (or Δ*CFI) values between models is negligible. Addressing this concern, Cheung and Rensvold (2002) recently examined the properties of 20 goodness-of-fit indexes within the context of invariance testing and suggested that the ΔCFI, ΔGamma hat, and/or ΔMcDonald's Noncentrality values provide the best information for determining evidence of measurement invariance. With respect to the ΔCFI (or Δ*CFI), they arbitrarily suggest that its difference value should not exceed .01. Given that their research on the topic is the most statistically grounded to date, this criterion of ΔCFI = .01 is likely to become a standard (at least in the short term) among researchers interested in a practical approach to multigroup invariance. To provide a different perspective regarding decisions related to the equality of measurement parameters across groups, in the present chapter, I follow this practical approach and base evidence of invariance on both model goodness-of-fit and *ΔCFI values of less than or equal to 0.01.

Testing for Invariance of Factor Loadings

First-Order Loadings

As is customary, the initial model, in testing for invariance, specified equality constraints on all (except those fixed to 1.00) first-order factor loadings of the BDI-II across Hong Kong and American adolescents. This analysis resulted in a very good fit to the data for this multisample model (i.e., S-B$\chi^2_{(353)}$ = 804.879; SRMR = .063; CFI = .940; RMSEA = .026; 90% C.I. = .024, .028). Comparison of fit between this model (i.e., Model 2) with that for the configural model (i.e., Model 1) yielded a Δ*CFI value of 0.010. Based on both of these criteria, we conclude that the first-order factor loadings are operating in the same way across the two groups of adolescents.

Second-Order Loadings

In testing for the invariance of second-order factor loadings, equality constraints are placed on all first-order as well as second-order loadings. The constraints portion of the input file is shown in Table 10.2. Results from this test again resulted in a well-fitting model (i.e., S-B$\chi^2_{(356)}$ = 809.570; SRMR = .073; CFI = .939; RMSEA = .026; 90% C.I. = .023, .028). The resulting difference in *CFI values between this model (i.e., Model 3) and the configural model (i.e., Model 1) was .011, this time arguing for the invariance of all first- and second-order factor loadings.

TABLE 10.2
Selected EQS Input: Testing Invariance of First- and Second-Order Factor Loadings

---

/TITLE
Testing for Invariance of BDI-II across HK and US Adolescents "HKUSInv2"
HK Adolescents (GROUP 1)
1st-order and 2nd Factor Loadings constrained equal
            .
            .
            .

/CONSTRAINTS
  (D2,D2) = (D1,D1)
  (1,V5,F1) = (2,V5,F1);
  (1,V6,F1) = (2,V6,F1);
  (1,V9,F1) = (2,V9,F1);
  (1,V10,F1) = (2,V10,F1);
  (1,V11,F1) = (2,V11,F1);
  (1,V12,F1) = (2,V12,F1);
  (1,V13,F1) = (2,V13,F1);
  (1,V14,F1) = (2,V14,F1);
  (1,V18,F1) = (2,V18,F1);
  (1,V8,F2) = (2,V8,F2);
  (1,V15,F2) = (2,V15,F2);
  (1,V17,F2) = (2,V17,F2);
  (1,V21,F2) = (2,V21,F2);
  (1,V23,F2) = (2,V23,F2);
  (1,V19,F3) = (2,V19,F3);
  (1,V22,F3) = (2,V22,F3);
  (1,V24,F3) = (2,V24,F3);
  (1,F1,F4) = (2,F1,F4);
  (1,F2,F4) = (2,F2,F4);
  (1,F3,F4) = (2,F3,F4);
/PRINT
  FIT = ALL;
/LMTEST
/END

Testing for Invariance of Intercepts

Observed Variable Intercepts

As discussed in chapter 9, intercepts at the first level of the factor structure represent the means of the observed variables. Given no indirect effects of the constant on the measured variables, each intercept value represents a direct effect and should equal the observed mean. Within the EQS framework, these parameters represent regression paths that lead from the Constant (V999) to each observed variable. In testing for the invariance of observed variable intercepts for a higher order model, equality constraints are imposed on (a) all invariant first-order factor loadings (except those fixed to 1.00), (b) all invariant second-order factor loadings, and (c) all observed variable intercepts (including those associated with variables fixed to 1.00). That is, these parameters are estimated in the first group and then constrained equal across the second group. Results for this test for invariance again yielded a very good fit to the multigroup data (i.e., S-B$\chi^2_{(376)}$ = 1092.765; SRMR = .074; CFI = .939; RMSEA = .032; 90% C.I. = .029, 0.034), with the difference between this model (i.e., Model 4) and the configural model (i.e., Model 1) again yielding a Δ*CFI value of 0.011. To assist in following this series of invariance tests, the partial input file for Model 4 is presented in Table 10.3; model specification for Group 2 is not included because it replicates that for Group 1.

Latent Factor Intercepts

One difficulty that commonly arises in the testing of latent factor intercepts (i.e., intercepts of first-order factors) is that the number of estimated intercepts exceeds the number of observed variables—a situation that is unacceptable in a single group because it leads to model under-identification (Bentler, 2005). In this case, for example, there are 23 intercepts (20 observed variable intercepts and three latent factor intercepts) and only 20 observed variables. Thus, this situation needs to be addressed before we can proceed in testing for the invariance of higher order intercepts. One approach to resolving this difficulty is to constrain the three observed variable intercepts associated with the reference variables (i.e., variables with factor loadings fixed to 1.0); the imposed constraint represents the estimated observed variable intercept value for Group 1. As such, the number of estimated intercepts is reduced from 23 to 20, thereby yielding a just-identified model that is testable. In the present case, these fixed intercepts are V999 → V7, V999 → V16, and V999 → V20; the constrained values are .502, .161, and .580, respectively.[5] With these three constraints in place, invariance of the three latent factor intercepts across the two groups can be tested.

Testing of this model (i.e., Model 5) again yielded a well-fitting model (i.e., S-B$\chi^2_{(376)}$ = 1092.747; SRMR = .074; CFI = .938; RMSEA = .032; 90% C.I. = .029; .034)[6] with negligible change from the previous model (i.e., Model 4), in which the observed variable intercepts were tested for invariance across groups. Comparison of this model with the configural model (i.e., Model 1) yielded a Δ*CFI value of .012.

---

[5]These values were obtained for Group 1 by estimating a model in which the first- and second-order factor loadings were constrained equal across groups but the observed variable intercepts were freely estimated.

[6]Readers may wonder why the number of df (i.e., 376) remains the same as those for Model 4 given that three additional parameters (the latent factor intercepts were estimated). This occurs because three parameters (the observed variable intercepts) were also constrained. As usual, these latent factor intercept parameters were estimated for Group 1 and constrained equal for Group 2.

TABLE 10.3

Selected EQS Input: Testing Invariance of Observed Variable Intercepts

/TITLE
Testing for Invariance of BDI-II across HK and US Adolescents "HKUSInv4"
1st- and 2nd-order factor loadings constrained equal
Observed variable intercepts constrained equal
/SPECIFICATIONS
DATA=' C:\EQS61\Files\Books\Data\BDIHK2C.ess ' ; Groups=2;
CASE=1460; VAR=44; ME=ML,ROBUST; ANAL=MOM; MA=RAW; FO= '(8X,20F1.0,20X)' ;
/LABELS
V1=Cultural; V2=Linkvar; V3=Gender; V4=Age; V5=1SAD; V6=2PESSM; V7=3FAIL; V8=4PLEASUR;
V9=5GUILT; V10=6PUNISH; V11=7SELFD; V12=8SELFCR; V13=9SUICIDE; V14=10CRY; V15=11AGITN;
V16=12INTRST; V17=13INDEC; V18=14WORTH; V19=15ENERGY; V20=16SLEEP; V21=17IRRIT;
V22=18APPET; V23=19CONCN; V24=20FATIG; V25=H1_2; V26=H2_2; V27=H3_2; V28=H4_2; V29=H5_2;
V30=H6_2; V31=H7_2; V32=H8_2; V33=H9_2; V34=H10_2; V35=H11_2; V36=H12_2; V37=H13_2;
V38=H14_2; V39=H15_2; V40=H16_2; V41=H17_2; V42=H18_2; V43=H19; V44=H20_2;

F1=NEGATT; F2=PERFDIFF; F3=SOMELEM; F4=DEPRESS;
/EQUATIONS
    V5 = *V999 + *F1 + E5;
    V6 = *V999 + *F1 + E6;
    V7 = *V999 + F1 + E7;
    V9 = *V999 + *F1 + E9;
    V10 = *V999 + *F1 + E10;
    V11 = *V999 + *F1 + E11;
    V12 = *V999 + *F1 + E12;
    V13 = *V999 + *F1 + E13;
    V14 = *V999 + *F1 + E14;
    V18 = *V999 + *F1 + E18;
      V8 = *V999 + *F2 + E8;
      V15 = *V999 + *F2 + E15;
      V16 = *V999 +F2 + E16 ;
      V17 = *V999 + *F2 + E17 ;
      V21 = *V999 + *F2 + E21 ;
      V23 = *V999 + *F2 + E23 ;
          V19 = *V999 + *F3 + E19 ;
          V20 = *V999 + F3 + E20 ;
          V22 = *V999 + *F3 + E22 ;
          V24 = *V999 + *F3 + E24 ;
    F1 = *F4 + D1;
    F2 = *F4 + D2;
    F3 = *F4 + D3;
/VARIANCES
    F4= 1.0;
    D1= *;
    D2= *;
    D3= *;
    E5 to E24 = *;
/CONSTRAINTS
    (D2,D2) = (D1,D1)
/END

TABLE 10.3

(Continued)

/TITLE
US Adolescents - Group 2

All specifications replicate those for Group 1 above

/CONSTRAINTS
```
(D2,D2)    =   (D1,D1)
(1,V5,F1)   =   (2,V5,F1);
(1,V6,F1)   =   (2,V6,F1);
(1,V9,F1)   =   (2,V9,F1);
(1,V10,F1)  =   (2,V10,F1);
(1,V11,F1)  =   (2,V11,F1);
(1,V12,F1)  =   (2,V12,F1);
(1,V13,F1)  =   (2,V13,F1);
(1,V14,F1)  =   (2,V14,F1);
(1,V18,F1)  =   (2,V18,F1);
(1,V8,F2)   =   (2,V8,F2);
(1,V15,F2)  =   (2,V15,F2);
(1,V17,F2)  =   (2,V17,F2);
(1,V21,F2)  =   (2,V21,F2);
(1,V23,F2)  =   (2,V23,F2);
(1,V19,F3)  =   (2,V19,F3);
(1,V22,F3)  =   (2,V22,F3);
(1,V24,F3)  =   (2,V24,F3);
(1,F1,F4)   =   (2,F1,F4);
(1,F2,F4)   =   (2,F2,F4);
(1,F3,F4)   =   (2,F3,F4);
(1,V5,V999)   =   (2,V5,V999);
(1,V6,V999)   =   (2,V6,V999);
(1,V7,V999)   =   (2,V7,V999);
(1,V9,V999)   =   (2,V9,V999);
(1,V10,V999)  =   (2,V10,V999);
(1,V11,V999)  =   (2,V11,V999);
(1,V12,V999)  =   (2,V12,V999);
(1,V13,V999)  =   (2,V13,V999);
(1,V14,V999)  =   (2,V14,V999);
(1,V18,V999)  =   (2,V18,V999);
(1,V8,V999)   =   (2,V8,V999);
(1,V15,V999)  =   (2,V15,V999);
(1,V16,V999)  =   (2,V16,V999);
(1,V17,V999)  =   (2,V17,V999);
(1,V21,V999)  =   (2,V21,V999);
(1,V23,V999)  =   (2,V23,V999);
(1,V19,V999)  =   (2,V19,V999);
(1,V20,V999)  =   (2,V20,V999);
(1,V22,V999)  =   (2,V22,V999);
(1,V24,V999)  =   (2,V24,V999);
```
/PRINT
  FIT = ALL;
/LMTEST
/END

TABLE 10.4
Tests for Invariance of BDI-II Hierarchical Structure: Goodness-of-Fit Statistics

Modal	S-Bχ^2	df	*CFI	SRMR	*RMSEA	*RMSEA 90% CI	Model Comparison	Δ*CFI
Model 1 Configural No constraints	707.494	336	.950	.036	.024	.022, .027	-------	
Model 2 First-order factor loadings invariant	804.879	353	.940	.063	.026	.024, .028	2 vs 1	.010
Model 3 First- and second-order factor loadings invariant	809.570	356	.939	.073	.026	.023, .028	3 vs 1	.011
Model 4 First- and second-order factor loadings; observed variable intercepts invariant	1092.765	376	.939	.074	.032	.029, .034	4 vs 1	.011
Model 5 First- and second-order factor loadings; observed variable and latent factor intercepts invariant	1092.747	376	.938	.074	.032	.029, .034	5 vs 1	.012

S-Bχ^2 = Satorra-Bentler Scaled Statistic; *CFI = Robust CFI; SRMR = Standardized Root Mean Square Residual; *RMSEA = Robust Root Mean Square Error of Approximation; 90% CI = 90% Confidence Interval.

As discussed previously in this chapter as well as in chapter 9, testing for invariance of the measurement component of a hypothesized model represents a necessary prerequisite to any testing for latent mean differences across groups. Clearly, these tests—as they bear on hypothesized structure of the BDI-II for Hong Kong and American adolescents—were extremely rigorous and yet yielded well-fitting models at each step of the invariance-testing hierarchy. Based on the practical approach to invariance testing whereby Δ*CFI values of less than or equal to 0.01 are considered indicative of invariance, we can conclude that items composing the BDI-II are operating equivalently across these two cultural groups of adolescents. These results are summarized in Table 10.4.

Testing for Latent Mean Differences

Provided with evidence of invariant factor loadings and intercepts, we now test for group differences in the latent factor means. Consistent with conditions underlying tests for latent mean differences related to first-order models, the same two conditions hold for second-order models. That is, first, equality constraints are placed on both the first-order and higher order factor loadings as well as on intercepts of both the observed variables and the first-order latent factors. Second, given that the latent factor intercepts have an arbitrary origin when intercepts of the observed variables are constrained equal, the latent factor means for one group must be fixed to zero (Bentler, 2005; and Byrne, 1994a, 1998, 2001). This group then operates as a reference group against which latent means for the other group(s) are compared. As a consequence, factor intercepts are interpretable only in a relative sense. Statistical significance associated with differences between the latent mean(s) for the reference group (i.e., fixed at 0.0) and those freely estimated for the other group(s) is determined on the basis of the z-statistic. We turn first to the test for differences in the lower order latent factor means.

First-Order Latent Factor Means

That a picture is worth a thousand words has probably never been more true than it is in understanding the link between intercepts and means. Figure 10.2 depicts this test as it pertains to first-order latent mean differences. It shows the hypothesized second-order CFA structure of the BDI-II but with the addition of both the observed variable and latent factor intercepts. The observed variable intercepts are represented by single-headed arrows leading from the Constant (V999) to each of the observed variables; the latent factor intercepts are represented by three single-headed curved arrows leading from the Constant to each of the first-order factors. The symbols associated with each parameter identify their status in this initial test for differences in the first-order latent means. With respect to the factor loadings and observed variable intercepts, the symbols [* =] signify that the parameter is estimated for one group (in this case, Group 1) and constrained equal for the other group. The symbols [* 0] associated with the latent factor intercepts represent the first-order latent factor means and indicate that these parameters are estimated in one group (Group 1) and fixed to zero for the other group. Table 10.5 shows the specification of these first-order latent factor means for each group.

As expected, results from this test of first-order latent mean differences yielded a well-fitting model (i.e., S-B$\chi^2_{(370)}$ = 1060.120; SRMR = .066; CFI = .939; RMSEA = .031; 90% C.I. = .029, .033). Given that the higher order factor loadings are not constrained equal in this first-order means test and therefore are estimated for both Groups 1 and 2 (compared with Model 5 in which these parameters for Group 2 were constrained equal to those of Group 1), there is the question of why the degrees of freedom are 370 rather than 373. Recall that in Model 5, the variable intercepts associated with the reference indicators were fixed for identification purposes. In the present model, these same intercepts are freely estimated rather than fixed, which accounts for the additional 3 df.

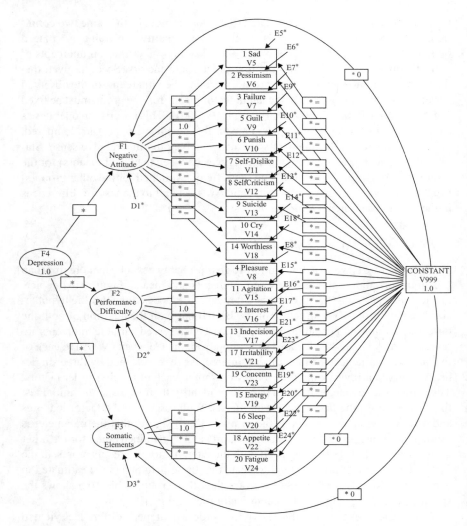

FIG. 10.2.   Mean structure model representing test for first-order latent factor mean differences.

Examination of the construct equations as shown in Table 10.6 reveals the three first-order latent means to be significantly different between the two cultural groups. Specifically, these findings suggest that scores on the Negative Attitude, Performance Difficulty, and Somatic Elements factors of the BDI-II are significantly higher for Hong Kong adolescents than for American adolescents, as indicated by the z-values of 3.363, 3.806, and 5.600, respectively.

TABLE 10.5

Selected EQS Input: Testing Latent Mean Differences in First-Order Factors

---

/TITLE

Testing for Latent mean Differences in 1st-order Factors "HKUSMeans1"
HK Adolescents - Group 1
.
.
.

/EQUATIONS
.
.
.

F1 = *V999 + *F4 + D1;
F2 = *V999 + *F4 + D2;
F3 = *V999 + *F4 + D3;
.
.
.

/TITLE

US Adolescents - Group 2
.
.
.

/EQUATIONS
.
.
.

F1 = 0.0 V999 + *F4 + D1;
F2 = 0.0 V999 + *F4 + D2;
F3 = 0.0 V999 + *F4 + D3;
.
.
.

/END

Second-Order Latent Factor Mean

We turn now to the higher order factor of (general) Depression and here is where we deal with the difficult situation noted at the beginning of this chapter. When a second-order model is added to a first-order factor model with a mean structure, an identification issue arises. Lubke et al. (2001) discussed this point as follows with regard to the equation for means μ_i in the ith group:

$$\mu_i = \nu_i + \Lambda_i \alpha_i + \Lambda_i \Gamma_i \kappa_i$$

where ν_i is the variable intercept vector, Λ_i is the first-order factor loading matrix, α_i is the vector of residual (see more below) first-order factor means, Γ_i is the

TABLE 10.6

Selected EQS Output: Group 1 Latent Mean Estimates for First-Order Factors

---

CONSTRUCT EQUATIONS WITH STANDARD ERRORS AND TEST STATISTICS
STATISTICS SIGNIFICANT AT THE 5% LEVEL ARE MARKED WITH @.
(ROBUST STATISTICS IN PARENTHESES)

```
NEGATT   =F1   =        .088*V999     +    .406*F4    + 1.000 D1
                        .026                .019
                       3.335@            21.255@
                 (      .026)         (    .019)
                 (     3.363@         (  21.057@

PERFDIFF=F2   =         .113*V999     +    .430*F4    + 1.000 D2
                        .030                .016
                       3.811@            27.596@
                 (      .030)         (    .019)
                 (     3.806@         (  22.259@

SOMELEM  =F3   =        .144*V999     +    .351*F4    + 1.000 D3
                        .026                .019
                       5.603@            18.785@
                 (      .026)         (    .019)
                 (     5.600@         (  18.227@
```

---

matrix of second-order factor loadings, and κ_i is the vector of second-order means. Lubke et al. state (p. 305) as follows:

> The model for the observed means, μ_i, as denoted in Equation 3 is not identified. As explained by Sörbom (1974), only group differences in latent means can be modeled, not the latent means in both groups. Estimation of the latent group differences can be accomplished by setting the latent means in one group equal to zero and v equal across groups. The estimated latent means in the other group then represent the latent mean differences between groups. In case of the second-order factor model, however, this does not yet yield unique estimates of the differences in latent means because there remains an indeterminancy between first- and second-order factor means. If mean differences in second order factors, κ, are estimated, only $(p - 1)$ elements of a p-dimensional vector of mean differences in first-order residuals, α, are identified (i.e., one element in α has to be fixed to zero). With these constraints, the parameters in α are interpreted as that part of the group differences on the tests which is not accounted for by the difference in the second-order factor.

In this subsection, I present you with three model specifications that attempt to address this identification problem. The first (Approach A), in principal, is analogous to the model proposed by Lubke et al. (2001) but is specified in a way that is more compatible with the approach taken by EQS in the computation of this analysis.[7] The second method of dealing with the problem (Approach B) places

---

[7]I am grateful to Peter Bentler for his explanation and detailing of the identification issue and for his proposed model specification as outlined in Approach A.

constraints on the observed variable intercepts. The third and last strategy proposed as a solution to the identification issue constrains the latent factor intercepts to zero; as such, this model argues that the first-order latent means do not exist. We begin examining this interesting series of models by discussing the model proposed by Bentler (Personal Communication, February 26, 2005).

Approach A

In describing this model, it is important to note that the notation differs from that used by Lubke et al. (2001). Specifically, we use α with a subscript to denote an intercept (or mean), with α_0 being the intercept of the variables, α_1 being the intercept of the first-order factors, and α_2 being the intercept (or mean) of the second-order factor(s). Then we start with the first-order model based on k factors η as:

$$y = \alpha_0 + \Lambda\eta + \varepsilon \tag{1}$$

and add the second-order model with r second-order factors ξ:

$$\eta = \alpha_1 + \Gamma\xi + \zeta \tag{2}$$

We now take expectations of the second-order model:

$$E(\eta) = \alpha_1 + \Gamma E(\xi) + E(\zeta)$$

and, as usual, assume that the residuals have zero expectation, giving:

$$E(\eta) = \alpha_1 + \Gamma\alpha_2 \tag{3}$$

Taking expectation of (1) recognizing that the expectation of ε is zero and substituting (3) into it yields:

$$E(y) = \alpha_0 + \Lambda(\alpha_1 + \Gamma\alpha_2)$$

or

$$\mu = \alpha_0 + \Lambda\alpha_1 + \Lambda\Gamma\alpha_2 \tag{4}$$

This is the mean structure of the model. It expresses the observed variable means in terms of the variable intercepts, the first-order factor intercepts, and the second-order factor mean. In a single group, this model is not identified because there are p variable means, p variable intercepts α_0, k first-order factor intercepts α_1, and r second-order factor means α_2. Thus, at least $(k + r)$ restrictions must be imposed on the model to have it identified. In a one-group model, typically α_1 and α_2 are simply set to zero for identification; however, alternatively one could

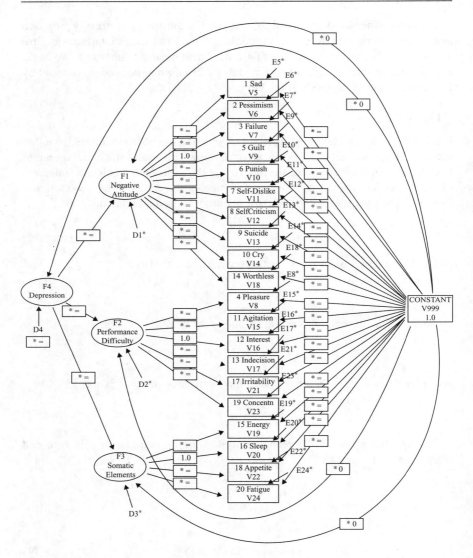

FIG. 10.3. Mean structure model representing test for second-order latent factor mean differences (Approach A). Although not explicitly shown here, F1, V999 = F4,V999.

fix $(k + r)$ elements in α_0 to identify the model. Also note that the mean structure in (3) is not identified, because there are k means $E(\eta)$ but $(k + r)$ intercepts explaining these means. This point shows up again in the multiple-group context.

Now we consider a two-group setup in which there are two sets of equations (1) to (4), one for each group. A superscript labels the group number. Without further discussion, we use Sörbom's (1974) proposal to fix the variable intercepts equal across groups and also fix latent factor intercepts to zero in one group. Thus, we have:

$$\mu^{(1)} = \alpha_0 \tag{5}$$
$$\mu^{(2)} = \alpha_0 + \Lambda\alpha_1^{(2)} + \Lambda\Gamma\alpha_2^{(2)} \tag{6}$$

For p variables and two groups, there are 2p observed means. The total number of parameters is $(p + k + r)$, which is typically less than 2p and therefore would seem to indicate that the mean structure is identified. But, in Group 2, Equation (6), there is still an identification problem at the level of the factors. There are k first-order factor means $E(\eta)$ but $(k + r)$ intercepts explaining those means. Thus, we must add at least r constraints to identify this model; if $r = 1$, with only a single second-order factor, one constraint is needed. The simplest constraint is to set $\alpha_2^{(2)}$, the second-order factor mean, to zero; then, all the mean-structure action is at the first-order level, even though a second-order factor model is involved (see Equation [2]). Other options are possible—for example, to set r equality constraints somewhere, such as between $\alpha_1^{(2)}$ and $\alpha_2^{(2)}$. All of these options are essentially arbitrary, although one constraint or another may be more meaningful or interpretable from a substantive point of view. It is relevant that testing for differences in first-order latent mean differences, as portrayed in Fig. 10.2, basically uses Equations (5) and (6) with $\alpha_2^{(2)} = 0$.

The simulated test for latent mean differences related to the higher order factor of depression based on Approach A is schematically presented in Fig. 10.3 and the related input file is shown in Table 10.7.

Review of this file reveals four key specifications that should be highlighted. First, in the /EQUATIONS paragraph, note that (a) the first-order latent factor means are freely estimated for Group 1 but constrained to 0.0 for Group 2; and, likewise, (b) the higher order latent mean is estimated for Group 1 but constrained to 0.0 for Group 2. Second, in the /CONSTRAINTS paragraph for Group 1, the latent factor intercept for F1 (F1,V999) is constrained equal to the latent factor intercept for F4 (F4,V999). Third, in the /CONSTRAINTS paragraph that follows specifications for Group 2, the higher order factor residual (D4) is constrained equal across the two groups, as are all first- and second-order factor loadings and all observed variable intercepts. In terms of the previous equations, this model uses Equations (5) and (6). Specifically, it fixes k $(=1)$ elements of $\alpha_2^{(2)}$ to be equal to some elements in $\alpha_1^{(2)}$; specifically, it constrains (F1 $\leftarrow$ V999) = (F4 $\leftarrow$ V999).

Results bearing on the test of this initial second-order model revealed a well-fitting model (i.e, S-B$\chi^2_{(373)} = 1063.726$; SRMR = .075; CFI = .939; RMSEA = .031; 90% C.I. = .029, .33) with a statistically significant difference in latent mean scores of overall depression between the two groups. Not surprisingly, these findings were consistent with those at the lower order level in determining a higher

TABLE 10.7

Selected EQS Input: Testing Latent Mean Differences in Second-Order Factor (Approach A)

```
/TITLE
Testing for Differences in Latent Mean for 2nd-order Factor "HKUSMeans2a"
HK Adolescents - Group 1
        .
        .
        .

/EQUATIONS
     V5 =  *V999 +  *F1 + E5;
     V6 =  *V999 +  *F1 + E6;
     V7 =  *V999 +  F1 + E7;
     V9 =  *V999 +  *F1 + E9;
    V10 =  *V999 +  *F1 + E10;
    V11 =  *V999 +  *F1 + E11;
    V12 =  *V999 +  *F1 + E12;
    V13 =  *V999 +  *F1 + E13;
    V14 =  *V999 +  *F1 + E14;
    V18 =  *V999 +  *F1 + E18;
          V8 =  *V999 +  *F2 + E8;
         V15 =  *V999 +  *F2 + E15;
         V16 =  *V999 +  F2 + E16   ;
         V17 =  *V999 +  *F2 + E17   ;
         V21 =  *V999 +  *F2 + E21   ;
         V23 =  *V999 +  *F2 + E23   ;
                 V19 =  *V999 +  *F3 + E19   ;
                 V20 =  *V999 +  F3 + E20   ;
                 V22 =  *V999 +  *F3 + E22   ;
                 V24 =  *V999 +  *F3 + E24   ;
     F1 =  *V999 +  1F4 + D1;
     F2 =  *V999 +  *F4 + D2;
     F3 =  *V999 +  *F4 + D3;
     F4 =  *V999 +  D4;
/VARIANCES
     D1=   *;
     D2=   *;
     D3=   *;
     D4=   *;
     E5 to E24 = *;
/CONSTRAINTS
     (D2,D2) = (D1,D1)
     (F1,V999) = (F4,V999);
/END
/TITLE
US Adolescents - Group 2
/EQUATIONS
        .
        .             Same as Group 1
        .
     F1 = 0.0 V999 +  F4 + D1;
     F2 = 0.0 V999 +  *F4 + D2;
     F3 = 0.0 V999 +  *F4 + D3;
     F4 = 0.0 V999 +  D4;
```

TABLE 10.7
(Continued)

/VARIANCES
    •
    •   Same as Group 1
    •

/CONSTRAINTS
   (D2,D2) = (D1,D1)
   (1,V5,F1) = (2,V5,F1);
   (1,V6,F1) = (2,V6,F1);
   (1,V9,F1) = (2,V9,F1);
   (1,V10,F1) = (2,V10,F1);
   (1,V11,F1) = (2,V11,F1);
   (1,V12,F1) = (2,V12,F1);
   (1,V13,F1) = (2,V13,F1);
   (1,V14,F1) = (2,V14,F1);
   (1,V18,F1) = (2,V18,F1);
   (1,V8,F2) = (2,V8,F2);
   (1,V15,F2) = (2,V15,F2);
   (1,V17,F2) = (2,V17,F2);
   (1,V21,F2) = (2,V21,F2);
   (1,V23,F2) = (2,V23,F2);
   (1,V19,F3) = (2,V19,F3);
   (1,V22,F3) = (2,V22,F3);
   (1,V24,F3) = (2,V24,F3);
   (1,V5,V999) = (2,V5,V999);
   (1,V6,V999) = (2,V6,V999);
   (1,V7,V999) = (2,V7,V999);
   (1,V9,V999) = (2,V9,V999);
   (1,V10,V999) = (2,V10,V999);
   (1,V11,V999) = (2,V11,V999);
   (1,V12,V999) = (2,V12,V999);
   (1,V13,V999) = (2,V13,V999);
   (1,V14,V999) = (2,V14,V999);
   (1,V18,V999) = (2,V18,V999);
   (1,V8,V999) = (2,V8,V999);
   (1,V15,V999) = (2,V15,V999);
   (1,V16,V999) = (2,V16,V999);
   (1,V17,V999) = (2,V17,V999);
   (1,V21,V999) = (2,V21,V999);
   (1,V23,V999) = (2,V23,V999);
   (1,V19,V999) = (2,V19,V999);
   (1,V20,V999) = (2,V20,V999);
   (1,V22,V999) = (2,V22,V999);
   (1,V24,V999) = (2,V24,V999);
   (1,F1,F4) = (2,F1,F4);
   (1,F2,F4) = (2,F2,F4);
   (1,F3,F4) = (2,F3,F4);
   (1,D4,D4) = (2,D4,D4)
/END

TABLE 10.8

Selected EQS Output: Group 1 Latent Mean Estimate for Second-Order Factor (Approach A)

CONSTRUCT EQUATIONS WITH STANDARD ERRORS AND TEST STATISTICS
STATISTICS SIGNIFICANT AT THE 5% LEVEL ARE MARKED WITH @.
(ROBUST STATISTICS IN PARENTHESES)

```
DEPRESS =F4    =       .044*V999 + 1.000 D4
                       .013
                      3.452@
                 (     .013)
                 (    3.495@
```

---

level of overall depression for Hong Kong adolescents compared with their American adolescent peers. These results are reported in Table 10.8.

For a different perspective in testing differences in the second-order latent factor mean, we turn to the next analytical approach.

Approach B

This strategy follows from the specification for Model 5 discussed previously in this chapter in which we constrained the three observed variable intercepts related to the reference indicator to the estimated value for this parameter for Group 1. This model is presented in Fig. 10.4 and the related input file is in Table 10.9.

Comparison of this model with the one shown in Fig. 10.2 reveals three major changes. First, whereas the three variable intercepts associated with the reference variables (V7, V16, and V20) were freely estimated for Group 1 and constrained equal for Group 2 in the test for latent mean differences related to the first-order factors, here they are fixed to the values of .502, .161, and .580, as described previously. The latent factor intercepts are freely estimated for Group 1 and constrained equal for Group 2, as indicated by the associated symbols of [*=]. Second, the mean of the higher order factor is represented by the uppermost regression path curving from the Constant to F4 and is therefore symbolized as [* 0]. Again, due to space limitations, only the most pertinent model specifications related to this test for mean difference in the higher order latent factor are included in Table 10.9. Review of this file reveals the fixed values assigned to the observed variable intercepts associated with the reference variables; these same values are specified for each group. Relatedly, in the /CONSTRAINTS paragraph, the same three parameters are not constrained equal across groups.

In contrast to the models shown in Figs. 10.2 and 10.3, this model does not use Equations (5) and (6). Rather, it uses:

$$\mu^{(1)} = \bar{\alpha}_0 + \Lambda\alpha_1 \tag{7}$$

$$\mu^{(2)} = \bar{\alpha}_0 + \Lambda\alpha_1 + \Lambda\Gamma\alpha_2^{(2)} \tag{8}$$

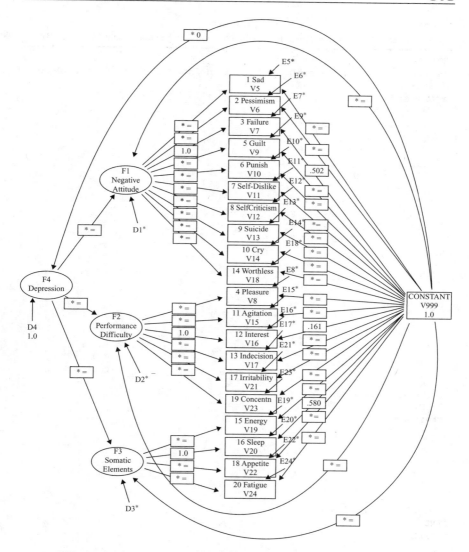

FIG. 10.4. Mean structure model representing test for second-order latent factor mean differences (Approach B).

where $\bar{\alpha}_0$ is α_0 with k intercepts taken at known values. In this model, there are $(p - k) + k + r$ intercept parameters in total. We can say that α_1 is identified in the first group because there are p means to estimate in that group and $(p - k + k = p)$ parameters to estimate; and $\alpha_2^{(2)}$ is identified because α_1 is identified through Group 1—hence, k first-order mean parameters can be used to estimate r second-order factor means in Group 2.

TABLE 10.9

Selected EQS Input: Testing Latent Mean Differences in Second-Order Factor (Approach B)

```
/TITLE
Testing for Latent Mean Differences in 2nd-order Factor "HKUSMeans2"
HK Adolescents - Group 1
/EQUATIONS
    V5  =  *V999 + *F1 + E5;
    V6  =  *V999 + *F1 + E6;
    V7  =  .502 V999 + F1 + E7;
    V9  =  *V999 + *F1 + E9;
    V10 =  *V999 + *F1 + E10;
    V11 =  *V999 + *F1 + E11;
    V12 =  *V999 + *F1 + E12;
    V13 =  *V999 + *F1 + E13;
    V14 =  *V999 + *F1 + E14;
    V18 =  *V999 + *F1 + E18;
        V8  =  *V999 + *F2 + E8;
        V15 =  *V999 + *F2 + E15;
        V16 =  .161 V999 + F2 + E16   ;
        V17 =  *V999 + *F2 + E17   ;
        V21 =  *V999 + *F2 + E21   ;
        V23 =  *V999 + *F2 + E23   ;
            V19 =  *V999 + *F3 + E19  ;
            V20 =  .580 V999 + F3 + E20  ;
            V22 =  *V999 + *F3 + E22  ;
            V24 =  *V999 + *F3 + E24  ;
    F1 = *V999 + *F4 + D1;
    F2 = *V999 + *F4 + D2;
    F3 = *V999 + *F4 + D3;
    F4 = *V999 + D4;
/VARIANCES
    D1= *;
    D2= *;
    D3= *;
    D4 = 1.0;
    E5 to E24 = *;
/CONSTRAINTS
  (D2,D2) = (D1,D1);
/END
/TITLE
US Adolescents - Group 2
/EQUATIONS
    .
    .
            Same as Group 1
    .
    .
    F1 = *V999 + *F4 + D1;
    F2 = *V999 + *F4 + D2;
    F3 = *V999 + *F4 + D3;
    F4 = 0.0 V999 + D4;
```

TABLE 10.9
(Continued)

```
/VARIANCES
     .
     .
     .

/CONSTRAINTS
    (D2,D2) = (D1,D1);
    (1,V5,F1) = (2,V5,F1);
    (1,V6,F1) = (2,V6,F1);
    (1,V9,F1) = (2,V9,F1);
    (1,V10,F1) = (2,V10,F1);
    (1,V11,F1) = (2,V11,F1);
    (1,V12,F1) = (2,V12,F1);
    (1,V13,F1) = (2,V13,F1);
    (1,V14,F1) = (2,V14,F1);
    (1,V18,F1) = (2,V18,F1);
    (1,V8,F2) = (2,V8,F2);
    (1,V15,F2) = (2,V15,F2);
    (1,V17,F2) = (2,V17,F2);
    (1,V21,F2) = (2,V21,F2);
    (1,V23,F2) = (2,V23,F2);
    (1,V19,F3) = (2,V19,F3);
    (1,V22,F3) = (2,V22,F3);
    (1,V24,F3) = (2,V24,F3);
    (1,V5,V999) = (2,V5,V999);
    (1,V6,V999) = (2,V6,V999);
    (1,V9,V999) = (2,V9,V999);
    (1,V10,V999) = (2,V10,V999);
    (1,V11,V999) = (2,V11,V999);
    (1,V12,V999) = (2,V12,V999);
    (1,V13,V999) = (2,V13,V999);
    (1,V14,V999) = (2,V14,V999);
    (1,V18,V999) = (2,V18,V999);
    (1,V8,V999) = (2,V8,V999);
    (1,V15,V999) = (2,V15,V999);
    (1,V17,V999) = (2,V17,V999);
    (1,V21,V999) = (2,V21,V999);
    (1,V23,V999) = (2,V23,V999);
    (1,V19,V999) = (2,V19,V999);
    (1,V22,V999) = (2,V22,V999);
    (1,V24,V999) = (2,V24,V999);
    (1,F1,V999) = (2,F1,V999);
    (1,F2,V999) = (2,F2,V999);
    (1,F3,V999) = (2,F3,V999);
    (1,F1,F4) = (2,F1,F4);
    (1,F2,F4) = (2,F2,F4);
    (1,F3,F4) = (2,F3,F4);
/END
```

TABLE 10.10

Selected EQS Output: Group 1 Latent Mean Estimate for Second-Order Factor (Approach B)

CONSTRUCT EQUATIONS WITH STANDARD ERRORS AND TEST STATISTICS
STATISTICS SIGNIFICANT AT THE 5% LEVEL ARE MARKED WITH @.
(ROBUST STATISTICS IN PARENTHESES)

DEPRESS =F4   =   .261*V999 + 1.000 D4
                     .058
                     4.523@
                     (.059)
                     (4.435@

Results bearing on this test again revealed a well-fitting model (i.e., $S\text{-}B\chi^2_{(375)} = 1075.284$; SRMR = .075; CFI = .938; RMSEA = .031; 90% C.I. = .029, .033) with a statistically significant difference in latent mean scores of overall depression between the two groups. Not surprisingly, these findings were consistent with those at the lower order level in determining a higher level of overall depression for Hong Kong adolescents compared with their American adolescent peers. These results are reported in Table 10.10.

Approach C

We now reanalyze the data in light of Approach C. This approach to testing for differences in the higher order latent mean specifies that in lieu of the fixed values assigned to the observed variable intercepts for V7, V16, and V20 in both groups, the three latent factor intercepts are fixed to zero for both groups. From an equation perspective, this model again uses Equations (5) and (6) but with $\alpha_1^{(2)} = 0$. The general support for this strategy is that it may provide a clearer interpretation of the findings. Essentially, this specification argues that the first-order latent means are nonexistent (i.e., they are fixed to zero). As such, the model hypothesizes that the single higher order factor mean is sufficient to account for mean differences across all BDI items and the three latent means are approximately equal in magnitude. The partial input file for this model is shown in Table 10.11 and its schematic representation is shown in Fig. 10.5.

Results based on this Approach C specification yielded results that basically mirrored those of Approach B in revealing a well-fitting model (i.e., $S\text{-}B\chi^2_{(375)} = 1075.425$; SRMR = 0.075; CFI = 0.939; RMSEA = 0.031; 90% C.I. = 0.029, .033). Review of findings related to the construct equations, reveals basically the same results as those for Approach B. These results are presented in Table 10.12.

It is interesting that all model testing results based on both Approach B and Approach C were basically identical. Thus, these two approaches can best be regarded as alternative strategies in testing the same model.

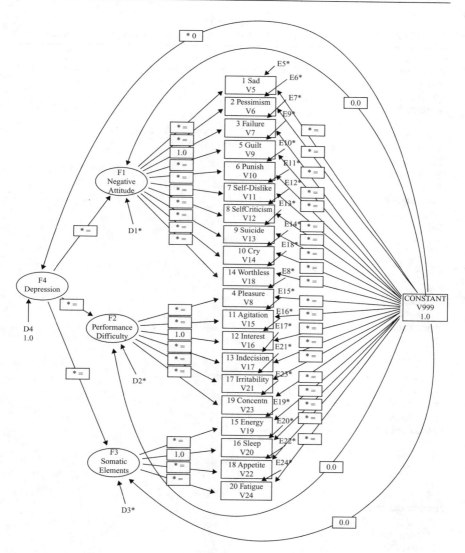

FIG. 10.5. Mean structure model representing test for second-order latent factor mean differences (Approach C).

TABLE 10.11

Selected EQS Input: Testing Latent Mean Differences in Second-Order Factor (Approach C)

```
/TITLE
Testing for Latent Mean Differences in 2nd-order Factor "HKUSMeans2"
Latent Factor Intercepts Fixed to 0.0 for Both Groups
HK Adolescents - Group 1
/EQUATIONS
       .
       .
F1 = 0.0 V999 + *F4 + D1;
F2 = 0.0 V999 + *F4 + D2;
F3 = 0.0 V999 + *F4 + D3;
F4 = *V999 + D4;
/VARIANCES
D1=  *;
D2=  *;
D3=  *;
D4 = 1.0;
E5 to E24 = *;
       .
       .

/TITLE
US Adolescents - Group 2
/EQUATIONS
       .
       .
       .
F1 = 0.0 V999 + *F4 + D1;
F2 = 0.0 V999 + *F4 + D2;
F3 = 0.0 V999 + *F4 + D3;
F4 = 0.0 V999 + D4;
/VARIANCES
D1=  *;
D2=  *;
D3=  *;
D4 = 1.0;
E5 to E24 = *;
/CONSTRAINTS
(D2,D2) = (D1,D1);
(1,V5,F1) = (2,V5,F1);
(1,V6,F1) = (2,V6,F1);
(1,V9,F1) = (2,V9,F1);
(1,V10,F1) = (2,V10,F1);
(1,V11,F1) = (2,V11,F1);
(1,V12,F1) = (2,V12,F1);
(1,V13,F1) = (2,V13,F1);
(1,V14,F1) = (2,V14,F1);
```

TABLE 10.11
(Continued)

```
(1,V18,F1) = (2,V18,F1);
(1,V8,F2)  = (2,V8,F2);
(1,V15,F2) = (2,V15,F2);
(1,V17,F2) = (2,V17,F2);
(1,V21,F2) = (2,V21,F2);
(1,V23,F2) = (2,V23,F2);
(1,V19,F3) = (2,V19,F3);
(1,V22,F3) = (2,V22,F3);
(1,V24,F3) = (2,V24,F3);
(1,V5,V999) = (2,V5,V999);
(1,V6,V999) = (2,V6,V999);
(1,V7,V999) = (2,V7,V999);
(1,V9,V999) = (2,V9,V999);
(1,V10,V999) = (2,V10,V999);
(1,V11,V999) = (2,V11,V999);
(1,V12,V999) = (2,V12,V999);
(1,V13,V999) = (2,V13,V999);
(1,V14,V999) = (2,V14,V999);
(1,V18,V999) = (2,V18,V999);
(1,V8,V999) = (2,V8,V999);
(1,V15,V999) = (2,V15,V999);
(1,V16,V999) = (2,V16,V999);
(1,V17,V999) = (2,V17,V999);
(1,V21,V999) = (2,V21,V999);
(1,V23,V999) = (2,V23,V999);
(1,V19,V999) = (2,V19,V999);
(1,V20,V999) = (2,V20,V999);
(1,V22,V999) = (2,V22,V999);
(1,V24,V999) = (2,V24,V999);
(1,F1,F4) = (2,F1,F4);
(1,F2,F4) = (2,F2,F4);
(1,F3,F4) = (2,F3,F4);
/END
```

TABLE 10.12
Selected EQS Output: Group 1 Latent Mean Estimate for Second-Order Factor (Approach C)

CONSTRUCT EQUATIONS WITH STANDARD ERRORS AND TEST STATISTICS
STATISTICS SIGNIFICANT AT THE 5% LEVEL ARE MARKED WITH @.
(ROBUST STATISTICS IN PARENTHESES)

```
DEPRESS =F4  =    .261*V999   + 1.000 D4
                  .058
                 4.523@
              (   .059)
              (  4.436@
```

This chapter outlined the major problem of identification encountered in testing for differences in the latent mean of a higher order factor, presented the series of equations associated with this test, and illustrated three approaches that can be used in conducting these analyses. Of the three strategies presented, Approach A is considered the one of preference. However, the other two approaches are nonetheless sound and do address the identification issue.

As in chapter 9, no attempt has been made to probe the substantive interpretations of these findings. Clearly, cultural considerations again come into play; therefore, knowledge of these factors is essential before meaningful interpretations of the findings can be made. Interested readers, however, may wish to review related discussion points in Byrne & Stewart (in press) and Byrne et al. (2004).

IV

Special Topics

11

Application 9:
Testing for Construct Validity:
The Multitrait–Multimethod
Model

The application illustrated in this chapter uses CFA procedures to test hypotheses bearing on construct validity. Specifically, hypotheses are tested within the framework of a multitrait–multimethod (MTMM) design by which multiple traits are measured by multiple methods. Following from the seminal work of Campbell and Fiske (1959), construct validity research typically focuses on the extent to which data exhibit evidence of (a) convergent validity, the extent to which different assessment methods concur in their measurement of the same trait (i.e., construct)—ideally, these values should be moderately high; (b) discriminant validity, the extent to which independent assessment methods diverge in their measurement of different traits—ideally, these values should demonstrate minimal convergence; and (c) method effects, an extension of the discriminant validity issue. Method effects represent bias that can derive from use of the same method in the assessment of different traits; correlations among these traits are typically higher than those measured by different methods.

Since its inception, the original MTMM design (Campbell & Fiske, 1959) has been the target of much criticism as methodologists uncovered a growing number of limitations in its basic analytical strategy (see, e.g., Marsh, 1988, 1989; and Schmitt & Stults, 1986). Although several alternative MTMM approaches have been proposed in the interim (for an early review, see Schmitt & Stults, 1986), the analysis of MTMM data within the framework of covariance structure modeling has gained the most prominence. Within this analytical context, some argue for the

325

superiority of the Correlated Uniqueness (CU) model (Kenny, 1976, 1979; Kenny & Kashy, 1992; and Marsh, 1989) whereas others support the general CFA model (Conway, Scullen, Lievens, & Lance, 2004; and Lance, Noble, & Scullen, 2002) or Composite Direct Product (CDP) model (Browne, 1984b; and Goffin, & Jackson, 1992). Nonetheless, review of the applied MTMM literature reveals that the general CFA model[1] has been and continues to be the method of choice (Kenny & Kashy, 1992; and Marsh & Grayson, 1995). The popularity of this approach likely derives from Widaman's (1985) seminal paper in which he proposed a taxonomy of nested-model comparisons. (For diverse comparisons of the CU, CDP, and general CFA models, see Bagozzi, 1993; Bagozzi & Yi, 1990, 1993; Byrne & Goffin, 1993; Coenders & Saris, 2000; Hernández & González-Romá, 2002; Lance et al., 2002; Marsh & Bailey, 1991; Marsh, Byrne, & Craven, 1992; Marsh & Grayson, 1995; Tomás, Hontangas, & Oliver, 2000; and Wothke, 1996.)

This application is taken from a study by Byrne and Bazana (1996) that was based on the general CFA approach to MTMM analysis. However, given increasing interest in the CU model in the intervening years, we also work through analysis based on this approach to MTMM data. The primary intent of the original study was to test for evidence of convergent validity, discriminant validity, and method effects related to four facets of perceived competence (i.e., social, academic, English, and mathematics) as measured by self, teacher, parent, and peer ratings for early and late preadolescents and adolescents in Grades 3, 7, and 11, respectively. For our purposes, however, we focus only on data for late preadolescents (Grade 7; n = 193). (For further elaboration of the sample, instrumentation, and analytic strategy, see Byrne & Bazana, 1996.)

Rephrased within the context of an MTMM design, the model of interest in this chapter is composed of four traits (i.e., social competence, academic competence, English competence, and mathematics competence) and four methods (i.e., self-ratings, teacher ratings, parent ratings, and peer ratings). A schematic portrayal of this model is presented in Fig. 11.1.

Before discussing this model, it is worthwhile to take a slight diversion in order that I can show you an option in the Diagrammer that can be helpful when working with a complex model that occupies a lot of page space. If there are many observed variables, for example, the user may want to alter the size of the rectangles encasing them. Of course, you can always do this by dragging on their object handles (see chap. 2), but the process becomes tedious. Thus, one alternate approach is to use the Preference option, which is made available with the EDIT menu, as shown in Fig. 11.2. Recall that in order To use the Diagrammer, you must always open a data file first; the partially shown data in Fig. 11.2 is pertinent to the current application.

---

[1]The term *general* is used to distinguish the generic CFA model from other special cases, such as the CU model (Marsh, 1989) that is described and illustrated later in this chapter.

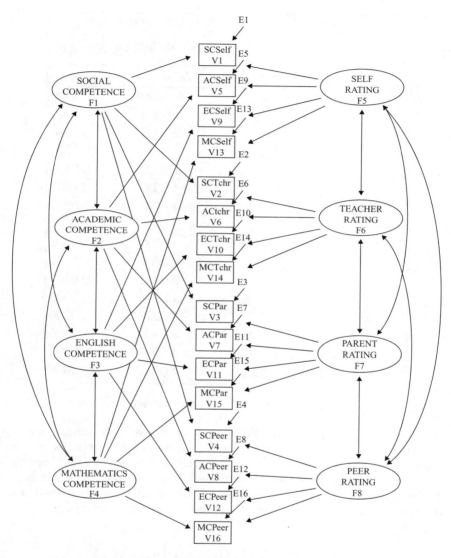

FIG. 11.1. Hypothesized MTMM general CFA model (Model 1: Correlated Traits/Correlated Methods).

After clicking the Preference option, the EQS Preference dialog box shown in Fig. 11.3 is presented. Here you see a host of options from which to choose in modifying various aspects of the program. For example, in the lower left-hand corner, one option changes the general font size, text color, and background color. However, we are interested in the Diagrammer option. Clicking on this tab triggers

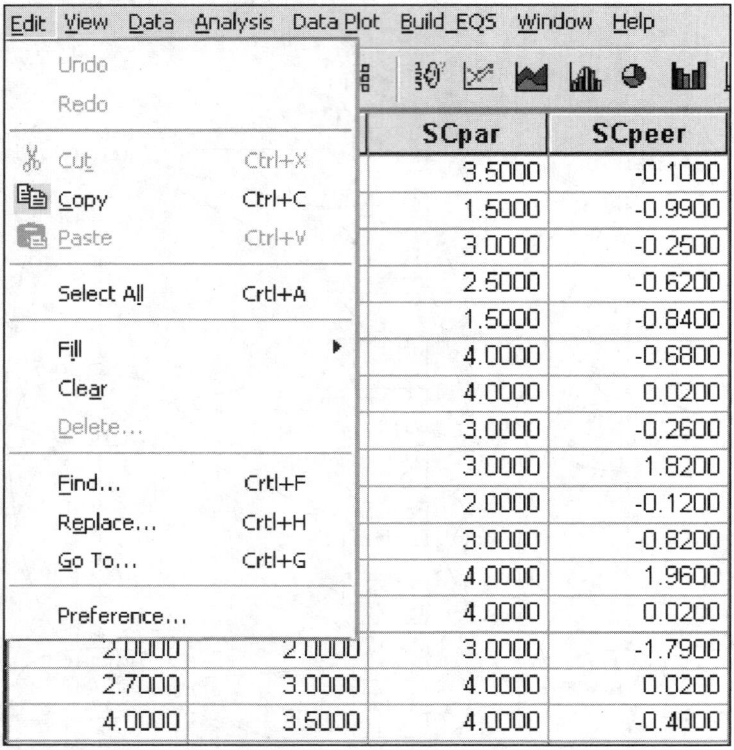

| Edit | View | Data | Analysis | Data Plot | Build_EQS | Window | Help |

	SCpar	SCpeer
Undo		
Redo		
✂ Cut Ctrl+X	3.5000	-0.1000
📋 Copy Ctrl+C	1.5000	-0.9900
📋 Paste Ctrl+V	3.0000	-0.2500
Select All Crtl+A	2.5000	-0.6200
	1.5000	-0.8400
Fill ▶	4.0000	-0.6800
Clear	4.0000	0.0200
Delete...	3.0000	-0.2600
Find... Crtl+F	3.0000	1.8200
Replace... Crtl+H	2.0000	-0.1200
Go To... Crtl+G	3.0000	-0.8200
	4.0000	1.9600
Preference...	4.0000	0.0200

2.0000	2.0000	3.0000	-1.7900
2.7000	3.0000	4.0000	0.0200
4.0000	3.5000	4.0000	-0.4000

FIG. 11.2.   EQS Edit menu showing Preference option.

the related dialog box presented in Fig. 11.4. As can be readily discerned, there are innumerable options from which to choose in making changes to the Diagrammer setup for any particular figure. Of primary interest is the capability to change the size of the rectangle for each observed variable. As shown in the lower right-hand corner of this dialog box focused on Object Size 'Variable' was selected and then the vertical and horizontal ruler tabs were used to select the desired size.[2]

THE GENERAL CFA APPROACH
TO MTMM ANALYSES

In testing for evidence of construct validity within the framework of the general CFA model, it has become customary to follow guidelines set forth by Widaman

---

[2]The size displayed is for demonstration purposes only and does not represent the actual size of the observed variable rectangles shown in Fig. 11.1.

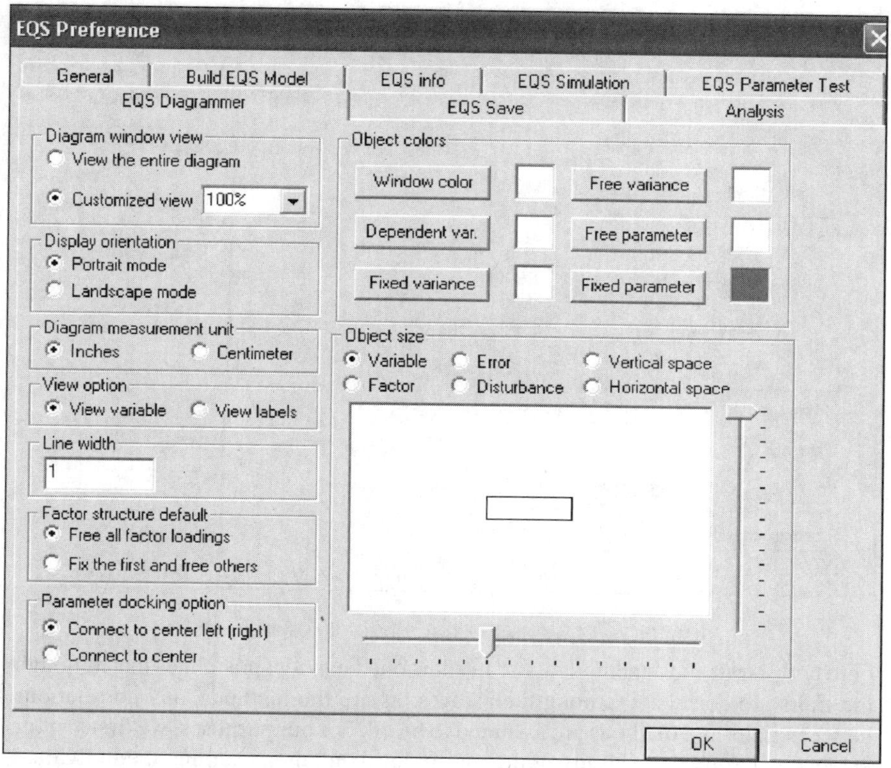

FIG. 11.3. EQS preference/DIAGRAMMER dialog box.

(1985). As such, the hypothesized MTMM model is compared with a nested series of more restrictive models in which specific parameters are either eliminated or constrained equal to zero or 1.0. The difference in χ^2 ($\Delta\chi^2$) (or analogously, the S-B $\Delta\chi^2$, as discussed in previous chapters) provides the yardstick by which to judge evidence of convergent and discriminant validity. Although these evaluative comparisons are made solely at the matrix level, the CFA format allows for an assessment of construct validity at the individual parameter level. Review of the literature bearing on the CFA approach to MTMM analyses indicates that assessment is typically formulated at both the matrix and the individual parameter levels; both are examined in the current application.

The MTMM model shown in Fig. 11.1 represents the hypothesized model and is the baseline against which all other alternatively nested models are compared in the process of assessing evidence of construct validity. Clearly, this CFA model represents a more complex structure than any of the CFA models examined thus far. This complexity arises primarily from the loading of each observed variable

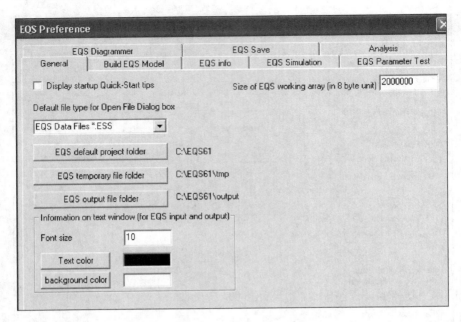

FIG. 11.4.   EQS Preference dialog box.

onto both a trait and a method factor. In addition, the model postulates that although the traits are correlated among themselves, as are the methods, any correlations between traits and mathods are assumed to be nil. For our purposes, we first test for evidence of construct validity at the matrix level and then examine the individual parameters. The four nested models described and tested in the current application represent those most commonly included in CFA MTMM analyses.

THE HYPOTHESIZED MODEL

Model 1: Correlated Traits/ Correlated Methods

The first model to be tested (Model 1) represents the hypothesized CFA model shown in Fig. 11.1 and is the baseline against which all alternative MTMM models are compared. As noted previously, because its specification includes both trait and method factors and allows for correlations among traits and methods, this model is typically the least restrictive.[3] The input file for this model is presented in Table 11.1.

---

[3] As a consequence of problems related to both the identification and estimation of CFA models, trait–method correlations cannot be freely estimated (Schmitt & Stults, 1986; and Widaman, 1985).

TABLE 11.1
EQS Input for MTMM Model 1: Correlated Traits/Correlated Methods

---

/TITLE
MTMM TEST FOR CONSTRUCT VALIDITY: 4 TRAITS AND 4 METHODS "mtmmctcm7i"
GRADE 7
MODEL 1: CORRELATED TRAITS/CORRELATED METHODS
/SPECIFICATIONS
DATA= ' C:\EQS61\files\books\data\ind7mt.ess ' ;
VARIABLES= 16; CASES= 193;
FO= ' (3F3.1,F5.2,3F3.1,F5.2,3F3.1,F5.2,3F3.1,F5.2) ' ;
METHOD=ML,ROBUST; MATRIX=RAW;
/LABELS
V1=SCSELF;   V2=SCTCH;   V3=SCPAR;   V4=SCPEER;
V5=ACSELF;   V6=ACTCH;   V7=ACPAR;   V8=ACPEER;
V9=ECSELF;   V10=ECTCH;   V11=ECPAR;   V12=ECPEER;
V13=MCSELF;   V14=MCTCH;   V15=MCPAR;   V16=MCPEER;
F1=SC; F2=AC; F3=EC; F4=MC; F5=SELF; F6=TCHR; F7=PAR; F8=PEER;
/EQUATIONS
V1= *F1+ *F5+ E1;
V2= *F1+ *F6+ E2;
V3= *F1+ *F7+ E3;
V4= *F1+ *F8+ E4;
    V5= *F2+ *F5 +E5;
    V6= *F2+ *F6 +E6;
    V7= *F2+ *F7 +E7;
    V8= *F2+ *F8 +E8;
        V9= *F3+ *F5 + E9;
        V10= *F3+ *F6+ E10;
        V11= *F3+ *F7+ E11;
        V12= *F3+ *F8+ E12;
            V13= *F4+ *F5+ E13;
            V14= *F4+ *F6+ E14;
            V15= *F4+ *F7+ E15;
            V16= *F4+ *F8+ E16;
/VARIANCES
F1 TO F8= 1.0;
E1 TO E16= *;
/COVARIANCES
F1 TO F4= *; F5 TO F8 = *;
/PRINT
FIT=ALL;
/END

THE EQS INPUT FILE

Although you will likely find this input file to be fairly straightforward, I wish first to clarify the names of the variables and then point out two important features regarding the specification of factor variances and covariances. Regarding the labeling mechanism, the variables SCSELF through SCPEER represent general Social Competence (SC) scores as derived from self, teacher, parent, and peer ratings. Relatedly, for each of the remaining traits (Academic SC, English SC, Math SC) there are ratings by self, teacher, parents, and peers. Two important specifications are worthy of note. First, in the /EQUATIONS paragraph, you will see that, unlike previous examples, all factor loadings are freely estimated. Recall from Chapter 5 that in the specification of model parameters, the user can estimate either a factor loading or the variance of its related factor but cannot estimate both; the rationale underlying this caveat is linked to the issue of model identification. In all previous examples, one factor loading in every set of congeneric measures has been fixed to 1.00 for this purpose. However, in MTMM models, interest focuses on the estimated factor loadings; thus, the alternative approach to model identification is implemented. Therefore, /VARIANCES paragraph, all factor variances have been constrained to equal 1.00. Second, as specified in the /COVARIANCES paragraph, all trait (F1 to F4) and method (F5 to F8) covariances are freely estimated. However, note that covariances among traits and methods have not been specified (F1 to F4 with F5 to F8).

THE EQS OUTPUT FILE

We first review the descriptive statistics for the sample data in the output file related to this model, shown in Table 11.2. An interesting aspect of these results is the elevated kurtosis associated only with peer ratings of the four SC facets. These findings notwithstanding, given that Mardia's normalized estimate (5.746) is < 6.00 (see Bentler, 2005), the data are considered normally distributed. Thus, all subsequent analyses are based on the ML rather than the robust χ^2 statistic.

The next set of results important to this output is the message that there are condition codes associated with (a) the covariance between F4 and F2 (SCPEER/SCTCH), which is constrained at upper bound; and (b) the variance of the error term related to ACSELF (E5), which is constrained at lower bound, as shown in Table 11.3. The upper-bound condition code indicates that the correlation of F4 and F2 exceeds the value of 1.00; thus, the program fixes the value at 1.00. The lower-bound condition reflects the situation that E5 is a boundary parameter; that is, its variance is close to zero. In programs such as LISREL and AMOS, these boundary parameters are typically estimated as negative variances. The EQS

TABLE 11.2

Selected EQS Output: Sample Statistics

UNIVARIATE STATISTICS

VARIABLE		SCSELF	SCTCH	SCPAR	SCPEER	ACSELF
MEAN		3.0321	2.9539	3.3010	-.1258	3.0052
SKEWNESS	(G1)	-.5480	-.2964	-1.0274	-.2382	-.1947
KURTOSIS	(G2)	-.4582	-.1606	.1531	5.3372	-.5261
STANDARD DEV.		.7083	.6857	.8089	1.1165	.5754

VARIABLE		ACTCH	ACPAR	ACPEER	ECSELF	ECTCH
MEAN		3.2492	3.5710	.0812	3.1192	3.1477
SKEWNESS	(G1)	-.8361	-1.3842	1.8462	-.4892	-.3917
KURTOSIS	(G2)	.0793	.8399	2.7544	-.4423	-.8750
STANDARD DEV.		.7339	.6407	1.0361	.5665	.7781

VARIABLE		ECPAR	ECPEER	MCSELF	MCTCH	MCPAR
MEAN		3.4119	.0407	2.9363	3.0772	3.3057
SKEWNESS	(G1)	-.9145	1.7502	-.4140	-.5469	-1.2255
KURTOSIS	(G2)	-.1554	3.0246	-.7072	-.5466	.4412
STANDARD DEV.		.6960	1.0501	.8207	.8563	.8808

VARIABLE		MCPEER
MEAN		.0511
SKEWNESS	(G1)	1.8624
KURTOSIS	(G2)	2.8473
STANDARD DEV.		1.0240

MULTIVARIATE KURTOSIS

MARDIA'S COEFFICIENT (G2,P) =   19.8515
NORMALIZED ESTIMATE =   5.7455

program, however, fixes such estimated values to zero, the rationale being that negative variances are meaningless and illogical.

It is now widely known that the estimation of improper estimates such as these is a common occurrence with applications of the general CFA model to MTMM data. Indeed, so pervasive is this problem that the estimation of a proper solution may be regarded as a rare find (see, e.g., Kenny & Kashy, 1992; Marsh, 1989). Although these results can be triggered by a number of factors, one likely cause in the case of MTMM models is the overparameterization of the model (Wothke, 1993); this condition likely occurs as a function of the complexity of specification. In addressing this conundrum, early research suggested a reparameterization of the model in the format of the CU model (Kenny, 1976, 1979; Kenny & Kashy, 1992; Marsh, 1989; Marsh & Bailey, 1991; and Marsh & Grayson, 1995). Alternative approaches

TABLE 11.3

Selected EQS Output: Evidence of Condition Code

PARAMETER	CONDITION CODE
F4,F2	CONSTRAINED AT UPPER BOUND
E5,E5	CONSTRAINED AT LOWER BOUND

TABLE 11.4

Selected EQS Output: Goodness-of-Fit Statistics for Model 1

```
PARAMETER ESTIMATES APPEAR IN ORDER,
NO SPECIAL PROBLEMS WERE ENCOUNTERED DURING OPTIMIZATION.

GOODNESS OF FIT SUMMARY FOR METHOD = ML

CHI-SQUARE =        78.480 BASED ON        77 DEGREES OF FREEDOM
PROBABILITY VALUE FOR THE CHI-SQUARE STATISTIC IS        .43165

FIT INDICES (BASED ON MODIFIED INDEPENDENCE MODEL)
-----------
BENTLER-BONETT        NORMED FIT INDEX =        .948
BENTLER-BONETT NON-NORMED FIT INDEX =        .998
COMPARATIVE FIT INDEX (CFI)          =        .999
ROOT MEAN-SQUARE RESIDUAL (RMR)      =        .038
STANDARDIZED RMR                     =        .052
ROOT MEAN-SQUARE ERROR OF APPROXIMATION (RMSEA)   =        .010
90% CONFIDENCE INTERVAL OF RMSEA   (           .000,        .042)
```

have appeared in the more recent literature including the use of multiple indicators (Eid, Lischetzke, Nussbeck, & Trierweiler, 2003; and Tomás, Hontangas, & Oliver, 2000) and the specification of equality constraints in the CU model (Coenders & Saris, 2000; and Corten, Saris, Coenders, van der Veld, Aalberts, & Kornelis, 2002). Because the CU model has become a topic of considerable interest and debate in recent years, I considered it worthwhile to include this model in the present chapter. However, given that (a) the CU model represents a special case of rather than a nested model within the general CFA framework, and (b) it is important to work through the nested-model comparisons proposed by Widaman (1985), I delay discussion and application of this model until later in the chapter.

Marsh, Byrne, and Craven (1992) showed that when improper solutions occur in CFA modeling of MTMM data, one approach to resolution of the problem is to impose an equality constraint between parameters with similar estimates. Thus, in an attempt to resolve the presence of at least the condition code related to E5, Model 1 was respecified such that this error variance was constrained equal to E9—the error term associated with ECSELF—because it also had a low estimated

TABLE 11.5
EQS Input for MTMM Model 2: No Traits/Correlated Methods

/TITLE
MTMM TEST FOR CONSTRUCT VALIDITY: 4 TRAITS AND 4 METHODS "mtmmntcm7"
GRADE 7
MODEL 2: NO TRAITS/CORRELATED METHODS
/SPECIFICATIONS
DATA=' C:\EQS61\files\books\data\ind7mt.ess ';
VARIABLES= 16; CASES= 193;
FO=' (3F3.1,F5.2,3F3.1,F5.2,3F3.1,F5.2,3F3.1,F5.2)';
METHOD=ML; MATRIX=RAW;
/LABELS
V1=SCSELF; V2=SCTCH; V3=SCPAR; V4=SCPEER;
V5=ACSELF; V6=ACTCH; V7=ACPAR; V8=ACPEER;
V9=ECSELF; V10=ECTCH; V11=ECPAR; V12=ECPEER;
V13=MCSELF; V14=MCTCH; V15=MCPAR; V16=MCPEER;
F1=SC; F2=AC; F3=EC; F4=MC; F5=SELF; F6=TCHR; F7=PAR; F8=PEER;
/EQUATIONS
V1= *F5+ E1;
V2= *F6+ E2;
V3= *F7+ E3;
V4= *F8+ E4;
      V5= *F5 +E5;
      V6= *F6 +E6;
      V7= *F7 +E7;
      V8= *F8 +E8;
          V9= *F5+ E9;
          V10= *F6+ E10;
          V11= *F7+ E11;
          V12= *F8+ E12;
              V13= *F5+ E13;
              V14= *F6+ E14;
              V15= *F7+ E15;
              V16= *F8+ E16;
/VARIANCES
F5 TO F8= 1.0;
E1 TO E16= *;
/COVARIANCES
F5 TO F8 = *;
/PRINT
FIT=ALL;
/END

TABLE 11.6
Selected EQS Output: Goodness-of-Fit Statistics for Model 2

GOODNESS OF FIT SUMMARY FOR METHOD = ML

CHI-SQUARE =   332.954 BASED ON   98 DEGREES OF FREEDOM
PROBABILITY VALUE FOR THE CHI-SQUARE STATISTIC IS   .00000

FIT INDICES

BENTLER-BONETT   NORMED FIT INDEX =   .777
BENTLER-BONETT NON-NORMED FIT INDEX =   .791
COMPARATIVE FIT INDEX (CFI)   =   .829
ROOT MEAN-SQUARE RESIDUAL (RMR)   =   .056
STANDARDIZED RMR   =   .087
ROOT MEAN-SQUARE ERROR OF APPROXIMATION (RMSEA)   =   .112
90% CONFIDENCE INTERVAL OF RMSEA   (.098,   .125)

---

value. This respecified model yielded a proper solution, the results of which are reported in Table 11.4.

As shown in Table 11.4, this reestimated model resulted in the message *PARAMETER ESTIMATES APPEAR IN ORDER*. Not only did this minor respecification resolve the error variance difficulty for the ACSELF variable, but it also resolved the overfitted factor covariance between Factor 2 (academic SC) and Factor 4 (math SC); this correlation is now 0.78.

The fit statistics related to this model indicate an almost perfect fit to the data (i.e., $\chi^2_{(11)} = 78.480$; SRMR = .052; CFI = .999; RMSEA = .010; 90% C.I. = .00, .042). Indeed, if additional parameters were added to the model as a result of post hoc analyses, the results would have been indicative of an overfitted model. However, because this was not the case, we can only presume that the model fits the data exceptionally well.

We turn now to the other MTMM models against which Model 1 is compared. In the interest of space, Only model specification input and goodness-of-fit statistical output are presented in tables for each.

Model 2: No Traits/Correlated Methods

Specification of parameters for this model is presented in Table 11.5 and the related output is in Table 11.6. Of major importance with this input file is the absence of trait factors. As a consequence, in the /EQUATIONS, /VARIANCES, and /COVARIANCES paragraphs, only Factors 5 through 8 are specified. As indicated by the goodness-of-fit statistics shown in Table 11.6, the fit for this model is extremely poor (i.e., $\chi^2_{(98)} = 332.954$; SRMR = .087; CFI = .829; RMSEA = .112; 90% C.I. = .098, .125). Comparisons between this model and Model 1, as well as all subsequent model comparisons, are presented in table format following review of each MTMM model.

TABLE 11.7

EQS Output for MTMM Model 3: Perfectly Correlated Traits/Freely Correlated Methods

---

/TITLE

MTMM TEST FOR CONSTRUCT VALIDITY: 4 TRAITS AND 4 METHODS "mtmmpctcm7"
GRADE 7

MODEL 3: PERFECTLY CORRELATED TRAITS/CORRELATED METHODS

/SPECIFICATIONS

DATA='C:\EQS61\files\books\data\ind7mt.ess';

VARIABLES= 16; CASES= 193;

FO=' (3F3.1,F5.2,3F3.1,F5.2,3F3.1,F5.2,3F3.1,F5.2)';

METHOD=ML; MATRIX=RAW;

/LABELS

V1=SCSELF; V2=SCTCH; V3=SCPAR; V4=SCPEER;

V5=ACSELF; V6=ACTCH; V7=ACPAR; V8=ACPEER;

V9=ECSELF; V10=ECTCH; V11=ECPAR; V12=ECPEER;

V13=MCSELF; V14=MCTCH; V15=MCPAR; V16=MCPEER;

F1=SC; F2=AC; F3=EC; F4=MC; F5=SELF; F6=TCHR; F7=PAR; F8=PEER;

/EQUATIONS

V1= *F1+ *F5+ E1;

V2= *F1+ *F6+ E2;

V3= *F1+ *F7+ E3;

V4= *F1+ *F8+ E4;

    V5= *F2+ *F5 +E5;

    V6= *F2+ *F6 +E6;

    V7= *F2+ *F7 +E7;

    V8= *F2+ *F8 +E8;

        V9= *F3+ *F5+ E9;

        V10= *F3+ *F6+ E10;

        V11= *F3+ *F7+ E11;

        V12= *F3+ *F8+ E12;

            V13= *F4+ *F5+ E13;

            V14= *F4+ *F6+ E14;

            V15= *F4+ *F7+ E15;

            V16= *F4+ *F8+ E16;

/VARIANCES

 F1 TO F8= 1.0;

 E1 TO E16= *;

/COVARIANCES

 F1 TO F4= 1.0; F5 TO F8 = *;

/PRINT

FIT=ALL;

/END

TABLE 11.8

Selected EQS Output: Goodness-of-Fit Statistics for Model 3

```
GOODNESS OF FIT SUMMARY FOR METHOD = ML

CHI-SQUARE =        206.951 BASED ON      82 DEGREES OF FREEDOM
PROBABILITY VALUE FOR THE CHI-SQUARE STATISTIC IS        .00000

FIT INDICES
-----------
BENTLER-BONETT     NORMED FIT INDEX =         .862
BENTLER-BONETT NON-NORMED FIT INDEX =         .867
COMPARATIVE FIT INDEX (CFI)          =        .909
ROOT MEAN-SQUARE RESIDUAL (RMR)      =        .045
STANDARDIZED RMR                     =        .071
ROOT MEAN-SQUARE ERROR OF APPROXIMATION (RMSEA)   =        .089
90% CONFIDENCE INTERVAL OF RMSEA   (        .074,        .104)
```

Model 3: Perfectly Correlated Traits/Freely Correlated Methods

Input specifications and output results for Model 3 are illustrated in Tables 11.7 and 11.8, respectively. As with Model 1, the hypothesized model, each observed variable loads on both a trait and a method factor. In contrast, however, correlations among the trait factors (F1 through F4) are fixed to 1.0, as indicated in the /COVARIANCES paragraph. Review of the goodness-of-fit results in Table 11.8 shows that the fit of this model (i.e., $\chi^2_{(82)} = 206.951$; SRMR = .071; CFI = .909; RMSEA = .089; 90% C.I. = .074, .104) is marginally good albeit substantially less well-fitting than was the case for Model 1.

Model 4: Freely Correlated Traits/ Uncorrelated Methods

As evident in review of the input file shown in Table 11.9, the only difference between this model and Model 1 is the absence of specified correlations among the method factors (F5 to F8) in the /COVARIANCES paragraph.[4] Turning to Table 11.10, you will note that estimation of this model resulted in a condition code related to the error term associated with ACSELF advising that the variance estimate for E5 had been fixed to lower bound (i.e., 0.0). Examination of the other error variance estimates revealed E7 (i.e., error associated with parent-perceived academic competence; ACPAR) to also have a small and nonsignificant estimate, although it had not been fixed to that value by the program. As a result, this model was reestimated with an equality constraint specified between E5 and E7. Results

---

[4]Alternatively, we could have specified a model in which the method factors were uncorrelated, indicating their zero correlation. Although both specifications provide the same yardstick by which to determine discriminant validity, the interpretation of results must necessarily be altered accordingly.

TABLE 11.9
EQS Input for MTMM Model 4: Freely Correlated Traits/Uncorrelated Methods

---

/TITLE
MTMM TEST FOR CONSTRUCT VALIDITY: 4 TRAITS AND 4 METHODS "mtmmctpcm7"
GRADE 7
MODEL 4: FREELY CORRELATED TRAITS/UNCORRELATED METHODS
/SPECIFICATIONS
DATA='C:\EQS61\files\books\data\ind7mt.ess';
VARIABLES= 16; CASES= 193;
FO=' (3F3.1,F5.2,3F3.1,F5.2,3F3.1,F5.2,3F3.1,F5.2)';
METHOD=ML; MATRIX=RAW;
/LABELS
V1=SCSELF;   V2=SCTCH;   V3=SCPAR;   V4=SCPEER;
V5=ACSELF;   V6=ACTCH;   V7=ACPAR;   V8=ACPEER;
V9=ECSELF;   V10=ECTCH; V11=ECPAR; V12=ECPEER;
V13=MCSELF; V14=MCTCH; V15=MCPAR; V16=MCPEER;
F1=SC; F2=AC; F3=EC; F4=MC; F5=SELF; F6=TCHR; F7=PAR; F8=PEER;
/EQUATIONS
V1= *F1+ *F5+ E1;
V2= *F1+ *F6+ E2;
V3= *F1+ *F7+ E3;
V4= *F1+ *F8+ E4;
    V5= *F2+ *F5 +E5;
    V6= *F2+ *F6 +E6;
    V7= *F2+ *F7 +E7;
    V8= *F2+ *F8 +E8;
        V9= *F3+ *F5+ E9;
        V10= *F3+ *F6+ E10;
        V11= *F3+ *F7+ E11;
        V12= *F3+ *F8+ E12;
            V13= *F4+ *F5+ E13;
            V14= *F4+ *F6+ E14;
            V15= *F4+ *F7+ E15;
            V16= *F4+ *F8+ E16;
/VARIANCES
F1 TO F8= 1.0;
E1 TO E16= *;
/COVARIANCES
F1 TO F4= *;
/PRINT
FIT=ALL;
/END

TABLE 11.10
Selected EQS Output: Goodness-of-Fit Statistics for Model 4

PARAMETER	CONDITION CODE
E5, E5	CONSTRAINED AT LOWER BOUND

GOODNESS OF FIT SUMMARY FOR METHOD = ML

CHI-SQUARE =   110.551 BASED ON   82 DEGREES OF FREEDOM
PROBABILITY VALUE FOR THE CHI-SQUARE STATISTIC IS   .01951

FIT INDICES

BENTLER-BONETT NORMED FIT INDEX =	.926	
BENTLER-BONETT NON-NORMED FIT INDEX =	.970	
COMPARATIVE FIT INDEX (CFI) =	.979	
ROOT MEAN-SQUARE RESIDUAL (RMR) =	.053	
STANDARDIZED RMR =	.071	
ROOT MEAN-SQUARE ERROR OF APPROXIMATION (RMSEA) =	.043	
90% CONFIDENCE INTERVAL OF RMSEA (.018,	.062)	

from this specification yielded the message *PARAMETER ESTIMATES APPEAR IN ORDER*. Goodness-of-fit results for this model revealed an exceptionally good fit to the data (i.e., $\chi^2_{(83)} = 111.791$; SRMR = .071; CFI = .979; RMSEA = .043; 90% C.I. = .018, .061).

TESTING CONSTRUCT VALIDITY (MATRIX LEVEL)

Comparison of Models

Now that goodness-of-fit results have been examined for each MTMM model, we turn to the task of determining evidence of construct validity. In this subsection, information is ascertained only at the matrix level by comparing particular pairs of models. Fit related to all four MTMM models is summarised in Table 11.11, and results of model comparisons are summarized in Table 11.12.

Evidence of Convergent Validity

As noted previously, one criterion of construct validity bears on the issue of convergent validity: the extent to which independent measures of the same trait are correlated (e.g., teacher and self-ratings of social competence). These values should be substantial and statistically significant (Campbell & Fiske, 1959). Using Widaman's (1985) paradigm, evidence of convergent validity can be tested by comparing a model in which traits are specified (Model 1) with one in which they are not (Model 2). The difference in χ^2 between the two models ($\Delta\chi^2$) provides the basis for judgment; a significant difference in χ^2 supports evidence of convergent validity. In an effort to provide indicators of nested-model

TABLE 11.11
Summary of Goodness-of-Fit Indexes for MTMM Models

Model	χ^2	df	SRMR	CFI	RMSEA	90% C.I.
1 Freely correlated traits;[a] freely correlated methods	78.48	77	.05	.99	.01	.000, .042
2 No traits; freely correlated methods	332.95	98	.09	.83	.11	.098, .125
3 Perfectly correlated traits; freely correlated methods	206.95	82	.07	.91	.09	.074, .104
4 Freely correlated traits;[b] uncorrelated methods	111.79	83	.07	.98	.04	.018, .061

[a]Represents respecified model with an equality constraint imposed between E5 and E9.
[b]Represents respecified model with an equality constraint imposed between E5 and E7.

TABLE 11.12
Differential Goodness-of-Fit Indexes for MTMM Nested Model Comparisons

Model Comparisons	Difference in		
	χ^2	df	CFI
Test of Convergent Validity			
Model 1[a] vs. Model 2 (traits)	254.47	21	.16
Test of Discriminant Validity			
Model 1[a] vs. Model 3 (traits)	128.47	5	.08
Model 1[a] vs. Model 4[b] (methods)	33.31	6	.02

[a]Represents respecified model with an equality constraint imposed between E5 and E9.
[b]Represents respecified model with an equality constraint imposed between E5 and E7.

comparisons more realistic than those based on the χ^2 statistic, Bagozzi and Yi (1990), Widaman (1985), and others examined differences in CFI values. However, until the work of Cheung and Rensvold (2002), these ΔCFI values served only in a heuristic sense as an evaluative base on which to determine evidence of convergent and discriminant validity. Cheung and Rensvold (2002) examined the properties of 20 goodness-of-fit indexes within the context of invariance testing and arbitrarily recommended that ΔCFI values should not exceed .01. Although the current application does not include tests for invariance, the same principle holds regarding the model comparisons. As shown in Table 11.12, the $\Delta\chi^2$ was highly significant (i.e., $\chi^2_{(21)} = 254.47$, p < .001) and the difference in practical fit (i.e., ΔCFI = .16) was substantial, thereby arguing for the tenability of this criterion.

Evidence of Discriminant Validity

Discriminant validity is typically assessed in terms of both traits and methods. In testing for evidence of trait discriminant validity, a researcher is interested in the extent to which independent measures of different traits are correlated; these values should be negligible. When the independent measures represent different methods, correlations bear on the discriminant validity of traits; when they represent the same method, correlations bear on the presence of method effects—another aspect of discriminant validity.

In testing for evidence of discriminant validity among traits, a model in which traits correlate freely (Model 1) is compared with one in which they are perfectly correlated (Model 3); the larger the discrepancy between the χ^2 and the CFI values, the stronger the support for evidence of discriminant validity. This comparison yielded a $\Delta\chi^2$ value that was statistically significant (i.e., $\chi^2_{(5)} = 128.47$, $p < .001$), and the difference in practical fit was fairly large (ΔCFI $= .08$), thereby suggesting only modest evidence of discriminant validity. As was noted for the traits (see Footnote 5), we could alternatively specify a model in which perfectly correlated method factors are specified; as such, a minimal $\Delta\chi^2$ would argue against evidence of discriminant validity.

Based on the same logic, albeit in reverse, evidence of discriminant validity related to method effects can be tested by comparing a model in which method factors are freely correlated (Model 1) with one in which the method factors are specified as uncorrelated (Model 4). In this case, a large $\Delta\chi^2$ (or substantial ΔCFI) argues for the lack of discriminant validity and, thus, for common method bias across methods of measurement. On the strength of both statistical (i.e., $\Delta\chi^2_{(6)} = 33.31$) and nonstatistical (i.e., ΔCFI $= .02$) criteria (see Table 6.14), it seems reasonable to conclude that evidence of discriminant validity for the methods was substantially stronger than it was for the traits.

TESTING CONSTRUCT VALIDITY
(PARAMETER LEVEL)

Examination of Parameters

A more precise assessment of trait- and method-related variance can be ascertained by examining individual parameter estimates. Specifically, the factor loadings and factor correlations of the hypothesized model (Model 1) provide the focus here. Because it is difficult to envision the MTMM pattern of factor loadings and correlations from the printout when more than six factors are involved, these values were put in table format to facilitate the assessment of convergent and discriminant validity. Factor loadings and correlations are summarized in Tables 11.13 and 11.14, respectively. (For a more extensive discussion of these MTMM findings, see Byrne & Bazana, 1996.)

Evidence of Convergent Validity

In examining individual parameters, convergent validity is reflected in the magnitude of the trait loadings. As indicated in Table 11.13, all trait loadings are

TABLE 11.13
Trait and Method Loadings for MTMM Model 1 (Correlated Traits; Correlated Methods)[a]

	SC	AC	EC	MC	SR	TR	PAR	PER
Self Ratings (SR)								
Social Competence	.87				.13[b]			
Academic Competence		.94			−.21[b]			
English Competence			.87		.41			
Mathematics Competence				.86	−.20[b]			
Teacher Ratings (TR)								
Social Competence	.41					.26		
Academic Competence		.42				.84		
English Competence			.42			.72		
Mathematics Competence				.51		.56		
Parent Ratings (PAR)								
Social Competence	.60						.34	
Academic Competence		.52					.69	
English Competence			.60				.44	
Mathematics Competence				.71			.51	
Peer Ratings (PER)								
Social Competence	.31							.39
Academic Competence		.37						.86
English Competence			.33					.63
Mathematics Competence				.40				.65

[a]Standardized estimates.
[b]Not statistically significant.

TABLE 11.14
Trait and Method Correlations for MTMM Model 1 (Correlated Ttraits; Correlated Methods)

Measures	Traits				Methods			
	SC	AC	EC	MC	SR	TR	PAR	PER
Social Competence (SC)	1.00							
Academic Competence (AC)	.37	1.00						
English Competence (EC)	.19	.84	1.00					
Mathematics Competence (MC)	.28	.78	.53	1.00				
Self Ratings (SR)					1.00			
Teacher Ratings (TR)					−.25[a]	1.00		
Parent Ratings (PAR)					.00[a]	.48	1.00	
Peer Ratings (PER)					−.05[a]	.34	.10[a]	1.00

[a]Not statistically significant.

statistically significant. However, in a comparison of factor loadings across traits and methods, the proportion of method variance exceeds trait variance for all but one of the teacher ratings (i.e., social competence) and all but one of the peer ratings (Mathematics Competenee).[5] Thus, although at first, evidence of convergent validity appeared to be fairly good at the matrix level, more in-depth examination at the individual parameter level reveals the attenuation of traits by method effects related to teacher and peer ratings, thereby tempering evidence of convergent validity (see Byrne & Goffin, 1993, regarding adolescents).

Evidence of Discriminant Validity

Discriminant validity bearing on particular traits and methods is determined by examining the factor correlation matrices. Although conceptually, correlations among traits should be negligible to satisfy evidence of discriminant validity, such findings are highly unlikely in general and with respect to psychological data in particular. Although these findings, as shown in Table 11.14, suggest that relations between perceived academic competence and the subject-specific perceived competencies of English and mathematics are most detrimental to the attainment of trait discriminant validity, they are nonetheless consistent with construct validity research in this area as it relates to late preadolescent children (Byrne & Worth Gavin, 1996).

Finally, examination of method factor correlations in Table 11.14 reflects on their discriminability and thus on the extent to which the methods are maximally dissimilar; this factor is an important underlying assumption of the MTMM strategy (Campbell & Fiske, 1959). Given the obvious dissimilarity of self, teacher, parent, and peer ratings, it is somewhat surprising to find a correlation of .48 between teacher and parent ratings of competence. One possible explanation is that except for minor editorial changes necessary in tailoring the instrument to either teacher or parent as respondent, the substantive content of all comparable items in the teacher and parent rating scales were identically worded; the rationale was to maximize responses by different raters of the same student.

THE CORRELATED UNIQUENESS
APPROACH TO MTMM ANALYSES

As discussed previously the CU model represents a special case of the general CFA model. Building on the early work of Kenny (1976, 1979), Marsh (1988, 1989) proposed this alternative MTMM model in answer to the numerous estimation and convergency problems encountered with analyses of general CFA models and, in

---

[5]Trait and method variance within the context of the general CFA MTMM model equals the factor loading squared.

particular, with the Correlated Traits/Correlated Methods model (i.e., Model 1 in this application). However, recent research has shown that this model is also not without problems, with researchers proposing a number of specification alternatives to the general CU model (see, e.g., Conway et al., 2004; Corten et al., 2002 and Lance et al., 2002). The hypothesized CU model tested here, however, is based on the originally postulated CU model (see, e.g., Kenny, 1976, 1979; Kenny & Kashy, 1992; and Marsh, 1989). A schematic representation of this model is shown in Fig. 11.5.

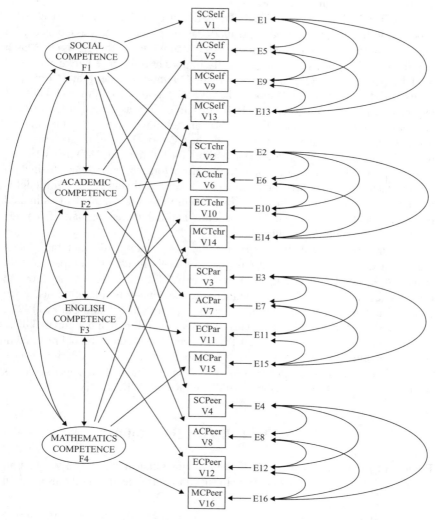

FIG. 11.5. Hypothesized MTMM correlated uniqueness model (Model 5).

Review of the model depicted in Fig. 11.5 shows that it embodies only the four correlated trait factors; in this aspect, it is consistent with the model shown in Fig. 11.4. The notably different feature about the CU model, however, is that although no method factors are specified per se, their effects are implied from the specification of correlated error terms (i.e., the uniquenesses)[6] associated with each set of observed variables embracing the same method. For example, as indicated in Fig. 11.5, all error terms associated with the self-rating measures of Social Competence are intercorrelated; likewise, those associated with teacher, parent, and peer ratings are also intercorrelated.

Consistent with the Correlated Traits/Uncorrelated Methods model (i.e., Model 4 in this application), the CU model assumes that effects associated with one method are uncorrelated with those associated with the other methods (Marsh & Grayson, 1995). However, one critically important difference between the CU model and both the Correlated Traits/Correlated Methods (Model 1) and Correlated Traits/No Methods (Model 4) models involves the assumed unidimensionality of the method factors. Whereas Models 1 and 4 implicitly assume that the method effects associated with a particular method are unidimensional (i.e., they can be explained by a single latent method factor), the CU model carries no such assumption (Marsh & Grayson, 1995). These authors further note (p. 185) that when an MTMM model includes more than three trait factors, this important distinction can be tested. However, when the number of traits equals three, the CU model is formally equivalent to the other two in the sense that the "number of estimated parameters and goodness-of-fit are the same, and parameter estimates from one can be transformed into the other."

Of course, from a practical perspective, the most important distinction between the CU model and Models 1 and 4 is that it typically results in a proper solution (Kenny & Kashy, 1992; Marsh, 1989; and Marsh & Bailey, 1991). Model 1, on the other hand, is now notorious for its tendency to yield inadmissible solutions, as we observed in the current application. As a case in point, Marsh and Bailey (1991), in their analyses of 435 MTMM matrices based on both real and simulated data, reported that whereas the Correlated Traits/Correlated Methods model resulted in improper solutions 77% of the time, the CU model yielded proper solutions nearly every time (98%). (For additional examples of the incidence of improper solutions with respect to Model 1, see Goffin, 1987; and Kenny & Kashy, 1992.)

THE HYPOTHESIZED MODEL

Review of the model depicted in Fig. 11.5 shows that there are only four trait factors and that these factors are hypothesized to correlate among themselves. In

---

[6]As noted in chapter 3, the term *uniqueness* is used in the factor-analytic sense to mean a composite of random and specific measurement error associated with a particular measuring instrument.

TABLE 11.15
EQS Input for MTMM Model 5: Correlated Uniquenesses

/TITLE
MTMM TEST FOR CONSTRUCT VALIDITY: 4 TRAITS AND 4 METHODS "mtmmunique7"
GRADE 7
MODEL 5: CORRELATED UNIQUENESSES
/SPECIFICATIONS
DATA=' C:\EQS61\files\books\data\ind7mt.ess ';
VARIABLES= 16; CASES= 193;
FO=' (3F3.1,F5.2,3F3.1,F5.2,3F3.1,F5.2,3F3.1,F5.2) ';
METHOD=ML; MATRIX=RAW;
/LABELS
V1=SCSELF; V2=SCTCH; V3=SCPAR; V4=SCPEER;
V5=ACSELF; V6=ACTCH;   V7=ACPAR; V8=ACPEER;
V9=ECSELF; V10=ECTCH; V11=ECPAR; V12=ECPEER;
V13=MCSELF; V14=MCTCH; V15=MCPAR; V16=MCPEER;
F1=SC; F2=AC; F3=EC; F4=MC; F5=SELF; F6=TCHR; F7=PAR; F8=PEER;
/EQUATIONS
V1= *F1 + E1;
V2= *F1 + E2;
V3= *F1 + E3;
V4= *F1 + E4;
    V5= *F2 + E5;
    V6= *F2 + E6;
    V7= *F2 + E7;
    V8= *F2 + E8;
        V9= *F3 + E9;
        V10= *F3 + E10;
        V11= *F3 + E11;
        V12= *F3 + E12;
            V13= *F4 + E13;
            V14= *F4 + E14;
            V15= *F4 + E15;
            V16= *F4 + E16;
/VARIANCES
F1 TO F4= 1.0;
E1 TO E16= *;
/COVARIANCES
F1 TO F4= *;
E1,E5 = *; E5,E9 = *; E9,E13 = *; E1,E9 = *; E5,E13 = *; E1,E13 = *;
E2,E6 = *; E6,E10 = *; E10,E14 = *; E2,E10 = *; E6,E14 = *; E2,E14 = *;
E3,E7 = *; E7,E11 = *; E11,E15 = *; E3,E11 = *; E7,E15 = *; E3,E15 = *;
E4,E8 = *; E8,E12 = *; E12,E16 = *; E4,E12 = *; E8,E16 = *; E4,E16 = *;
/PRINT
FIT=ALL;
/END

addition, the correlated error terms associated with each set of observed variables are derived from the same measuring instrument (i.e., sharing the same method of measurement). The EQS input file for this model specification is shown in Table 11.15.

THE EQS INPUT FILE

The major feature to note in this file is the specification of clustered error terms in the /COVARIANCES paragraph. Each line of error covariance specifications represents one set of uniquenesses specific to one particular method. As with Model 1, the traits are specified as freely estimated as are their intercorrelations; the model, however, is completely devoid of method factors.

THE EQS OUTPUT FILE

We turn now to selected sections of the EQS output file pertinent to this CU model. Review of Table 11.16 shows that consistent with past reported results (e.g., Kenny & Kashy, 1992; and Marsh & Bailey, 1991), this model resulted in no problematic parameter estimates and represents an excellent fit to the data (i.e., $\chi^2_{(74)} = 96.476$; SRMR = .07; CFI = .984; RMSEA = .040; 90% C.I. = .009; .060).

Assessment of convergent and discriminant validity related to the CU model can be accomplished in the same way as it is for the general CFA model when focused at the individual parameter level. As shown in Table 11.17, evidence related to the convergent validity of the traits was—not surprisingly—substantial. Although all parameters were similar in terms of their substantiality to those presented for

TABLE 11.16
Selected EQS Output: Goodness-of-Fit Statistics for Model 5

```
PARAMETER ESTIMATES APPEAR IN ORDER,
NO SPECIAL PROBLEMS WERE ENCOUNTERED DURING OPTIMIZATION.
```

GOODNESS OF FIT SUMMARY FOR METHOD = ML

```
CHI-SQUARE =          96.476 BASED ON       74 DEGREES OF FREEDOM
PROBABILITY VALUE FOR THE CHI-SQUARE STATISTIC IS          .04080
```

FIT INDICES
```
------------
BENTLER-BONETT      NORMED FIT INDEX =       .936
BENTLER-BONETT NON-NORMED FIT INDEX =       .974
COMPARATIVE FIT INDEX (CFI)          =       .984
ROOT MEAN-SQUARE RESIDUAL (RMR)      =       .053
STANDARDIZED RMR                     =       .071
ROOT MEAN-SQUARE ERROR OF APPROXIMATION (RMSEA)      =       .040
90% CONFIDENCE INTERVAL OF RMSEA   (        .009,          .060)
```

TABLE 11.17

Trait Loadings for MTMM Model 5 (Correlated Uniquenesses)[a]

	SC	AC	EC	MC
Self Ratings				
Social Competence	.76			
Academic Competence		.77		
English Competence			.68	
Mathematics Competence				.74
Teacher Ratings				
Social Competence	.46			
Academic Competence		.59		
English Competence			.58	
Mathematics Competence				.63
Parent Ratings				
Social Competence	.68			
Academic Competence		.65		
English Competence			.72	
Mathematics Competence				.80
Peer Ratings				
Social Competence	.36			
Academic Competence		.42		
English Competence			.41	
Mathematics Competence				.44

[a] Standardized estimates.

TABLE 11.18

Trait Correlations for MTMM Model 5 (Correlated Uniquenesses)

	Traits			
Measures	SC	AC	EC	MC
Social Competence (SC)	1.00			
Academic Competence (AC)	.36	1.00		
English Competence (EC)	.17	.87	1.00	
Mathematics Competence (MC)	.33	.80	.59	1.00

Model 1 in Table 11.13, there are interesting differences between the two models. Whereas the self-rating estimates for Model 1 are higher than those for the CU model, all other rating estimates are higher for the CU model than for Model 1.

We now look at the factor correlations as they relate to the traits; these estimates are presented in Table 11.18. Review of these values shows that all estimated values are statistically significant and of similar magnitude across Model 1 and the CU model.

Method effects in the CU model are determined by the degree to which the error terms are correlated with one another (Kenny & Kashy, 1992). In contrast to Model 1, there is no assumption that the method factor remains the same for all measures embracing the same method. Rather, as Kenny and Kashy (1992, p. 169) explain, "In the Correlated Uniqueness model, each measure is assumed to have its own method effect, and the covariances between measures using the same method assess the extent to which there is a common method factor." In other words, as Kenny and Kashy further note, whereas the general CFA MTMM model assumes that method effects are invariant across traits, the CU model allows for the multidimensionality of method effects. (For critiques of these effects, see Conway et al., 2004; and Lance et al., 2002; to understand the substance of these correlated error terms, see Saris & Aalberts, 2003). It is interesting that in Table 11.19, the strongest method effects are clearly associated with teacher ratings of the three academic competencies and with peer ratings of all four competencies under study. Indeed, from a substantive standpoint, these findings seem perfectly reasonable.

In concluding this chapter, it is worthwhile to underscore Marsh and Grayson's (1995, p. 198) recommendation regarding the analysis of MTMM data. As they emphasize, "MTMM data have an inherently complicated structure that will not be fully described in all cases by any of the models or approaches typically considered. There is, apparently, no 'right' way to analyze MTMM data that works in all situations." Consequently, Marsh and Grayson (1995), supported by Cudeck (1989), strongly advised that in the study of MTMM data, researchers should always consider alternative modeling strategies. In particular, Marsh and Grayson (1995) suggested an initial examination of data within the framework of the original Campbell–Fiske guidelines. This analysis should be followed by the testing of a subset of at least four CFA models (including the CU model); for example, the five models considered in the current application would constitute an appropriate subset. Finally, given that the Composite Direct Product Model[7] is designed to test for the presence of multiplicative rather than additive effects, it should also be included in the MTMM analysis alternative approach strategy. (For a critique of this approach, see Corten et al., 2002.) In evaluating results from each of the covariance structure models noted herein, Marsh and Grayson (1995) cautioned that in addition to technical considerations such as convergence to proper solutions and goodness-of-fit, researchers should strongly emphasize substantive interpretations and theoretical framework.

---

[7]Whereas CFA models assume that test scores represent the sum of trait and method components (i.e., additive effects), the Composite Direct Product Model assumes that they derive from the product of the trait and method components (i.e., multiplicative effects).

TABLE 11.19

Error Correlations for MTMM Model 5 (Correlated Uniquenesses)

	SCSelf	ACSelf	ECSelf	SCTchr	ACTchr	ECTchr	SCPar	ACPar	ECPar	SCPeer	ACPeer	ECPeer
SCSelf	1.00											
ACSelf	.34	1.00										
ECSelf	.38	.39	1.00									
MCSelf	.07^a	.56	.17									
SCTchr				1.00								
ACTchr				.24	1.00							
ECTchr				.13^a	.68	1.00						
MCTchr				.05^a	.51	.39						
SCPar							1.00					
ACPar							.22	1.00				
ECPar							.17^a	.25	1.00			
MCPar							.18^a	.47	.16^a			
SCPeer										1.00		
ACPeer										.36	1.00	
ECPeer										.28	.58	1.00
MCPeer										.21	.65	.43

^{a}Not statistically significant.

351

12

Application 10:
Testing for Change Over
Time: The Latent Growth
Curve Model

Behavioral scientists have long been intrigued with the investigation of change. From a general perspective, questions of interest in such inquiry might be: "Do the rates at which children learn differ in accordance with their interest in the subject matter?" From a more specific perspective, such questions might include: "To what extent do perceptions of ability in particular school subjects change over time?" and "Does the rate at which self-perceived ability in math and/or science change differ for adolescent boys and girls?" Answers to questions of change such as these necessarily demand repeated measurements on a sample of individuals at multiple points in time. This chapter addresses these types of change-related questions.

The application demonstrated herein is based on a study by Byrne and Crombie (2003) in which self-ratings of perceived ability in math, language, and science were measured for 601 adolescents in a three-year period that targeted Grades 8, 9, and 10. In this chapter, however, we focus on subscale scores related only to the subject areas of math and science. Consistent with most longitudinal research, some subject attrition occurred during the three-year period: 101 cases were lost, thereby leaving 500 complete-data cases. In the original study, we addressed this issue of missingness by employing a multiple-sample missing-data model that involved three time-specific groups.[1] However, because the primary focus of this

---

[1] Group 1 ($n = 500$) represented subjects for whom complete data were available across the three-year time span; Group 2 ($n = 543$) represented subjects for whom data were available only for Years 2

352

chapter is to walk you through a basic understanding and application of a simple latent growth curve (LGC) model, as well as in the interest of space and expediency, the current example is based only on the group with complete data across all three time points.[2] Nonetheless, readers are urged to become familiar with the pitfalls that might be encountered when working with incomplete data in the analysis of LGC models (Duncan & Duncan, 1994, 1995; and Muthén, Kaplan, & Hollis, 1987) and to study the procedures involved in working with a missing-data model (Byrne & Crombie, 2003; Duncan & Duncan, 1994, 1995; and Duncan, Duncan, Strycker, Li, & Alpert, 1999). In EQS, this can be as simple as adding MISSING= ML (see chap. 9, for example). For an elaboration of missing-data issues in general, see Byrne (2001), Little & Rubin (1987), and Muthén et al. (1987).

Historically, researchers typically based analyses of change on two-wave panel data, a strategy that Willett and Sayer (1994) deemed inadequate because of limited information. As they noted (p. 363), "When true development follows an interesting trajectory over time, 'snapshots' of status taken before and after are unlikely to reveal the intricacies of individual change." Addressing this weakness in longitudinal research, Willett (1988) and others (Bryk & Raudenbush, 1987; Rogosa, Brandt, & Zimowski, 1982; and Rogosa & Willett, 1985) outlined methods of individual growth modeling that in contrast capitalized on the richness of multiwave data, thereby allowing for more effective testing of systematic interindividual differences in change. (For a comparative review of the many advantages of LGC modeling over the former approach to the study of longitudinal data, see Tomarken & Waller, 2005.)

In a novel extension of this earlier work, researchers (e.g., McArdle & Epstein, 1987; Meredith & Tisak, 1990; and Muthén, 1991) showed how individual growth models can be tested using the analysis of mean and covariance structures within the framework of SEM. Considered within this context, it has become customary to refer to such models as latent growth curve (LGC) models. Given its many appealing features (for elaboration, see Willett & Sayer, 1994) together with the ease in which researchers can tailor its basic structure for use in innovative applications (see, e.g., Cheong, MacKinnon, & Khoo, 2003; Duncan, Duncan, Okut, Strycker, & Li, 2002; Hancock, Kuo, & Lawrence, 2001; and Li, Duncan, Duncan, McAuley, Chaumeton, & Harmer, 2001), it seems evident that LGC modeling has the potential to revolutionize analyses of longitudinal research.

In this chapter, the topic of LGC modeling is introduced via three gradations of conceptual understanding. First, I present a general overview of measuring change in individual growth over time. Next, I illustrate the testing of an LGC model that measures change in perceptions of math and science ability for adolescents during

---

and 3; and Group 3 ($n = 601$) represented subjects for whom data were available only for Year 1 of the study.

[2]In this case, however, the same pattern of results replicates those based on the multigroup missing-data model.

a three-year period from Grades 8 through 10. Finally, I demonstrate the addition of gender to the LGC model as a possible time-invariant predictor of change that may account for any heterogeneity in the individual growth trajectories (i.e., intercept and slope) of perceived ability in math and science.

MEASURING CHANGE IN INDIVIDUAL GROWTH OVER TIME: THE GENERAL NOTION

In answering questions of individual change related to one or more domains of interest, a representative sample of individuals must be observed systematically over time and their status in each domain measured on several temporally spaced occasions (Willett & Sayer, 1994). However, several conditions may also need to be met. First, the outcome variable representing the domain of interest must be of a continuous scale. Second, although the time lag between occasions can be either evenly or unevenly spaced, both the number and the spacing of these assessments must be the same for all individuals. Third, when the focus of individual change is structured as an LGC model with analyses conducted using an SEM approach, data must be obtained for each individual on three or more occasions. Finally, the sample size must be large enough to allow for the detection of person-level effects (Willett & Sayer, 1994). Moreover, when analyses entail SEM and researchers want to use robust statistics to correct for non-normal distributions, sample-size requirements become even more critical. Accordingly, one would expect minimum sample sizes of not less than two hundred at each time point (Boomsma, 1985; and Boomsma & Hoogland, 2001).

THE HYPOTHESIZED MODEL

Willett and Sayer (1994) noted that the basic building blocks of the LGC model comprise two underpinning submodels that they termed *Level 1* and *Level 2* models. The Level 1 model can be viewed as a "within-person" regression model that represents individual change over time with respect to (in the present example) two single outcome variables: Perceived Ability in Math and Perceived Ability in Science. The Level 2 model can be viewed as a "between-person" model that focuses on interindividual differences in change with respect to these outcome variables. We turn now to the first of these two submodels which addresses the issue of intra-individual change.

Modeling Intra-Individual Change

The first step in building an LGC model is to examine the within-person growth trajectory. In the present case, this task translates into determining for each individual the direction and extent to which his or her score in Self-Perceived Ability in Math and Science changes from Grades 8 through 10. Of critical importance in most appropriately specifying and testing the LGC model, however, is that the shape of the growth trajectory be known a priori. If the trajectory of hypothesized change is considered linear (a typical assumption underlying LGC modeling in practice), then the specified model includes two growth parameters: (a) an intercept parameter representing an individual's score on the outcome variable at Time 1, and (b) a slope parameter representing the individual's rate of change over the time period of interest. Within the context of our work here, the intercept represents an adolescent's Perceived Ability in Math and Science at the end of Grade 8; the slope represents the rate of change in this value during the three-year transition from Grades 8 through 10. As reported in Byrne and Crombie (2003), this assumption of linearity was tested and found to be tenable.[3] (For an elaboration of tests of underlying assumptions, see Byrne & Crombie, 2003; and Willett & Sayer, 1994.)

Of the many advantages in testing for individual change within the framework of a SEM over other longitudinal strategies, two are of primary importance. First, this approach is based on the analysis of mean and covariance structures and, as such, can distinguish group effects observed in means from individual effects observed in covariances. Second, a distinction can be made between observed and unobserved (or latent) variables in the specification of models. This allows for both the modeling and estimation of measurement error. With these basic concepts, we turn to Fig. 12.1, in which the hypothesized multiple-domain model to be tested in this first application is presented schematically.

Focus first on the six observed variables enclosed in rectangles at the bottom of the path diagram. Each variable constitutes a subscale score at one of three time points, with the first three (V16, V31, and V44) representing Perceived Math Ability and the latter three (V18, V33, and V46) representing Perceived Science Ability. Of course, associated with each is their matching random measurement error term (E). Moving up to the middle portion of the diagram, we find two latent factors associated with each of these constructs: Factors 1 and 2 represent the intercept and slope, respectively, for Perceived Math Ability; and likewise Factors 3 and 4 for Perceived Science Ability. In contrast to previous models presented thus far, the disturbance terms (D1–D4) take on a somewhat different connotation in LGC models. Interpreted within this context, they represent individual differences in the intercept and linear growth trajectories, respectively. Finally, at the top of the diagram we see the Constant variable with its typical EQS labeling of V999. As discussed in chapters 9 and 10, in keeping with the Bentler–Weeks representation system of EQS, this variable provides the mechanism by which a covariance structure is transformed into a mean and covariance (or moment) structure.

---

[3]If, on the other hand, the growth trajectory were considered nonlinear, the hypothesized model would include a third parameter representing curvature (for elaboration on this parameterization, see Byrne & Crombie, 2003; and Duncan et al., 1999). Fitting a nonlinear model such as a polynomial model requires more time points of measurement (Bentler, 2005).

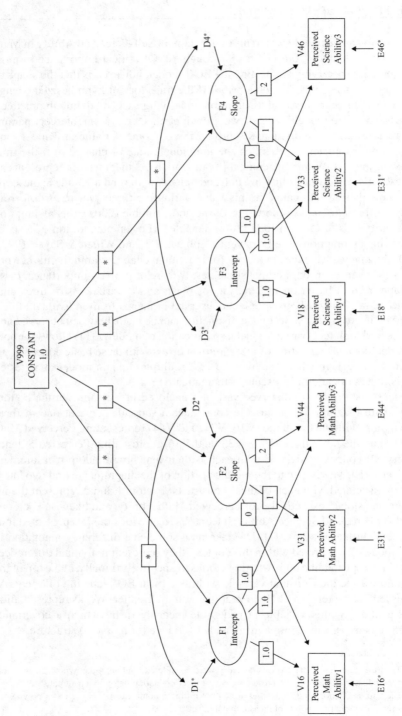

FIG. 12.1. Hypothesized multiple-domain latent growth curve model.

Let's turn now to the modeled paths in the diagram. As usual, the arrows leading from F1 and F2 to each of the related observed variables represent the regression of Perceived Math Ability scores onto both the Intercept and Slope at each of three time points; likewise for the regression paths related to Perceived Science Ability. In contrast, the arrows leading from the Constant to each of the Intercept and Slope factors represent the average intercept (or starting point of the growth curve) and average linear growth coefficient, respectively. As usual, the arrows leading from the E's to the observed variables represent the influence of random measurement error and, as stated previously, those from the D's represent the impact of individual differences in the intercept and linear growth trajectories, respectively. Finally, the modeled covariance between D1 and D2 and between D3 with D4 is assumed in the specification of an LGC model. The numerical values assigned to the regression paths leading from the Intercept and Slope factors to the observed variables are explained later in this chapter.

The primary focus in this subsection is to model intra-individual change. Within the framework of SEM, this focus is captured by the measurement model, the portion of a model that incorporates only linkages between the observed variables and their underlying unobserved factors. As you are well aware by now, of primary interest in any measurement model is the strength of the factor loadings or regression paths linking the observed and unobserved variables. As such, the only parts of the model in Fig. 12.1 that are relevant in the modeling of intraindividual change are the four factors (i.e., two intercepts and two slopes), the regression paths linking the six observed variables to these factors, the variances and covariances among the factors as given by the D's, and the related measurement errors associated with these observed variables.

We now consider this measurement model within a statistical framework. However, for simplicity, I present this summary pertinent to only one of the constructs: Perceived Math Ability (the same basic principles apply to the Perceived Science Ability construct). Accordingly, the measurement model as shown in Fig. 12.1 and expressed in matrix format is represented by the following regression equation:

$$\begin{bmatrix} \text{Perceived Math Abil1} \\ \text{Perceived Math Abil2} \\ \text{Perceived Math Abil3} \end{bmatrix} = \begin{bmatrix} 1 & 0 \\ 1 & 1 \\ 1 & 2 \end{bmatrix} \begin{bmatrix} \text{Intercept} \\ \text{Slope} \end{bmatrix} + \begin{bmatrix} \text{E16} \\ \text{E31} \\ \text{E44} \end{bmatrix} \qquad (1)$$

Essentially, this is an ordinary factor analysis model with two special features. First, all the loadings are fixed—there are no unknown factor loadings. Second, the particular pattern of fixed loadings plus the mean structure allows for interpretation of the factors as intercept and slope factors. As in all factor models, this equation states that each adolescent's Perceived Math Ability score at each of three time points (i.e., Time 1 = 0, Time 2 = 1 and Time 3 = 2) is a function of three distinct components: (a) a factor-loading matrix of constants (1, 1, 1) and known time values (0, 1, 2) that remain invariant across all individuals, multiplied by (b) an

LGC vector containing individual-specific and unknown factors, herein called individual growth parameters (Intercept and Slope), plus (c) a vector of individual-specific and unknown errors of measurement. Whereas the LGC vector represents the within-person true change in Perceived Math Ability over time, the error vector represents the within-person noise that erodes these true change values (Willett & Sayer, 1994).

In preparing for a transition from the modeling of intra-individual change to the modeling of interindividual change, it is important to briefly review the basic concepts underlying the analyses of mean and covariance structures in SEM. When population means are of no interest in a model, analysis is based only on covariance structure parameters. As such, all scores are considered deviations from their means; thus, the constant term (represented as α in a regression equation) equals zero. Given that mean values played no part in the specification of the Level 1 (or within-person) portion of the LGC model, only the analysis of covariance structures is involved. However, in the Level 2 (or between-person) portion of the model, interest focuses on mean values associated with the Intercept and Slope factors; these values, in turn, influence the means of the observed variables. Because both levels are involved in the modeling of interindividual differences in change, analyses are now based on both mean and covariance structures. Again, this explanation is limited to the Perceived Math Ability construct.

Modeling Interindividual Differences in Change

Level 2 argues that over and above hypothesized linear change in Perceived Math Ability over time, trajectories necessarily vary across adolescents as a consequence of different intercepts and slopes. Within the SEM framework, this portion of the model reflects the "structural model" component that, in general, portrays relations among unobserved factors and postulated relations among their associated residuals. Within the more specific LGC model, however, this structure is limited to the regression paths linking the Constant to the Intercept and Slope factors (F1,V999; F2,V999) along with their related residuals, as reflected in the upper tier of the model shown in Fig. 12.1. Expressed in simple matrix terms, this portion of the model is summarized as follows:

$$\begin{bmatrix} \text{Intercept} \\ \text{Slope} \end{bmatrix} = \text{Constant} \begin{bmatrix} F1,V999 \\ F2,V999 \end{bmatrix} + \begin{bmatrix} D_1 \\ D_2 \end{bmatrix} \qquad (2)$$

This equation clarifies that each factor is decomposed into a mean and a deviation from mean. The means carry information about average intercept and slope values; the residuals carry individual differences in intercept and slope. The specification of these parameters makes possible the estimation of interindividual differences in change. The key element in this specification is the Constant term because it provides the mechanism for transforming the covariance structure of the measurement (Level 1) model into the mean structure needed for analysis of the structural (Level 2) model. Specifically, in modeling and testing mean and covariance structures, as is the case here, analysis must be based on the moment matrix that is made possible by the inclusion of the Constant in the model specification. As discussed in chapters 9 and 10, this variable is always taken as an independent variable that has no variance and no covariance with other variables in the model.

Within the usual context of SEM specification, the model in Fig. 12.1 would convey the notion that both the Intercept and Slope factors are predicted by the Constant but with some degree of error as captured by the residual terms (D1, D2). Furthermore, these residuals are hypothesized to covary (D1, D2). However, in the special case of an LGC model, as noted previously, the residuals call for a different interpretation. Specifically, they represent individual differences in the intercept and slope parameters. These differences derive from deviations between the individual growth parameters and their respective population means (or average intercept and slope values).

We now reexamine Equation (2) albeit in more specific terms to clarify information bearing on possible differences in change across time. Within the context of the first construct, Perceived Ability in Math, interest focuses on five parameters that are key to determining between-person differences in change: two factor means (F1,V999 and F2,V999), two factor residual variances (D1 and D2), and one residual covariance (D1 and D2). The factor means represent the average population values for the intercept and slope and answer the question, "What is the population mean starting point and mean increment in Perceived Math Ability from Grades 8 through 10?" The factor residuals represent deviations of the individual intercepts and slopes from their population means, thereby reflecting population interindividual differences in the initial (Grade 8) Perceived Math Ability scores and the rate of change in these scores, respectively. Addressing the issue of variability, these key parameters answer the question, "Are there interindividual differences in the starting point and growth trajectories of Perceived Math Ability in the population?" Finally, the residual covariance represents the population covariance between any deviations in initial status and rate of change and answers the question, "Do students who start higher (or lower) in Perceived Math Ability tend to grow at higher (or lower) rates in that ability?"

Testing for Interindividual Differences in Change

Reviewing the hypothesized model in Fig. 12.1, we now focus on the assigned numerical values and asterisks. Numerical values are assigned only to the paths flowing from the Intercept and Slope factors to the observed variables; these paths of course represent fixed parameters in the model. The 1's specified for the paths flowing from the Intercept factor to each observed variable indicate that each is constrained to a value of 1.0. This constraint reflects the fact that the intercept value remains constant across time for each individual (Duncan, Duncan, Stryker, Li, & Alpert, 1999). The values of 0, 1, and 2 assigned to the Slope parameters represent Years 1, 2, and 3, respectively. These constraints address the issue of model identification; they also ensure that the second factor can be interpreted as a slope.

Three important points are of interest with respect to these fixed slope values. First, technically speaking, the first path (assigned a zero value) is really nonexistent and therefore has no effect. Although it would be less confusing to simply eliminate this parameter, it has become customary to include this path in the model, albeit with an assigned value of zero (Bentler, 2005). Second, these values represent equal time intervals (i.e., one year) between measurements; had data collection taken place at unequal intervals, the values would need to be calculated accordingly (e.g., 6 months = .5). Third, the choice of fixed values assigned to the Intercept and Slope factor loadings is somewhat arbitrary because any linear transformation of the time scale is usually permissible, and the specific coding of time chosen determines the interpretation of both factors. The Intercept factor is tied to a time scale (Duncan et al., 1999) because any shift in fixed loading values on the Slope factor necessarily modifies the scale of time bearing on the Intercept factor that, in turn, influences interpretations (Duncan et al., 1999). Relatedly, the variances and correlations among factors in the model change depending on the chosen coding. Here, the "initial value" coding is used, but there are other possibilities. Fourth, as indicated by the assigned asterisks, the paths flowing from the Constant to each factor is freely estimated. These parameters are typically unknown and, as noted previously, represent the average intercept (or starting point) and average linear growth coefficients. Finally, the variances of both the random measurement error and disturbance terms are estimated along with the disturbance covariances.

Before moving on, it may be instructive to examine Fig. 12.1 taking into account the points just presented. By path tracing in Fig. 12.1, starting with V999 and going down to the three Perceived Math Ability variables, we see that because of the fixed 1.0 Intercept (F1) loadings, the path V999 → F1 would reproduce precisely the mean of the Time 1 variable score. This score represents the mean initial level because the V999 → F2 path cannot be traced to the Time 1 variable. However, V999 → F2 is precisely the increment in means from Time 1 to Time 2 because its factor-loading multiplier is 1.0. The increment in means from Time 1 to Time 3 is 2.0 (times V999 → F2) due to the F2 → Time 3 loading. Hence, the mean slope, the V999 → F2 path, shows the mean change in Perceived Math Ability from occasion to occasion.

With a general understanding of LGC modeling and as it bears on the hypothesized multidimensional model in particular, we now direct our focus on analyses related to this model. We first review the EQS input file shown in Table 12.1.

TABLE 12.1
EQS Input for Hypothesized Model

```
/TITLE
  LGC Model of Perceived Math & Science Abilities "lgcmsG1"
  Based in Group 1 (Complete Data)
/SPECIFICATIONS
  DATA='c:\eqs61\files\books\data\LGC.Group1.ess';
  VARIABLES=46; CASES=500;
  METHODS=ML,ROBUST; MATRIX=RAW; ANALYSIS=MOMENT;
  DEL=467;
/LABELS
  V1=SUBJECT; V2=GENDER; V3=SCHTYPE; V4=MATGRDS1; V5=SCIGRDS1;
  V6=ENGGRDS1; V7=MATH04S1; V8=MATH05S1; V9=MATH06S1; V10=LANG04S1;
  V11=LANG05S1; V12=LANG06S1; V13=SCI04S1; V14=SCI05S1; V15=SCI06S1;
  V16=M_ABILS1; V17=L_ABILS1; V18=S_ABILS1; V19=MATGRDS2; V20=SCIGRDS2;
  V21=ENGGRDS2; V22=MATH04S2; V23=MATH05S2; V24=MATH06S2; V25=LANG04S2;
  V26=LANG05S2; V27=LANG06S2; V28=SCI04S2; V29=SCI05S2; V30=SCI06S2;
  V31=M_ABILS2; V32=L_ABILS2; V33=S_ABILS2; V34=MATGRDS3; V35=SCIGRDS3;
  V36=ENGGRDS3; V37=MATH04S3; V38=LANG04S3; V39=LANG05S3; V40=LANG06S3;
  V41=SCI04S3; V42=SCI05S3; V43=SCI06S3; V44=M_ABILS3; V45=L_ABILS3;
  V46=S_ABILS3;
/EQUATIONS
  V16 =  + 1F1  + 0F2  + 1E16;
  V31 =  + 1F1  + 1F2  + 1E31;
  V44 =  + 1F1  + 2F2  + 1E44;
  F1  =  + *V999 + 1D1;
  F2  =  + *V999 + 1D2;
  V18 =  + 1F3  + 0F4  + 1E18;
  V33 =  + 1F3  + 1F4  + 1E33;
  V46 =  + 1F3  + 2F4  + 1E46;
  F3  =  + *V999 + 1D3;
  F4  =  + *V999 + 1D4;
/VARIANCES
  V999 = 1.00;
  E16 = *;
  E31 = *;
  E44 = *;
  E18 = *;
  E33 = *;
  E46 = *;
  D1  = *;
  D2  = *;
  D3  = *;
  D4  = *;
/COVARIANCES
  D1,D2 = *; D3,D4 = *;
/PRINT
  FIT=ALL;
/LMTEST
  SET=PDD;
/END
```

THE EQS INPUT FILE

By now, model specifications in this file should be fairly straightforward, but we review the /EQUATIONS paragraph nonetheless. First, for each set of observed variables, note that Factor 1 (the Intercept) is fixed to a value of 1.0 at each of the three time points, whereas Factor 2 (the Slope) has fixed values of 0, 1, and 2 for Occasions 1, 2, and 3, respectively. Second, consistent with the path diagram, each of the four factors is regressed onto the Constant (V999) and these paths are freely estimated. In the /COVARIANCES paragraph, consistent with theory and underlying assumptions associated with LGC modeling, the disturbance terms related to the intercept and slope for both Perceived Math Ability and Perceived Science Ability are free to covary. Finally, review of the /LMTEST specification shows that the search for modification indexes is limited to possible correlations between pairs of disturbances (PDD). Realistically, this is the only modification that makes sense within the current context. We now discuss the related EQS output.

THE EQS OUTPUT FILE

Before reviewing goodness-of-fit of the hypothesized model, a brief overview of the related descriptive statistics is presented in Table 12.2. Not surprisingly, the initial reaction may be that nothing too exciting is going on here, and you will be quite correct in your perception. My interest in showing you these results is to draw your attention to the univariate and multivariate normality of the data. Univariately, variables are not too skewed or kurtotic, but there is some nonzero multivariate kurtosis. This is an opportunity to show that when data are fairly multivariate normal, any difference between the usual ML χ^2 statistic and the S-Bχ^2 statistic is minimal, as should be the case for the other fit statistics.

Turning to Table 12.3 in which the goodness-of-fit statistics are reported, we do find a slight difference between the usual $\chi^2_{(11)}$ (174.757) and corrected S-B$\chi^2_{(11)}$ (144.452) statistics. However, of primary concern is the obvious poor fit of the model, as indicated by the *CFI value of .800 (CFI = .815). Added to these model-fit results are an SRMR = .213 and the *RMSEA value of .156 (RMSEA = .173). Clearly, this model is misspecified in a very major way. For answers to this substantial misspecification, we review the LM Test statistics in Table 12.4.

Review of LM Test Univariate Incremental χ^2 statistics shows that not including a covariance between the intercept terms related to Perceived Math Ability and Perceived Science Ability accounts for most of the misspecification. Although misspecified covariance between the two slopes is also noted here, the LMχ^2 value is substantially less than the value associated with the intercepts. Given the substantive reasonableness of this residual covariance—together with Willet and Sayer's (1996) caveat that in multiple-domain LGC models, covariation among

TABLE 12.2

Selected EQS Output for Hypothesized Model: Descriptive Statistics

---

SAMPLE STATISTICS BASED ON COMPLETE CASES

UNIVARIATE STATISTICS

VARIABLE		M_ABILS1	S_ABILS1	M_ABILS2	S_ABILS2	M_ABILS3
MEAN		5.1162	4.7442	4.9973	4.9138	4.7669
SKEWNESS	(G1)	-.9833	-.4256	-.7506	-.7435	-.6518
KURTOSIS	(G2)	.8756	-.1277	.0534	.4142	-.3769
STANDARD DEV.		1.2324	1.1952	1.3184	1.2623	1.4798

VARIABLE		S_ABILS3	V999
MEAN		4.9973	1.0000
SKEWNESS	(G1)	-.8615	.0000
KURTOSIS	(G2)	.6890	.0000
STANDARD DEV.		1.2399	.0000

MULTIVARIATE KURTOSIS

```
MARDIA'S COEFFICIENT (G2,P) =     10.1996
NORMALIZED ESTIMATE =             11.6270
```

TABLE 12.3

Selected EQS Output for Hypothesized Model: Goodness-of-Fit Statistics

---

GOODNESS OF FIT SUMMARY FOR METHOD = ML

```
CHI-SQUARE =      174.757 BASED ON      11 DEGREES OF FREEDOM
PROBABILITY VALUE FOR THE CHI-SQUARE STATISTIC IS        .00000
```

FIT INDICES (BASED ON COVARIANCE MATRIX ONLY, NOT THE MEANS)

```
BENTLER-BONETT      NORMED FIT INDEX =        .808
BENTLER-BONETT NON-NORMED FIT INDEX =         .691
COMPARATIVE FIT INDEX (CFI)          =        .815
ROOT MEAN-SQUARE RESIDUAL (RMR)      =        .352
STANDARDIZED RMR                     =        .213
ROOT MEAN-SQUARE ERROR OF APPROXIMATION (RMSEA)   =        .173
90% CONFIDENCE INTERVAL OF RMSEA  (        .150,        .195)
```

GOODNESS OF FIT SUMMARY FOR METHOD = ROBUST

```
SATORRA-BENTLER SCALED CHI-SQUARE = 144.4517 ON 11 DEGREES OF FREEDOM
PROBABILITY VALUE FOR THE CHI-SQUARE STATISTIC IS        .00000
```

FIT INDICES (BASED ON COVARIANCE MATRIX ONLY, NOT THE MEANS)

```
BENTLER-BONETT      NORMED FIT INDEX =        .791
BENTLER-BONETT NON-NORMED FIT INDEX =         .667
COMPARATIVE FIT INDEX (CFI)          =        .800
ROOT MEAN-SQUARE ERROR OF APPROXIMATION (RMSEA)   =        .156
90% CONFIDENCE INTERVAL OF RMSEA  (        .134,        .179)
```

TABLE 12.4
Selected EQS Output for Hypothesized Model: Modification Indexes

		CUMULATIVE MULTIVARIATE STATISTICS			UNIVARIATE INCREMENT			
							HANCOCK'S SEQUENTIAL	
STEP	PARAMETER	CHI-SQUARE	D.F.	PROB.	CHI-SQUARE	PROB.	D.F.	PROB.
1	D3,D1	112.022	1	.000	112.022	.000	11	.000
2	D4,D2	121.531	2	.000	9.510	.002	10	.485

TABLE 12.5
Selected EQS Output for Model 2: Goodness-of-Fit Statistics

```
GOODNESS OF FIT SUMMARY FOR METHOD = ML

CHI-SQUARE =          45.550 BASED ON         10 DEGREES OF FREEDOM
PROBABILITY VALUE FOR THE CHI-SQUARE STATISTIC IS           .00000

FIT INDICES (BASED ON COVARIANCE MATRIX ONLY, NOT THE MEANS)
-----------
BENTLER-BONETT      NORMED FIT INDEX =       .952
BENTLER-BONETT NON-NORMED FIT INDEX =        .925
COMPARATIVE FIT INDEX (CFI)          =       .960
ROOT MEAN-SQUARE RESIDUAL (RMR)      =       .080
STANDARDIZED RMR                     =       .047
ROOT MEAN-SQUARE ERROR OF APPROXIMATION (RMSEA)     =        .084
90% CONFIDENCE INTERVAL OF RMSEA (         .060,        .110)

GOODNESS OF FIT SUMMARY FOR METHOD = ROBUST

SATORRA-BENTLER SCALED CHI-SQUARE =        37.9880 ON         10 DEGREES OF FREEDOM
PROBABILITY VALUE FOR THE CHI-SQUARE STATISTIC IS           .00004

FIT INDICES (BASED ON COVARIANCE MATRIX ONLY, NOT THE MEANS)
-----------
BENTLER-BONETT      NORMED FIT INDEX =       .947
BENTLER-BONETT NON-NORMED FIT INDEX =        .921
COMPARATIVE FIT INDEX (CFI)          =       .958
ROOT MEAN-SQUARE ERROR OF APPROXIMATION (RMSEA)     =        .075
90% CONFIDENCE INTERVAL OF RMSEA (         .051,        .101)
```

the growth parameters across domains (as reflected in their residual terms) should be considered—Model 2 was modified to address these concerns. Goodness-of-fit results for this respecified model are shown in Table 12.5.

Of primary interest is the difference that the incorporation of just one residual covariance can make to a model! We now have a well-fitting model with a *CFI value of .958 (CFI = .960). Furthermore, the SRMR has dropped to .047 and the *RMSEA to .075 (RMSEA = .084). However, we need to check on the residual covariance of D4,D2 noted in our review of the LM Test statistics related to the hypothesized model (see Table 12.4). To check all estimated residual covariances, we also need to review the status of their statistical significance. Results related to both the estimates and LM Test values are reported in Table 12.6.

Review of these results shows that although the residual covariances between the intercept and slope for Perceived Math Ability (D2,D1) and between the intercepts for both Perceived Math Ability and Perceived Science Ability (D3,D1)

TABLE 12.6

Selected EQS Output for Model 2: Residual Estimates and Modification Indexes

COVARIANCES AMONG INDEPENDENT VARIABLES

STATISTICS SIGNIFICANT AT THE 5% LEVEL ARE MARKED WITH @.

```
                 E                                    D
                ---                                  ---
                      I  D2  -  F2                       -.278*I
                      I  D1  -  F1                         .070 I
                      I                                  -3.947@I
                      I                                (  .076)I
                      I                                ( -3.631@I
                      I                                        I
                      I  D3  -  F3                         .515*I
                      I  D1  -  F1                         .053 I
                      I                                   9.677@I
                      I                                (  .055)I
                      I                                ( 9.370@I
                      I                                        I
                      I  D4  -  F4                        -.057*I
                      I  D3  -  F3                         .061 I
                      I                                    -.926 I
                      I                                (  .065)I
                      I                                ( -.871)I
                      I
```

	CUMULATIVE MULTIVARIATE STATISTICS				UNIVARIATE INCREMENT			
							HANCOCK'S SEQUENTIAL	
STEP	PARAMETER	CHI-SQUARE	D.F.	PROB.	CHI-SQUARE	PROB.	D.F.	PROB.
1	D4,D2	9.962	1	.002	9.962	.002	10	.444

are statistically significant, the residual covariance between the intercept and slope for Perceived Science Ability (D4,D3) is nonsignificant. Turning next to the LM Test results, we observe that the residual covariance between the slopes of the two constructs remains a misspecified parameter in the model. Again, given the substantive rationality of a covariance between the slopes of two closely related subject areas, the model was respecified with this parameter (D4,D2) freely estimated. In addition, the nonsignificant residual covariance between the intercept and slope for Perceived Science Ability (D4,D3) was deleted from the model. Goodness-of-fit results for Model 3 are reported in Table 12.7.

Not surprisingly, with the incorporation of this second residual covariance, the fit of the model is further improved and now represents an exceptionally well-fitting model, as exemplified by a *CFI value of .970 (CFI = .971). These values are further supported by a SRMR value of .046 and a *RMSEA value of .063 (RMSEA = .072).

Having determined a well-fitting model, we are ready to review the substantive results of the analysis. These unstandardized estimates, as reported in the EQS output file, are presented in Table 12.8.

TABLE 12.7

Selected EQS Output for Model 3: Goodness-of-Fit Statistics

```
GOODNESS OF FIT SUMMARY FOR METHOD = ML

CHI-SQUARE =         35.530 BASED ON       10 DEGREES OF FREEDOM
PROBABILITY VALUE FOR THE CHI-SQUARE STATISTIC IS         .00010

FIT INDICES (BASED ON COVARIANCE MATRIX ONLY, NOT THE MEANS)
-----------
BENTLER-BONETT      NORMED FIT INDEX =       .963
BENTLER-BONETT NON-NORMED FIT INDEX =       .947
COMPARATIVE FIT INDEX (CFI)         =       .971
ROOT MEAN-SQUARE RESIDUAL (RMR)     =       .078
STANDARDIZED RMR                    =       .046
ROOT MEAN-SQUARE ERROR OF APPROXIMATION (RMSEA)     =       .072
90% CONFIDENCE INTERVAL OF RMSEA  (         .047,        .098)

GOODNESS OF FIT SUMMARY FOR METHOD = ROBUST

SATORRA-BENTLER SCALED CHI-SQUARE =      29.9213 ON       10 DEGREES OF FREEDOM
PROBABILITY VALUE FOR THE CHI-SQUARE STATISTIC IS         .00088

FIT INDICES (BASED ON COVARIANCE MATRIX ONLY, NOT THE MEANS)
-----------
BENTLER-BONETT      NORMED FIT INDEX =       .959
BENTLER-BONETT NON-NORMED FIT INDEX =       .944
COMPARATIVE FIT INDEX (CFI)         =       .970
ROOT MEAN-SQUARE ERROR OF APPROXIMATION (RMSEA)     =       .063
90% CONFIDENCE INTERVAL OF RMSEA  (         .038,        .090)
```

Given that the measurement equations represented only fixed parameters, there is little of interest in this section. Of major importance, however, are the construct equations found next in the output file. The loading of the Constant (V999) onto each factor, of course, represents the latent factor score means. Here we see that all of the intercepts are statistically significant. Findings reveal the average score for Perceived Science Ability (4.760) is slightly lower than is the case for Perceived Math Ability (5.122). However, whereas adolescents' average Self-Perceived Math Ability decreased during a three-year period from Grades 8 through 10 (as indicated by the value of −0.164), average Self-Perceived Science Ability increased (0.125).

In the Variance section of the output file, all residual terms associated with the intercept and slope for each Perceived Ability domain (i.e., the D's) are statistically significant. These findings reveal strong interindividual differences in both the initial scores of Self-Perceived Ability in Math and Science at Time 1 and in their change over time, as the adolescents progressed from Grades 8 through 10. Such evidence of interindividual differences provides powerful support for further investigation of variability related to the growth trajectories. In particular, the incorporation of predictors in the model can serve to explain their variability. Of somewhat less importance substantively, albeit important methodologically, all random measurement error terms are also statistically significant.

We turn now to the Residual Covariances, review the within-domain residual covariance—that is, the covariance between the intercept and slope related to the

TABLE 12.8

Selected EQS Output for Model 3: Unstandardized Estimates

MEASUREMENT EQUATIONS WITH STANDARD ERRORS AND TEST STATISTICS
STATISTICS SIGNIFICANT AT THE 5% LEVEL ARE MARKED WITH @.
(ROBUST STATISTICS IN PARENTHESES)

M_ABILS1=V16 =   1.000 F1   + 1.000 E16

S_ABILS1=V18 =   1.000 F3   + 1.000 E18

M_ABILS2=V31 =   1.000 F1   + 1.000 F2   + 1.000 E31

S_ABILS2=V33 =   1.000 F3   + 1.000 F4   + 1.000 E33

M_ABILS3=V44 =   1.000 F1   + 2.000 F2   + 1.000 E44

S_ABILS3=V46 =   1.000 F3   + 2.000 F4   + 1.000 E46

CONSTRUCT EQUATIONS WITH STANDARD ERRORS AND TEST STATISTICS
STATISTICS SIGNIFICANT AT THE 5% LEVEL ARE MARKED WITH @.
(ROBUST STATISTICS IN PARENTHESES)

```
    F1    =F1 =   5.122*V999    + 1.000 D1
                   .054
                 94.000@
                 (   .054)
                 ( 94.000@

    F2    =F2 =  -.164*V999     + 1.000 D2
                   .032
                 -5.102@
                 (   .032)
                 ( -5.102@

    F3    =F3 =   4.760*V999    + 1.000 D3
                   .051
                 92.930@
                 (   .051)
                 ( 92.930@

    F4    =F4 =   .125*V999     + 1.000 D4
                   .030
                  4.145@
                 (   .030)
                 (  4.145@
```

VARIANCES OF INDEPENDENT VARIABLES

STATISTICS SIGNIFICANT AT THE 5% LEVEL ARE MARKED WITH @.

```
                    E                              D
                   ---                            ---

E16 -M_ABILS1             .207*I  D1  -  F1            1.283*I
                          .099 I                        .127 I
                         2.083@I                      10.063@I
                       (  .098)I                      (  .150)I
                       ( 2.108@I                      ( 8.554@I
                             I                              I
```

(Continued)

TABLE 12.8
(Continued)

```
E18 -S_ABILS1          .824*I D2  -  F2              .256*I
                       .070 I                        .056 I
                     11.720@I                       4.556@I
                     (  .070)I                     (  .059)I
                     ( 11.796@I                     ( 4.306@I
                          I                             I
E31 -M_ABILS2          .680*I D3  -  F3              .630*I
                       .061 I                        .065 I
                     11.173@I                       9.742@I
                     (  .075)I                     (  .065)I
                     (  9.089@I                     ( 9.640@I
                          I                             I
E33 -S_ABILS2          .784*I D4  -  F4              .093*I
                       .064 I                        .031 I
                     12.200@I                       2.970@I
                     (  .077)I                     (  .035)I
                     ( 10.213@I                     ( 2.617@I
                          I                             I
E44 -M_ABILS3          .971*I                          I
                       .130 I                          I
                      7.498@I                          I
                     (  .141)I                         I
                     (  6.911@I                        I
                          I                             I
E46 -S_ABILS3          .615*I                          I
                       .102 I                          I
                      6.005@I                          I
                     (  .109)I                         I
                     (  5.671@I                        I
                          I                             I
```

COVARIANCES AMONG INDEPENDENT VARIABLES

STATISTICS SIGNIFICANT AT THE 5% LEVEL ARE MARKED WITH @.

```
          E                            D
          ---                          ---
                  I D2  -  F2              -.249*I
                  I D1  -  F1               .070 I
                  I                       -3.540@I
                  I                      (  .076)I
                  I                      ( -3.277@I
                  I                             I
                  I D3  -  F3               .483*I
                  I D1  -  F1               .054 I
                  I                        8.872@I
                  I                      (  .057)I
                  I                      ( 8.454@I
                  I                             I
                  I D4  -  F4               .056*I
                  I D2  -  F2               .017 I
                  I                        3.232@I
                  I                      (  .020)I
                  I                      ( 2.871@I
                  I                             I
```

same construct. As expected, the estimated covariance between the intercept and slope for Perceived Math Ability is statistically significant. The negative estimate of $-.249$ suggests that for adolescents whose Self-Perceived Math Ability scores were high in Grade 8, their rate of increase in scores during the three-year period from Grades 8 through 10 was lower than for adolescents whose Self-Perceived Math Ability scores were lower at Time 1. In other words, Grade 8 students who perceived themselves as being less able than their peers in math made the greater gains. A negative correlation between initial status and possible gain is an old phenomenon in psychology known as the Law of Initial Values.

Turning to the first between-domain residual covariance (D3,D1), we observe a strong association between the intercepts of Perceived Ability in Math and in Science (.483), a finding that appears reasonable. In contrast, the residual covariance between the slopes for Perceived Ability in Math and in Science, although statistically significant, is small (.056). Nonetheless, review of the standardized coefficients in Table 12.9 shows this correlation ($r = .37$), together with the other between-domain residual ($r = .54$) and within-domain residual ($r = -.44$), to be moderately high.

TABLE 12.9
Selected EQS Output for Model 3: Standardized Solution

```
STANDARDIZED SOLUTION:                                          R-SQUARED

M_ABILS1=V16  =   .928 F1   +  .373 E16                             .861
S_ABILS1=V18  =   .658 F3   +  .753 E18                             .433
M_ABILS2=V31  =   .863 F1   +  .386 F2   +  .629 E31                .605
S_ABILS2=V33  =   .647 F3   +  .248 F4   +  .721 E33                .480
M_ABILS3=V44  =   .750 F1   +  .670 F2   +  .653 E44                .574
S_ABILS3=V46  =   .625 F3   +  .479 F4   +  .617 E46                .619
     F1   =F1   =   .000*V999 +1.000 D1                             .000
     F2   =F2   =   .000*V999 +1.000 D2                             .000
     F3   =F3   =   .000*V999 +1.000 D3                             .000
     F4   =F4   =   .000*V999 +1.000 D4                             .000

CORRELATIONS AMONG INDEPENDENT VARIABLES
-----------------------------------------
                    E                          D
                   ---                        ---

                        I  D2   -   F2           -.435*I
                        I  D1   -   F1                 I
                        I                             I
                        I  D3   -   F3            .537*I
                        I  D1   -   F1                 I
                        I                             I
                        I  D4   -   F4            .366*I
                        I  D2   -   F2                 I
                        I                             I
```

GENDER AS A TIME-INVARIANT
PREDICTOR OF CHANGE

As discussed previously, when provided with evidence of interindividual differences, we can then ask whether and to what extent one or more predictors might explain this heterogeneity. For our purposes here, we ask whether statistically significant heterogeneity in the individual growth trajectories (i.e., intercept and slope) of Perceived Ability in Math and in Science can be explained by gender as a time-invariant predictor of change. As such, we might ask two questions: "Do self-perceptions of ability in math and science differ for adolescent boys and girls at Time 1 (Grade 8)?" and "Does the rate at which self-perceived ability in math and science change over time differ for adolescent boys and girls?" To answer these questions, the predictor variable Gender must be incorporated into the Level 2 (or structural) part of the model. This predictor model represents an extension of the final best-fitting multiple-domain model (Model 3) and is shown schematically in Fig. 12.2.

Of importance regarding the path diagram displayed in Fig. 12.2 are the newly added components. The first of these is the regression path leading from the Constant to the predictor variable of Gender. Essentially, this path represents the intercept on the variable of Gender. However, this path can be more intuitively understood by reviewing the following standard regression equation:

$$y = a + b1x1 + b2x2 + \cdots + e \tag{3}$$

where the intercept "a" is the coefficient for the regression of a variable on a constant. As such, we can rewrite Equation (3) equivalently as follows:

$$y = a1 + b1x1 + b2x2 + \cdots + e \tag{4}$$

where "1" is the constant "variable."

The regression of a variable on a constant is an intercept when the variable is an independent variable; otherwise, it is the mean of the variable. Relatedly, the path flowing from the Constant to the variable of Gender in Fig. 12.2 essentially represents a simpler version of the standard regression equation that can be stated as follows:

$$y = a1 + e \tag{5}$$

where, y = Gender; a = the path leading from the Constant to Gender, with the Constant equal to 1; and E47 = e.

The second set of new components comprises the regression paths that flow from Gender to the Intercept and Slope factors associated with each Perceived Ability domain. These regression paths are of primary interest in this predictor

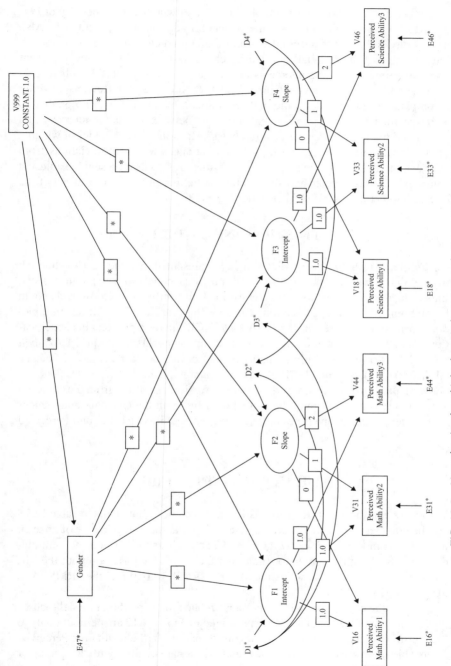

FIG. 12.2. Hypothesized multiple-domain latent growth curve predictor model.

371

model because they hold the key to the question of whether the trajectory of Perceived Ability in Math and in Science differs for adolescent boys and girls. Also noteworthy is the fact that with the addition of a predictor variable to the model, interpretation of the residuals necessarily changes; these residuals now represent variation remaining in the intercepts and slopes after all variability in their prediction by Gender has been explained (Willett & Keiley, 2000). Rephrased within a comparative framework, in the multiple-domain model in which no predictors were specified, the residuals represent deviations between the factor intercepts and slopes and their population means. In contrast, for this current model in which a predictor variable is specified, the residual variances represent deviations from their conditional population means. As such, these residuals represent the adjusted values of factor intercepts and slopes after partialling out the linear effect of the Gender predictor variable (Willett & Keiley, 2000).

THE EQS INPUT FILE

The EQS input file for this predictor model is presented in Table 12.10. Although most of this file remains the same as for the previous model (with no predictor), two important aspects related to parameter estimations for this predictor model should be highlighted. First, specifications are based on the final best-fitting multiple-domain model. As a result, the /COVARIANCES paragraph contains specifications for the two between-domain residual covariances (D1,D3 and D2,D4) albeit no specification for a within-domain residual covariance for Perceived Science Ability (D3,D4). Second, the /EQUATIONS paragraph now incorporates the Gender variable. In particular, observe that the regression path flows from the Constant (V999) to Gender (V47) and the paths flow from both the Constant and Gender to the intercept and slope for both Perceived Math Ability (F1, F2) and Perceived Science Ability (F3, F4).

THE EQS OUTPUT FILE

We now review the results from the testing of this model. Shown first in Table 12.11 are the goodness-of-fit statistics. It is interesting that there is evidence of an even better fitting model (*CFI = .975; CFI = .975) than was the case for the multiple-domain model with no predictor (note that the CFI value based on both the ML and robust χ^2 values is now identical). The SRMR is .039 and the *RMSEA is .056 (RMSEA = .062).

Because the content of major importance related to the predictor model focuses on the variable of Gender, the results presented in Table 12.12 are pertinent only to the construct equations that contain this information. In the results for Perceived Math Ability, we see that Gender was found to be a statistically significant predictor

TABLE 12.10
EQS Input for Predictor Model

```
/TITLE
 LGC Model of Perceived Math & Science Abilities "msG1gen"
 With Gender as Predictor
 Based on Group 1 (Complete Data)
 Based on Model 3
/SPECIFICATIONS
 DATA='c:\eqs61\files\books\data\LGC.Group1.ess';
 VARIABLES=46; CASES=500;
 METHODS=ML,ROBUST; MATRIX=RAW; ANALYSIS=MOMENT;
 DEL=467;
/LABELS
 V1=SUBJECT;   V2=GENDER;  V3=SCHTYPE;  V4=MATGRDS1;  V5=SCIGRDS1;
 V6=ENGGRDS1;  V7=MATH04S1; V8=MATH05S1; V9=MATH06S1;  V10=LANG04S1;
 V11=LANG05S1;  V12=LANG06S1; V13=SCI04S1; V14=SCI05S1; V15=SCI06S1;
 V16=M_ABILS1;  V17=L_ABILS1; V18=S_ABILS1; V19=MATGRDS2; V20=SCIGRDS2;
 V21=ENGGRDS2;  V22=MATH04S2; V23=MATH05S2; V24=MATH06S2; V25=LANG04S2;
 V26=LANG05S2;  V27=LANG06S2; V28=SCI04S2; V29=SCI05S2; V30=SCI06S2;
 V31=M_ABILS2;  V32=L_ABILS2; V33=S_ABILS2; V34=MATGRDS3; V35=SCIGRDS3;
 V36=ENGGRDS3;  V37=MATH04S3; V38=LANG04S3; V39=LANG05S3; V40=LANG06S3;
 V41=SCI04S3; V42=SCI05S3; V43=SCI06S3; V44=M_ABILS3; V45=L_ABILS3;
 V46=S_ABILS3;
/EQUATIONS
 V47 = *V999 + E47;
 V16 =   + 1F1  + 0F2  + 1E16;
 V31 =   + 1F1  + 1F2  + 1E31;
 V44 =   + 1F1  + 2F2  + 1E44;
 F1  =   + *V999 + *V47 + 1D1;
 F2  =   + *V999 + *V47 + 1D2;
 V18 =   + 1F3  + 0F4  + 1E18;
 V33 =   + 1F3  + 1F4  + 1E33;
 V46 =   + 1F3  + 2F4  + 1E46;
 F3  =   + *V999 + *V47 + 1D3;
 F4  =   + *V999 + *V47 + 1D4;
/VARIANCES
 V999 = 1.00;
 E16 = *;
 E31 = *;
 E44 = *;
 E18 = *;
 E33 = *;
 E46 = *;
 D1  = *;
 D2  = *;
 D3  = *;
 D4  = *;
/COVARIANCES
 D1,D2 = *; D1,D3 = *; D2,D4 = *;
/PRINT
 FIT=ALL;
/END
```

TABLE 12.11
Selected EQS Output for Predictor Model

```
GOODNESS OF FIT SUMMARY FOR METHOD = ML

CHI-SQUARE =          35.279 BASED ON        12 DEGREES OF FREEDOM
PROBABILITY VALUE FOR THE CHI-SQUARE STATISTIC IS          .00042

FIT INDICES (BASED ON COVARIANCE MATRIX ONLY, NOT THE MEANS)
-----------
BENTLER-BONETT      NORMED FIT INDEX =          .964
BENTLER-BONETT NON-NORMED FIT INDEX =          .947
COMPARATIVE FIT INDEX (CFI)          =          .975
ROOT MEAN-SQUARE RESIDUAL (RMR)      =          .066
STANDARDIZED RMR                     =          .039
ROOT MEAN-SQUARE ERROR OF APPROXIMATION (RMSEA)       =          .062
90% CONFIDENCE INTERVAL OF RMSEA (          .039,          .087)

GOODNESS OF FIT SUMMARY FOR METHOD = ROBUST
SATORRA-BENTLER SCALED CHI-SQUARE =        30.5457 ON       12 DEGREES OF FREEDOM
PROBABILITY VALUE FOR THE CHI-SQUARE STATISTIC IS       .00231

FIT INDICES (BASED ON COVARIANCE MATRIX ONLY, NOT THE MEANS)
-----------
BENTLER-BONETT      NORMED FIT INDEX =          .962
BENTLER-BONETT NON-NORMED FIT INDEX =          .947
COMPARATIVE FIT INDEX (CFI)          =          .975
ROOT MEAN-SQUARE ERROR OF APPROXIMATION (RMSEA)       =          .056
90% CONFIDENCE INTERVAL OF RMSEA (          .031,          .81)
```

of both initial status (.551) and rate of change (−.145). Given a coding of "0" for females and "1" for males, these findings suggest that whereas Self-Perceived Ability in Math was on average higher for boys than for girls at Time 1 by .551, the rate of change in this perception for boys from Grades 8 through 10 was slower than it was for girls by a value of −.145. (The negative coefficient indicates that boys had the lower slope.)

Results again revealed Gender as a significant predictor of Perceived Science Ability in Grade 8, with boys showing higher scores on average by a value of .233 than girls. On the other hand, rate of change was indistinguishable between boys and girls as indicated by its nonsignificant estimate.

In conclusion, I draw from the work of Willett and Sayer (1994, 1996) in highlighting several important features captured by the LGC modeling approach to the investigation of change. First, the methodology can accommodate from 3 to 30 waves of longitudinal data equally well. Willett (1988, 1989) showed, however, that the more waves of data collected, the more precise is the estimated growth trajectory and the higher is the reliability for the measurement of change. Second, there is no requirement that the time lag between each wave of assessments be equivalent. Indeed, LGC modeling can easily accommodate irregularly spaced measurements, but with the caveat that all subjects are measured on the same set of occasions. Third, individual change can be represented by either a linear or a nonlinear growth trajectory. Although linear growth is typically assumed by default, this assumption is easily tested and the model respecified to address

TABLE 12.12

Selected EQS Output for Predictor Model

CONSTRUCT EQUATIONS WITH STANDARD ERRORS AND TEST STATISTICS
STATISTICS SIGNIFICANT AT THE 5% LEVEL ARE MARKED WITH @.
(ROBUST STATISTICS IN PARENTHESES)

```
F1   =F1   =     .551*V47    +   4.851*V999 + 1.000 D1
                 .106                .075
                 5.178@           64.938@
            (    .107)        (      .080)
            (   5.149@        (    60.367@

F2   =F2   =    -.145*V47    -     .092*V999 + 1.000 D2
                 .064                .045
                -2.280@           -2.057@
            (    .064)        (      .045)
            (  -2.283@        (    -2.042@

F3   =F3   =     .233*V47    +   4.645*V999 + 1.000 D3
                 .102                .071
                 2.289@           65.027@
            (    .103)        (      .072)
            (   2.269@        (    64.344@

F4   =F4   =     .013*V47    +     .118*V999 + 1.000 D4
                 .060                .042
                 .213              2.804@
            (    .061)        (      .042)
            (    .211)        (     2.788@
```

curvilinearity if necessary. Fourth, in contrast to traditional methods used in measuring change, LGC models allow not only for the estimation of measurement error variances, but also for their autocorrelation and fluctuation across time in the event that tests for the assumptions of independence and homoscedasticity are untenable. Fifth, multiple predictors of change can be included in the LGC model. They may be fixed, as in the specification of Gender in this chapter, or time-varying (see, e.g., Byrne in press; and Willett & Keiley, 2000). Finally, the three key statistical assumptions associated with this application of LGC modeling (i.e., linearity, independence of measurement error variances, and homoscedasticity of measurement error variances), although not demonstrated in this chapter, can be easily tested via a comparison of nested models (see e.g., Byrne & Crombie, 2003).

To close this chapter on LGC modeling, readers should be aware that multilevel models provide an alternate way to study change with structural models. Singer and Willett (2003) provide an excellent discussion that focuses primarily on the Higher Linear Modeling approach.

13

Application 11:
Testing for Within- and
Between-Level Variance:
The Multilevel Model

In this final chapter, we examine SEM as it applies to multiple models drawn from a single data set. In contrast to the multigroup models illustrated in Part 3 that involved data from separate data sets, the multigroup model explored in this chapter is based on a single population that is hierarchically structured. Such models are termed *multilevel* because the data lend themselves to more than one level of analyses. The most common examples of hierarchically structured data are (a) students nested within schools, (b) patients nested within clinics, (c) employees nested within organizations, (d) children and adults nested within families, and the like. Such hierarchical structures are often termed *nested data* or *clustered data*. In essence, however, hierarchical structures may involve more than two levels of analysis. Building on these previous examples, data could be extended to include schools nested within districts and districts nested within states, or employees nested within departments, departments nested within organizations, organizations nested within regions, and so on. Beyond these examples, however, Hox (2002) showed that hierarchical structures also can include repeated measures within individuals or respondents within clusters, as in cluster sampling.

The application illustrated in this chapter represents a two-level multilevel CFA model based on data drawn from the Longitudinal Study of American Youth (Miller, Kimmel, Hoffer, & Nelson, 1999). We test for differences in quantitative skills and self-esteem within and across schools for Grade 7 adolescents. Before examining these analyses, however, a brief overview of multilevel modeling in general is presented.

OVERVIEW OF MULTILEVEL MODELING

In the past decade, multilevel modeling has been increasingly recognized as one of the most proficient means for investigating hierarchical data. Despite growing awareness, however, progress in the practical application of multilevel modeling has lagged far behind the substantive theory to which it is grounded. I think it safe to say that this lengthy delay in the use of multilevel modeling can be directly linked to the inability of existing SEM software packages to adequately address the complications associated with these analyses. As a consequence, researchers working with hierarchical data have been forced to disregard the rich source of potential information provided by such data and limit their investigations to single-level analyses, which are either on the lowest level of measurement (e.g., students) or on the highest level of measurement (e.g., schools). Rephrased differently, researchers need to either disaggregate or aggregate variables from their nested data to enable single-level analyses (Heck, 2001). These inappropriate analyses of hierarchically structured data, not surprisingly, led to several analytic and interpretation difficulties, a topic to which we now turn.

Single-Level Analyses of Hierarchically Structured Data: Related Problems

Consequences arising from single-level analyses of hierarchical data lead to problematic repercussions at both the individual (lower) and group (higher) levels; these arise from the disaggregation and aggregation approaches to the analyses, respectively.

Disaggregation Approach

In the disaggregation approach, analyses focus on the individual (e.g., student, lower) level of the hierarchy. At least two major analytic difficulties occur at this lower level when nested data are treated as a single unit. First, the underlying assumption that all observations are totally independent is violated. This assumption holds that all individuals within similar subunits and/or organizations share no common characteristics or perceptions (Heck, 2001), which of course, is totally unrealistic. Indeed, Muthén and Satorra (1995) argued that the more pronounced these similarities are among individuals within groups, the more biased are the parameter estimates, standard errors, and (ultimately) associated tests for significance. Second, the assumption that all random errors in the equation are independent, normally distributed, and homoscedastic—an important postulation associated with efficient estimation—is violated (Bryk & Raudenbush, 1992). Heck (2001) noted that such violation is often the case in single-level analysis of hierarchical data because it implies that no systematic influence of variables at the higher level is expected. As a consequence, all higher level influence is incorporated into the model error terms (Kreft & deLeeuw, 1998). In reality, however, the errors within each lower level group are dependent rather than independent because they are common to every individual within this group. Random error components of multilevel models, then, are more complex than single-level models.

Aggregation Approach

This approach to the analyses focuses on the group or higher level of the hierarchy. As such, organizations (e.g., schools) form the unit of analysis and the individual data are used to develop mean scores on the variables as they relate to each organization (Heck, 2001). Again, there are at least two limitations with these higher level analyses. First, because all variability present within each organizational unit is reduced to a single mean, any determined differences found at the higher level appear stronger than would be the case if within-organizational (i.e., individual) variability were also incorporated into the analysis (Kaplan & Elliott, 1997). Second, in situations in which the individual-level data for particular variables (e.g., socioeconomic status) may be meager in some groups, the attainment of efficient estimates is made more difficult, thereby resulting in less efficient prediction equations for these groups (Bryk & Raudenbush, 1992).

Multiple Level Analyses of Hierarchically Structured Data: Multilevel Modeling

Unlike the single-level analyses discussed previously, multilevel modeling allows the researcher to consider both levels of the hierarchically structured data simultaneously. In particular, it enables the partitioning of total variance into within- and between-group components and allows separate structural models to be specified. For example, in the case of students nested within schools, this means that the total covariance matrix, Σ, is partitioned into a within-covariance matrix (Σ_W) and a between-covariance matrix (Σ_B). The Σ_W matrix represents covariation (i.e., individual differences at the student level in, say, algebra achievement) and their correlates, controlling for variation across schools. In contrast, the Σ_B matrix represents covariation at the school level (i.e., differences across schools in, say, school climate or teaching quality) and their correlates (Bentler, 2005). Σ_W and Σ_B may have similar or totally different model structures. For each student, the total score is decomposed into an individual component (i.e., individual deviation from the group mean) and a group component (i.e., the disaggregated school group mean), and it is via this individual decomposition that the separate within- and between-groups covariance matrices are computed (Heck, 2001; and Hox, 2002). Not surprisingly, the related effects are termed *within-cluster* and *between-cluster* effects (Bentler, 2005). If a mean structure is needed, it is used to model the between-group means.

Analytic approaches to the estimation of multilevel models appear to involve mainly three different procedures: maximum likelihood (ML), Muthén's (1994) approximate estimator (MUML), and hierarchical linear modeling (HLM), where ML is commonly used (Hox, 2002). Given evidence that ML estimation with unbalanced groups—clusters of unequal sample size—can lead to incorrect χ^2 values, fit indexes, and standard errors (Kaplan, 1998; and Muthén, 1994), Muthén developed a limited ML method of estimation (MUML) that addressed this difficulty. More recently, ML estimation has been the norm. To ensure estimates with desirable asymptotic properties, the ML approach demands large sample sizes, especially at the highest level of a hierarchical structure (Yuan & Bentler, 2002, 2004b; Heck, 2001; and Hox, 2002). In fact, Bentler (2005) suggests that, ideally, there should be perhaps hundreds of units at the higher level (e.g., schools).

The EQS program allows for parameter estimation using each of these three different analytic approaches. However, unlike other current SEM programs, EQS can compute ML estimation in the face of unbalanced group sizes. Based on the work of Liang and Bentler (2004), EQS handles all estimation by means of the EM algorithm. Of the three analytic approaches to multilevel modeling performed by EQS, analyses based on the ML approach are the most straightforward and easily handled for two-level data (see, e.g., Bentler & Liang, 2003a, 2003b; and Liang & Bentler, 2004). Nonetheless, the two-stage approach to analyses implemented by EQS (Chou, Bentler, & Pentz, 2000) can, in principle, handle any number of levels (Bentler, 2005).

Following this introductory synopsis of multilevel modeling, we now examine the application under study in this chapter. Further details related to multilevel analyses emerge as we work through its various stages with respect to the current data. However, for more comprehensive coverage of the theory, related issues, and practice of multilevel modeling, readers are referred to four excellent sources: Heck (2001), Hox (2002), Reise & Duan (2003), and Tomarken & Waller (2005).

THE HYPOTHESIZED MODEL

As an aid to conceptualizing the multilevel model, McArdle and Hamagami (1996) suggested that researchers think of it as a typical multisample analysis. The rationale underlying this proposal stems from the fact that analyses focus on the estimation of two unstructured matrices, Σ_W and Σ_B, each of which represents a separate model. Although the standard statistical assumption of independent groups cannot be made, such a model can nonetheless be thought of as a two-group multigroup model (Bentler, 2005). Thus, specification of a multilevel model in EQS replicates any other two-group setup using this program, with one set of specifications for the within-level structure and one set for the between-level structure.

As stated at the beginning of this chapter, the data used in illustrating this multi-level model are drawn from the Longitudinal Study of American Youth conducted by Miller et al. (1999). The extrapolated variables for purposes of illustration represent measures of Quantitative Skills and Self-Esteem as they pertain to Grade 7 adolescents. Specific to this postulated two-level multilevel model, 2,673 students comprise the lower level and 52 schools comprise the higher level.[1] To facilitate conceptualization of this model, let's now turn to the schematic representation of this hypothesized model shown in Fig. 13.1.

Figure 13.1 shows that the within- and between-level models are identical in representing a three-factor CFA model. At each of two levels, the two-level structure represents a three-factor CFA model. The extrapolated variables comprising the data consist of four designed to measure quantitative skill and six to measure self-esteem. Specifically, the observed variables for quantitative skill represent interval scores for basic math, algebra, geometry, and quantitative literacy; the variables, as coded in the original data set, are BAS7, ALG7, GEO7, and QLIT7, respectively.[2] The self-esteem variables represent six of ten items composing the Rosenberg (1965) Self-Esteem Scale; they are labeled RSES1 through RSES6. These item variables are structured on a 1-to-5 scale, with 1 = *strongly agree* and 5 = *strongly disagree*. Based on results of the preanalyses of these data, the self-esteem items were found to measure two factors, termed Global Self-Esteem (F2) and Self-Derogation (F3), with Items 1 through 4 (RSES1–RSES4) loading on Global Self-Esteem and Items 5 and 6 (RSES5–RSES6) loading on Self-Derogation. Based on the same preanalyses, the three factors were found to be correlated.

Before testing for the validity of the hypothesized model shown in Fig. 13.1, however, I wish first to review the preliminary analyses conducted while also taking the opportunity to illustrate additional features of the EQS program.

Preliminary Analyses

Reverse Coding of Data

An important consideration with respect to the self-esteem items used herein is that the stems of Items 5 and 6 are negatively worded (i.e., RSES5: "I wish I respected myself more" and RSES6: "I feel I am a failure"). Thus, to maintain consistency of response direction with the other four items, it is of interest to reverse-code RSES5 and RSES6. In this regard, EQS has a very slick way to perform a recode of data. Unlike most statistical programs that require the need for variable transformation, which can often mean the specification of numerous

---

[1] The full sample of students was 3,116. However, at the time of writing this book, EQS was not yet capable of handling the issue of missing data for multilevel models.

[2] The original variable names appear in the EQS input and output files, to be discussed shortly.

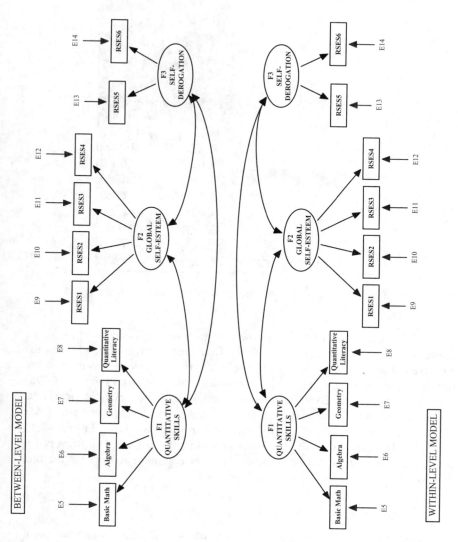

FIG. 13.1. Hypothesized two-level multilevel model.

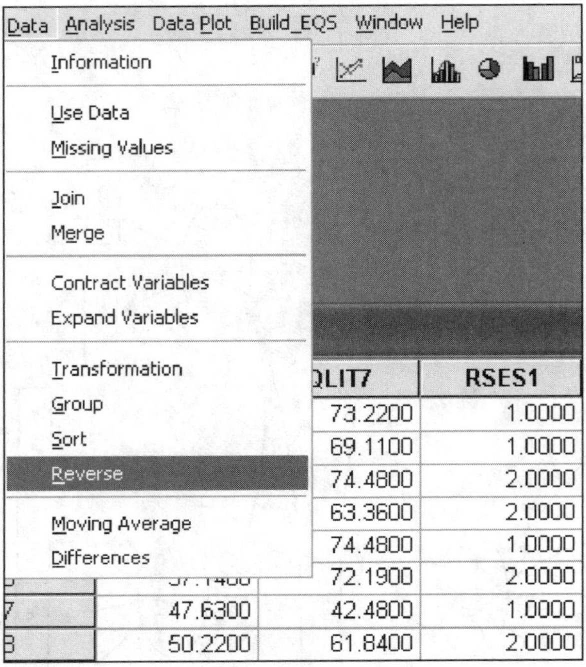

Data	Analysis	Data Plot	Build EQS	Window	Help
Information					
Use Data					
Missing Values					
Join					
Merge					
Contract Variables					
Expand Variables					
Transformation			QLIT7	RSES1	
Group			73.2200	1.0000	
Sort			69.1100	1.0000	
Reverse			74.4800	2.0000	
Moving Average			63.3600	2.0000	
Differences			74.4800	1.0000	
			72.1900	2.0000	
7		47.6300	42.4800	1.0000	
8		50.2200	61.8400	2.0000	

FIG. 13.2. Data drop-down menu with Reverse coding option selected.

If and *Else* statements, EQS allows the user to reverse all codes with a single click. To initiate this process, click on the Data drop-down menu and select the Reverse option shown highlighted in Fig. 13.2. The Reverse option triggers the opening of the Reverse Category Coding dialog box, as shown in Fig. 13.3. This box offers two options. By default, the program reverses only the numerical code. However, the user can also reverse the code labels by selecting Reverse Code Name. Once the variable is selected (here it is RSES5, as shown in Fig. 13.3), click OK. The user remains at this box to choose another variable for reversal if necessary. Clicking DONE implements the reverse coding, after which the box closes.

Exploratory Factor Analysis

Although the Self-Esteem Scale was originally designed as a unidimensional scale, there is substantial literature that has shown it to actually represent two factors (for a review, see Byrne, 1996), one representing Global Self-Esteem and the other a related but independent construct that is labeled Self-Derogation. Because of this discrepancy, then, I considered it important to determine if the six items included

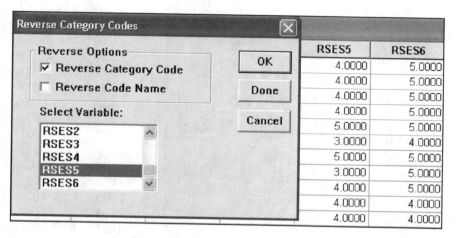

FIG. 13.3. Reverse Category Codes dialog box.

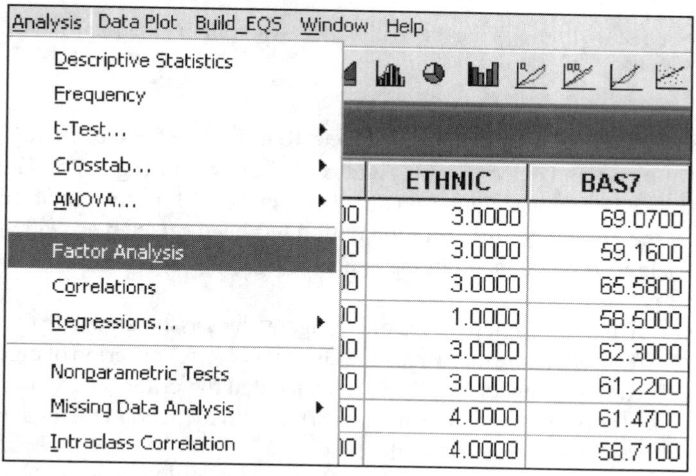

FIG. 13.4. Analysis drop-down menu with Factor Analysis option selected.

in the Miller et al. (1999) study were best described by a one- or two-factor model. Thus, an EFA of these items was conducted using Direct Oblimin rotation.

EQS provides two extraction methods that are fast and reliable: Principal Components Analysis and Equal Prior Instant Communalities (EPIC). Bentler and Wu (2002) posited that these methods typically yield a very good approximation of the more complex methods available in such statistical packages as SPSS for Windows. They further noted that if the variables are used subsequently to model

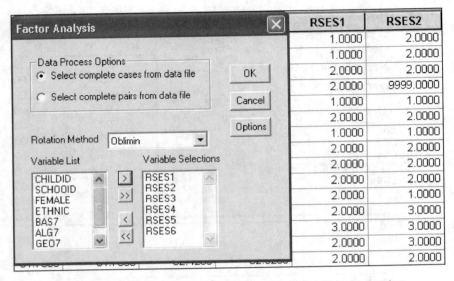

	RSES1	RSES2
	1.0000	2.0000
	1.0000	2.0000
	2.0000	2.0000
	2.0000	9999.0000
	1.0000	1.0000
	2.0000	2.0000
	1.0000	1.0000
	2.0000	2.0000
	2.0000	2.0000
	2.0000	2.0000
	2.0000	1.0000
	2.0000	3.0000
	3.0000	3.0000
	2.0000	3.0000
	2.0000	2.0000

FIG. 13.5.   Factor Analysis dialog box with direct Oblimin rotation selected.

latent variables, EPIC is the preferred choice. To initiate an EFA, click the Analysis drop-down menu and select Factor Analysis, as shown in Fig. 13.4. This action opens the Factor Analysis dialog box depicted in Fig. 13.5. Review of this figure shows that the Direct Oblimin rotation option has been selected as well as the six RSES variables to be included in the analysis. Clicking OK yields the Scree Plot shown in Fig. 13.6.

This plot displays the relative size of the eigenvalues associated with the correlation matrix. The dotted line represents the Guttman–Kaiser criterion of eigenvalues greater than 1.00. Review of Fig. 13.6 indicates that the criterion, in this case, includes two factors (i.e., two eigenvalues > 1.00), with the second factor accounting for substantially less variance than the first.

To retrieve the analytic results of this EFA, click the Factor Analysis option shown circled at the top of the plot in Fig. 13.6. The key results of interest here are summarized in Table 13.1. For substantially more information related to both the program options and related output, readers are referred to the user's guide (Bentler & Wu, 2002) and the manual (Bentler, 2005).

Review of Table 13.1 shows that consistent with the Scree Plot, there are two eigenvalues greater than 1.00, the first one substantially larger than the second. In the rotated factor loadings, we find that (as expected) RSES1 through RSES4 load on Factor 1 and RSES5 and RSES6 load on Factor 2. In both cases, the loadings are clearly delineated and substantial. Finally, the Factor Correlation Matrix reveals that the correlation between the two factors is moderately strong, at .413.

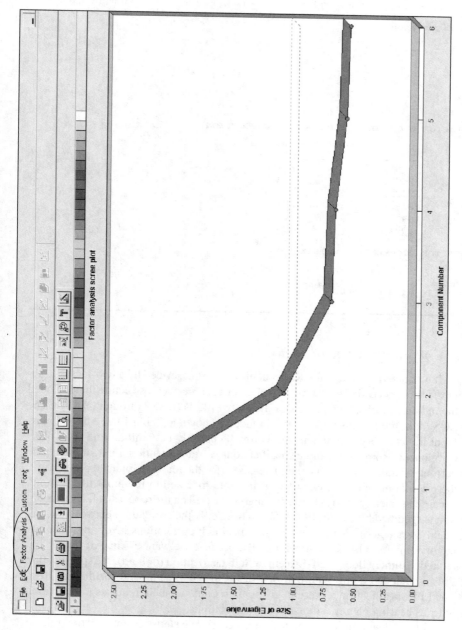

FIG. 13.6.   Graph of factor analysis Scree Plot.

385

TABLE 13.1

Selected EQS Output for Exploratory Factor Analysis of Self-Esteem Items (RSES)

Eigenvalues

1	2.343
2	1.099
3	0.708
4	0.682
5	0.594
6	0.575

FACTOR LOADINGS (DIRECT OBLIMIN SOLUTION)

	FACTOR 1	FACTOR 2
RSES1	0.592	0.052
RSES2	0.645	-0.072
RSES3	0.609	-0.020
RSES4	0.566	0.091
RSES5	-0.062	0.603
RSES6	0.131	0.509

FACTOR CORRELATION MATRIX

	FACTOR 1	FACTOR 2
FACTOR 1	1.000	
FACTOR 2	0.413	

Confirmatory Factor Analyses

It was determined that the RSES items are best described by a two-factor structure; I then proceeded to test for the validity of a three-factor structure that included
the indicator variables measuring quantitative skills (BAS7 through QLIT7). The
EQS input file for this hypothesized model is shown in Table 13.2. Although this
input file is a very simple one and you will certainly be familiar with each of its
components, some of the input specifications warrant attention. First, although the
current example is based on complete cases (for the reason explained previously),
the original number of cases (3,116) remains specified in the input file. Second,
because I typically always begin my analyses based on the robust statistics, this option is specified here (ML, ROBUST). Third, only the correlation between Factors
2 and 3 (as determined in the EFA) is specified; correlations involving the other
factors remain to be determined. Finally, because we want to know if Factor 1 is
related to either Global Self-Esteem or Self-Derogation (or both), the specification
PFF is included along with that of PEE in the SET command for the LM Test.
The PFF specification represents a Phi matrix and, as such, requests modification
indexes bearing on any omitted factor correlations.

Table 13.3 summarizes the univariate descriptive statistics, information related
to multivariate kurtosis, and a notation on the number of cases for which data

TABLE 13.2
EQS Input for Hypothesized CFA Model

/TITLE
Testing for Validity of 3-Factor CFA "MLEVELCFA"
/SPECIFICATIONS
DATA='c:\eqs61\files\books\data\lsayredr.ess';
VARIABLES=14; CASES=3116;
METHOD=ML,ROBUST; ANALYSIS=COVARIANCE; MATRIX=RAW;
/LABELS
V1=CHILDID; V2=SCHOOLID; V3=FEMALE; V4=ETHNIC; V5=BAS7;
V6=ALG7; V7=GEO7; V8=QLIT7; V9=RSES1; V10=RSES2;
V11=RSES3; V12=RSES4; V13=RSES5; V14=RSES6;
/EQUATIONS
V5 =   F1 + E5;
V6 =   *F1 + E6;
V7 =   *F1 + E7;
V8 =   *F1 + E8;
V9 =   F2 + E9;
V10 = *F2 + E10;
V11 = *F2 + E11;
V12 = *F2 + E12;
V13 =   F3 + E13;
V14 = *F3 + E14;
/VARIANCES
F1 to F3 = *;
E5 to E14 = *;
/COVARIANCES
F2,F3 = *;
/PRINT
FIT=ALL;
/LMTEST
SET=PFF,PEE;
/END

are complete (i.e., 2,673). Review of the descriptive statistics shows that there is virtually no evidence of any substantial univariate skewness or kurtosis. The normalized estimate of Mardia's multivariate kurtosis is 21.568. With the large case contributions to kurtosis (Mardia's coefficient is the average of such scores), it is likely that outlying cases may be more of a problem than bad distributions. However, we do not want to eliminate cases from this sample. The Robust option could be used to handle this situation but, because there are only 52 schools, this method may not work reliably; thus, ML statistics are used.

Review of the goodness-of-fit statistics in Table 13.4 as they relate to this initial CFA model shows that it is very well fitting (i.e., CFI = .950; SRMR = .080; RMSEA= .061). However, the LM Test statistics in Table 13.5 reveal a substantial misspecification regarding parameter F3,F1, the covariance between Quantitative

TABLE 13.3

Selected EQS Output for Hypothesized CFA Model: Descriptive Statistics and Related Information

SAMPLE STATISTICS BASED ON COMPLETE CASES

UNIVARIATE STATISTICS

VARIABLE	BAS7	ALG7	GEO7	QLIT7	RSES1
MEAN	50.8142	50.4744	50.5493	50.6730	1.9065
SKEWNESS (G1)	.2830	.2895	1.1180	.5653	1.0319
KURTOSIS (G2)	-.5063	-.6185	1.1665	-.5003	1.3309
STANDARD DEV.	10.2059	10.0425	10.3981	10.1711	.8549

VARIABLE	RSES2	RSES3	RSES4	RSES5	RSES6
MEAN	2.1646	2.0524	2.2091	2.0535	1.1358
SKEWNESS (G1)	.6555	.9033	.7918	-.0790	.7785
KURTOSIS (G2)	.3910	.9220	.2542	-.9126	-.2895
STANDARD DEV.	.9147	.8921	1.0075	1.1827	1.1529

MULTIVARIATE KURTOSIS

MARDIA'S COEFFICIENT (G2,P) =   12.9252
NORMALIZED ESTIMATE =   21.5675

CASE NUMBERS WITH LARGEST CONTRIBUTION TO NORMALIZED MULTIVARIATE KURTOSIS:

CASE NUMBER	1411	1998	2022	2112	2610
ESTIMATE	2859.7468	2326.7302	2963.9467	2318.3765	2311.1209

COVARIANCE MATRIX TO BE ANALYZED: 10 VARIABLES (SELECTED FROM 14 VARIABLES)
                                       BASED ON 2673 CASES.

TABLE 13.4

Selected EQS Output for Hypothesized CFA Model: Goodness-of-Fit Statistics

GOODNESS OF FIT SUMMARY FOR METHOD = ML

CHI-SQUARE =   366.869 BASED ON   34 DEGREES OF FREEDOM
PROBABILITY VALUE FOR THE CHI-SQUARE STATISTIC IS   .00000

FIT INDICES

BENTLER-BONETT NORMED FIT INDEX =	.945	
BENTLER-BONETT NON-NORMED FIT INDEX =	.933	
COMPARATIVE FIT INDEX (CFI) =	.950	
ROOT MEAN-SQUARE RESIDUAL (RMR) =	.985	
STANDARDIZED RMR =	.080	
ROOT MEAN-SQUARE ERROR OF APPROXIMATION (RMSEA) =	.061	
90% CONFIDENCE INTERVAL OF RMSEA (.055,	.066)	

TABLE 13.5

Selected EQS Output for Hypothesized CFA Model: Modification Indexes

		CUMULATIVE MULTIVARIATE STATISTICS			UNIVARIATE INCREMENT		HANCOCK'S SEQUENTIAL	
STEP	PARAMETER	CHI-SQUARE	D.F.	PROB.	CHI-SQUARE	PROB.	D.F.	PROB.
1	F3,F1	200.439	1	.000	200.439	.000	34	.000
2	E11,E10	230.402	2	.000	29.963	.000	33	.619
3	E14,E12	240.837	3	.000	10.435	.001	32	1.000
4	E6,E5	250.469	4	.000	9.632	.002	31	1.000
5	E14,E6	258.494	5	.000	8.025	.005	30	1.000
6	E14,E5	265.933	6	.000	7.440	.006	29	1.000
7	E13,E10	271.525	7	.000	5.592	.018	28	1.000

TABLE 13.6

Selected EQS Output for CFA Model 2: Modification Indexes

		CUMULATIVE MULTIVARIATE STATISTICS			UNIVARIATE INCREMENT		HANCOCK'S SEQUENTIAL	
STEP	PARAMETER	CHI-SQUARE	D.F.	PROB.	CHI-SQUARE	PROB.	D.F.	PROB.
1	F2,F1	37.590	1	.000	37.590	.000	33	.267
2	E11,E10	70.847	2	.000	33.257	.000	32	.406
3	E8,E7	85.411	3	.000	14.564	.000	31	.995
4	E14,E12	97.575	4	.000	12.165	.000	30	.998
5	E13,E9	106.740	5	.000	9.165	.002	29	1.000
6	E14,E6	115.116	6	.000	8.376	.004	28	1.000

Literacy and Self-derogation. With an LM Test χ^2 value of 200.439 compared to the remaining univariate incremental values, it is evident that the model requires respecification that includes the estimation of this parameter.

The model was modified accordingly and, again, the LM Test statistics revealed misspecification regarding the last possible factor covariance between Quantitative Skills and Self-esteem; these values are shown in Table 13.6. Although there is also evidence of misspecification involving error covariances, it is best not to include these parameters in the model for at least two reasons: (a) the model is already well fitting (i.e., CFI = .982; SRMR = .044; RMSEA = .037), and (b) to do so runs the risk of overparameterizing the model, with the risk of capitalization on chance factors. A final model that included the two additional factor covariances revealed an extremely well-fitting model, as indicated by the goodness-of-fit statistics reported in Table 13.7. As shown in Table 13.8, all three factor correlations were statistically significant, albeit the relation between Factor 1 (Quantitative Skills) and Factor 2 (Global Self-Esteem) is small ($r = -.152$).

TABLE 13.7

Selected EQS Output for CFA Model 3: Goodness-of-Fit Statistics

---

GOODNESS OF FIT SUMMARY FOR METHOD = ML

CHI-SQUARE =   113.443 BASED ON   32 DEGREES OF FREEDOM
PROBABILITY VALUE FOR THE CHI-SQUARE STATISTIC IS   .00000

FIT INDICES

BENTLER-BONETT   NORMED FIT INDEX =   .983
BENTLER-BONETT NON-NORMED FIT INDEX =   .983
COMPARATIVE FIT INDEX (CFI)   =   .988
ROOT MEAN-SQUARE RESIDUAL (RMR)   =   .479
STANDARDIZED RMR   =   .023
ROOT MEAN-SQUARE ERROR OF APPROXIMATION (RMSEA)   =   .031
90% CONFIDENCE INTERVAL OF RMSEA (.025,   .037)

TABLE 13.8

Selected EQS Output for CFA Model 3: Unstandardized and Standardized Factor Covariances

---

COVARIANCES AMONG INDEPENDENT VARIABLES

STATISTICS SIGNIFICANT AT THE 5% LEVEL ARE MARKED WITH @.
```
                             I F2  -    F2              -.747*I
                             I F1  -    F1               .124 I
                             I                         -6.034@I
                             I                       (   .123)I
                             I                       ( -6.064@I
                             I                              I
                             I F3  -    F3             -1.691*I
                             I F1  -    F1               .185 I
                             I                         -9.159@I
                             I                       (   .187)I
                             I                       ( -9.049@I
                             I                              I
                             I F3  -    F3               .113*I
                             I F2  -    F2               .013 I
                             I                          8.958@I
                             I                       (   .014)I
                             I                       ( 7.979@I
                             I                              I
```

CORRELATIONS AMONG INDEPENDENT VARIABLES

```
                             I F2  -    F2             -.152*I
                             I F1  -    F1                  I
                             I                              I
                             I F3  -    F3             -.408*I
                             I F1  -    F1                  I
                             I                              I
                             I F3  -    F3              .461*I
                             I F2  -    F2                  I
                             I                              I
```

A Word of Caution

Although the EFA and CFA models are good, this may have been due to luck. Analyses were based on all students without considering school differences. We mixed within and between scores of variance and certainly could have obtained confusing results. However, as observed in Fig. 13.1, the same type of three-factor model is expected to hold at both levels; hence, analysis of the overall data might be only minimally distorting.

Testing for Validity of the Hypothesized Multilevel Model

Having established the validity of the three-factor model that forms the basic structure of the multilevel model, we now test for the validity of this multilevel structure. To build the input file for this model, the interactive approach using BUILD_EQS was chosen. Thus, before reviewing the entire EQS input file, I believe that it may be instructive to walk you through this procedure as it relates to a multilevel model.

THE EQS INPUT FILE

As illustrated in chapter 2, as soon as the BUILD_EQS menu drops down and Title/Specifications is selected, the user is presented with the EQS Model Specifications dialog box, where the program has completed information related to the number of variables and cases. In this case, as shown in Fig. 13.7, there are 14 variables and 3,116 cases. Below this information, in the Analysis section on the left side of the dialog box, Multilevel Analysis is an option. Selecting this option automatically triggers the presentation of the Additional Specifications Option dialog box displayed in Fig. 13.8 (the checkmark does not remain active in the first dialog box). In the section labeled Multilevel Options (see Fig. 13.7 overlay to the right), three different analytic approaches are available, as described previously in this chapter. Consistent with the analyses used in this chapter, ML is selected. In the same section, the cluster variable also must be identified, which, in this case, is SCHOOLID (i.e., each school had its own identification label). After selecting Continue under Type of Analysis, checkmarks appear next to Multisample Analysis and Multilevel Analysis as shown in Fig. 13.8. Clicking OK completes specifications for this section of the input file.

Captured in the upper part of Fig. 13.9 is the input file completed thus far. The last line in the /SPECIFICATIONS paragraph is pertinent to the multilevel analysis. As such, we note that the procedure is based on the ML option, with V2 (SCHOOLID) serving as the cluster variable. The lower portion of the figure displays the Build Equations dialog box, where three factors have been specified.

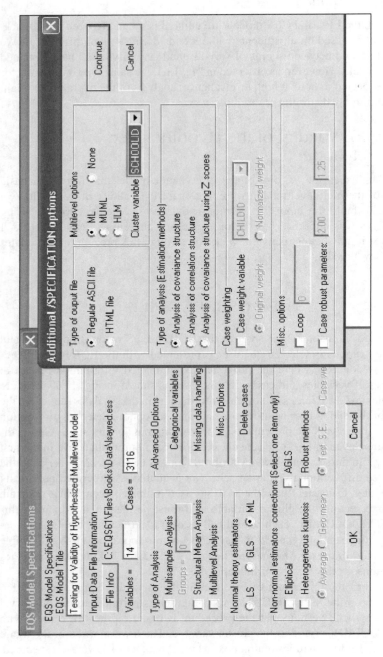

FIG. 13.7. EQS Model Specifications dialog box showing Additional/SPECIFI-CATION Options dialog box for a multilevel model using the ML approach.

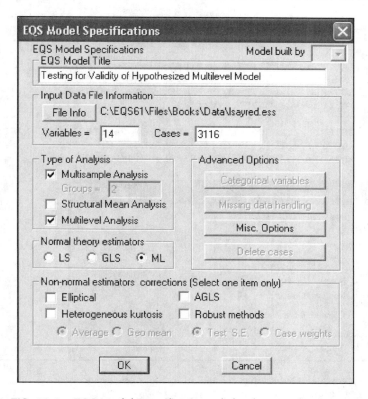

FIG. 13.8.   EQS Model Specifications dialog box confirming multilevel analysis.

Of importance here is the notation that these equations relate only to the Within Level (specified beneath the Cancel button). Continuing with these specifications, Figs. 13.10 and 13.11 illustrate the selection of variables to be included in the equations and specifics related to loadings of the observed variables onto the factors, respectively. Finally, Fig. 13.12 displays the Build Variances/Covariances dialog box, in which the specification of factor covariances is shown, with respect to the three factors.

At this point in construction of the input file, all measurement equation, variance, and covariance specifications have been specific for the Within Level. Once these have been completed, the program automatically presents, the EQS Model Specifications dialog box again. This second box is shown in Fig. 13.13, albeit this time labeled at the top of the dialog box as Between Level. After clicking OK, the user is again presented with the two Build Equations and one Build Variances/Covariances dialog boxes. Given that it is the same model, the same specifications are repeated.

```
/TITLE
Testing for Validity of Hypothesized Multilevel Model
/SPECIFICATIONS
DATA='C:\EQS61\Files\Books\Data\lsayred.ess';
VARIABLES=14; CASES=3116; GROUPS=2;
METHOD=ML; ANALYSIS=COVARIANCE; MATRIX=RAW;
MULTILEVEL=ML; CLUSTER=V2;
/LABELS
V1=CHILDID; V2=SCHOOLID; V3=FEMALE; V4=ETHNIC; V5=BAS7;
V6=ALG7; V7=GEO7; V8=QLIT7; V9=RSES1; V10=RSES2;
V11=RSES3; V12=RSES4; V13=RSES5; V14=RSES6;
/END
```

Build Equations

Type of Equation Building

○ Adopt Equations from Factor Analysis
Factor Loading Filter   0.5

● Create New Equations
Number of Variables: 14
Number of Factors: 3

○ Compare Covariance Matrices

Special Instructions
☐ Structured Means   ☐ Use All Variables

OK

Cancel

Within Level

FIG. 13.9. Completed multilevel model specifications and Build Equations dialog box.

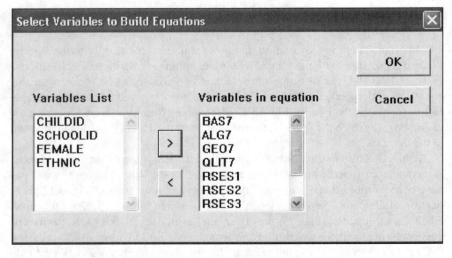

Select Variables to Build Equations

OK

Cancel

Variables List

CHILDID
SCHOOLID
FEMALE
ETHNIC

>

<

Variables in equation

BAS7
ALG7
GEO7
QLIT7
RSES1
RSES2
RSES3

FIG. 13.10. Select Variables to Build Equations dialog box.

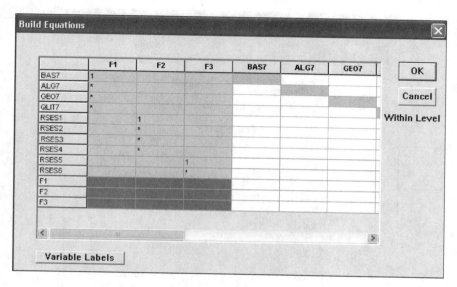

FIG. 13.11.   Build Equations dialog box.

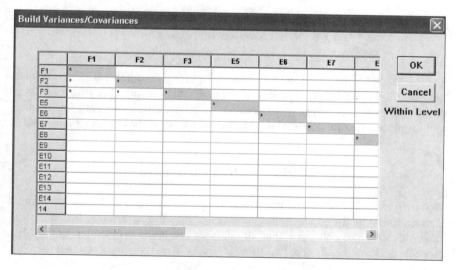

FIG. 13.12.   Build Variances/Covariances dialog box.

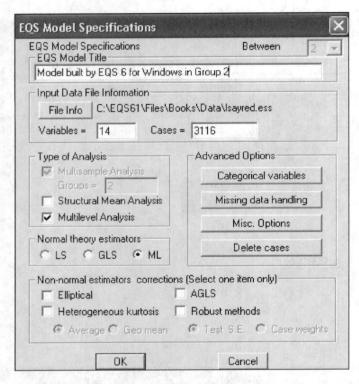

FIG. 13.13. EQS Model Specifications dialog box for between-level analysis.

The multilevel input file is now complete and shown in Table 13.9. Note that the /SPECIFICATION paragraph now indicates that the model is structured as a multisample model having two groups and two conditional statements: one related to the multilevel estimation method (ML) and the other to the cluster variable (V2).

THE EQS OUTPUT FILE

We turn now to the findings related to testing of the hypothesized multilevel model. Presented first in Table 13.10 is a summary of the cluster variable, which in this case is School ID; note also, that all analyses are based on Bentler–Liang ML procedures. Here we observe that there are 52 clusters, which means that there is a sample size of 52 schools available for analyses of the modeled between-level structure. As specified in the output, the sample size relative to each school appears on the left; the ID associated with each school appears on the right. School #304, for example, has a sample size of thirteen student participants. In another example,

TABLE 13.9

EQS Input for Two-Level Multilevel Model

```
/TITLE
Testing for Validity of Hypothesized Multilevel Model "MLEVEL1"
Level 1 - Within-Level
/SPECIFICATIONS
DATA='c:\eqs61\files\books\data\lsayredr.ess';
VARIABLES=14; CASES=3116; GROUPS=2;
METHOD=ML; ANALYSIS=COVARIANCE; MATRIX=RAW;
MULTILEVEL=ML; CLUSTER==V2;
/LABELS
V1=CHILDID; V2=SCHOOLID; V3=FEMALE; V4=ETHNIC; V5=BAS7;
V6=ALG7; V7=GEO7; V8=QLIT7; V9=RSES1; V10=RSES2;
V11=RSES3; V12=RSES4; V13=RSES5; V14=RSES6;
/EQUATIONS
V5  =    1F1 + E5;
V6  =    *F1 + E6;
V7  =    *F1 + E7;
V8  =    *F1 + E8;
V9  =    1F2 + E9;
V10 =    *F2 + E10;
V11 =    *F2 + E11;
V12 =    *F2 + E12;
V13 =    1F3 + E13;
V14 =    *F3 + E14;
/VARIANCES
F1 = *;
F2 = *;
F3 = *;
E5 = *;
E6 = *;
E7 = *;
E8 = *;
E9 = *;
E10 = *;
E11 = *;
E12 = *;
E13 = *;
E14 = *;
/COVARIANCES
F2,F3 = *;
F3,F1 = *;
F2,F1 = *;
/END
/TITLE
Level 2 - Between-Level
/LABELS
V1=CHILDID; V2=SCHOOLID; V3=FEMALE; V4=ETHNIC; V5=BAS7;
V6=ALG7; V7=GEO7; V8=QLIT7; V9=RSES1; V10=RSES2;
V11=RSES3; V12=RSES4; V13=RSES5; V14=RSES6;
```

(Continued)

TABLE 13.9

(Continued)

```
/EQUATIONS
V5  =    1F1 + E5;
V6  =    *F1 + E6;
V7  =    *F1 + E7;
V8  =    *F1 + E8;
V9  =    1F2 + E9;
V10 =    *F2 + E10;
V11 =    *F2 + E11;
V12 =    *F2 + E12;
V13 =    1F3 + E13;
V14 =    *F3 + E14;
/VARIANCES
F1  = *;
F2  = *;
F3  = *;
E5  = *;
E6  = *;
E7  = *;
E8  = *;
E9  = *;
E10 = *;
E11 = *;
E12 = *;
E13 = *;
E14 = *;
/COVARIANCES
F2,F3 = *;
F3,F1 = *;
F2,F1 = *;
/PRINT
FIT=ALL;
/END
```

Schools #120, #136, and #308 each have 49 students participating in the study. As noted earlier in this chapter, The Bentler–Liang ML approach to the analyses is able to take this sample variability into account in the calculation of the χ^2 statistic and goodness-of-fit indexes and in the estimating of parameters.

The model-based intraclass correlations appear below the Cluster Summary in Table 13.10. Indeed, the intraclass correlations are the "pièce de résistance" of multilevel modeling in that they can alert the user to whether in fact there is any rationale for conducting analyses at the higher level of the model. It is entirely possible that there may be no between-cluster effects at all, as indicated by very small intraclass correlation coefficients; as such, there is no reason to model within and between levels of the structure. The obvious question is: How small is small? To answer this question, Muthén (1997) states that typically, coefficient values in

TABLE 13.10

Selected EQS Output for Hypothesized Multilevel Model: Cluster Statistics

FOR BENTLER-LIANG MAXIMUM LIKELIHOOD ANALYSIS, THERE ARE 52 CLUSTERS.
CLUSTERS ARE DETERMINED BY VARIABLE 2

SIZE (S)	CLUSTER ID WITH SIZE S					
13	304					
16	305					
33	307					
35	303					
37	116					
39	114					
41	138					
44	122	132				
45	144					
46	108	118				
47	117	134				
48	106					
49	120	136	308			
50	102	105	111	142	145	
51	101	141	147			
52	126	128	301			
53	109	121	131	135		
54	110	112	119	124	139	146
55	123	129	133	137	143	
56	103	127	130			
57	140					
66	104					
83	302					
90	309					
111	115					

AVERAGE CLUSTER SIZE IS 51.404

MODEL-BASED INTRACLASS CORRELATIONS

BAS7	ALG7	GEO7	QLIT		
.157	.069	.114	.151		
RSES1	RSES2	RSES3	RSES4	RSES5	RSES6
.007	.008	.012	.019	.013	.030

PARAMETER ESTIMATES APPEAR IN ORDER,
NO SPECIAL PROBLEMS WERE ENCOUNTERED DURING OPTIMIZATION.

survey data tend to range from .0 to .5; when values of 0.1 or larger are combined with group sizes exceeding 15, the multilevel structure of the data should be modeled.

Intraclass correlations point to the proportion of variance explained by the grouping structure in the population (Hox, 2002). They are considered, most appropriately, as the proportion of between (or group) variance compared with total variance. In other words, they represent a ratio of variances such that between-cluster variance is divided by the sum of within- and between-cluster variance on a given variable (Bentler, 2005). Accordingly, this ratio is summarized as follows:

$$\text{Intraclass Correlation} = \frac{\sigma_B^2}{\sigma_W^2 + \sigma_B^2}$$

The results in Table 13.10 show that whereas the intraclass correlations for the Quantitative Skills measures are substantial, those for Global Self-Esteem and Self-Derogation are very small indeed, thereby sending a clear message that it is not necessary to model these variables as a multilevel structure.[3]

Table 13.11 summarizes only the within-level parameter estimates of particular interest; all are shown to be statistically significant. Although not shown in the table, all error variances were also statistically significant. Noteworthy, however, is the correlation between Factor 1 (Quantitative Skills) and Factor 2 (Global Self-Esteem), which—although statistically significant—indicates a minimal relation between the two constructs.

Table 13.12 reports findings related to the same parameters but this time as they relate to the between-level estimates. As for the within-level component, all factor loadings are shown to be statistically significant. However, findings for the factor variances are far less glowing. Given our knowledge of the intraclass correlations and taking into account the substantially smaller sample size at this level, it is not surprising that both factor variances related to the Rosenberg Self-Esteem Scale are not statistically significant. In total, only the factor variance for Quantitative Skills (F1) and the factor covariance between Quantitative Skills and Self-Derogation (F3,F1) are statistically significant. However, we probably should not get excited about this covariance (F3,F1), as the variance of F3 is not much larger than zero. Results bearing on the error variances were also poor; of the ten parameters estimated, only two (E7,E8) were significant. Indeed, the variance for E5 (BAS7) was so low that the program fixed its value at 0.0, thereby leading to the Condition Code noted at the top of the first page of the output.

Goodness-of-fit related to this hypothesized model, reported in Table 13.13, shows it to be extremely well fitting as indicated by a CFI of .991, a SRMR of .020, and a RMSEA of .020.

Regardless of the excellent fit of this model to the data, it is clear that the postulated structure as a multilevel model is unrealistic. For didactic purposes, it is worthwhile to modify this model so that the between-level model specifies only one factor: Quantitative Skills. Although this idea appears straightforward, it is

---

[3]To compute data-based intraclass correlations prior to conducting a multilevel analysis, click on Analysis in the toolbar and then select Intraclass Correlation from the drop-down menu (see, e.g., Fig. 13.4).

TABLE 13.11
Selected EQS Output for Hypothesized Multilevel Model: Within-Level Parameter Estimates

MEASUREMENT EQUATIONS WITH STANDARD ERRORS AND TEST STATISTICS
STATISTICS SIGNIFICANT AT THE 5% LEVEL ARE MARKED WITH @.

```
BAS7   =V5  =    1.000 F1     + 1.000 E5

ALG7   =V6  =     .613*F1     + 1.000 E6
                  .024
                25.562@

GEO7   =V7  =     .752*F1     + 1.000 E7
                  .024
                31.413@

QLIT7  =V8  =     .869*F1     + 1.000 E8
                  .023
                37.105@

RSES1  =V9  =    1.000 F2     + 1.000 E9

RSES2  =V10 =    1.024*F2     + 1.000 E10
                  .048
                21.506@

RSES3  =V11 =     .964*F2     + 1.000 E11
                  .046
                21.138@

RSES4  =V12 =    1.140*F2     + 1.000 E12
                  .053
                21.697@

RSES5  =V13 =    1.000 F3     + 1.000 E13

RSES6  =V14 =    2.075*F3     + 1.000 E14
                  .222
                 9.329@
```

VARIANCES OF INDEPENDENT VARIABLES
`-----------------------------------`

```
                V                            F
                ---                          ---
                          I F1 -  F1            66.749*I
                          I                      2.682 I
                          I                     24.889@I
                          I                          I
                          I F2 -  F2              .289*I
                          I                      .019 I
                          I                    14.871@I
                          I                          I
                          I F3 -  F3              .184*I
                          I                      .027 I
                          I                     6.929@I
```

(Continued)

TABLE 13.11
(Continued)

COVARIANCES AMONG INDEPENDENT VARIABLES

V		F
I F2 - F2		-.645*I
I F1 - F1		.112 I
I		-5.743@I
I		I
I F3 - F3		-1.332*I
I F1 - F1		.162 I
I		-8.213@I
I		I
I F3 - F3		.101*I
I F2 - F2		.012 I
I		8.161@I
I		I

CORRELATIONS AMONG INDEPENDENT VARIABLES

V		F
I F2 - F2		-.147*I
I F1 - F1		I
I		I
I F3 - F3		-.380*I
I F1 - F1		I
I		I
I F3 - F3		.439*I
I F2 - F2		I
I		I

not exactly the case. At the present time, EQS requires that all variables specified in the within-level model also be specified in the between-level model (Bentler, Pers. Comm., January 30, 2005). However, one way around this constraint is to specify the estimation of only the error variances associated with the Self-Esteem and Self-Derogation variables (i.e., RSES1 through RSES6). This respecification for the between-level model (i.e., Model 2) is shown in Table 13.14 and the model is schematically portrayed in Fig. 13.14.

Selected results from this analysis, and the goodness-of-fit statistics are summarized in Tables 13.15 and 13.16, respectively. Turning first to the parameter estimates, again you will note the same persistent Condition Code reported for E5. As expected, all estimated factor loadings for the Quantitative Skills factor are statistically significant, as is the factor variance. However, note that the error variances associated with V7 (GEO7) and V8 (QLIT7) are again the only ones related to the Quantitative Skills factor that are statistically significant, meaning that the factor explained essentially all variance in BAS7 (V5) and ALG7 (V6).

TABLE 13.12

Selected EQS Output for Hypothesized Multilevel Model: Between-Level Parameter Estimates

PARAMETER	CONDITION CODE
E5,E5	CONSTRAINED AT LOWER BOUND

MEASUREMENT EQUATIONS WITH STANDARD ERRORS AND TEST STATISTICS
STATISTICS SIGNIFICANT AT THE 5% LEVEL ARE MARKED WITH @.

```
BAS7   =V5  =    1.000 F1    + 1.000 E5

ALG7   =V6  =     .639*F1    + 1.000 E6
                  .049
                13.116@

GEO7   =V7  =     .806*F1    + 1.000 E7
                  .062
                12.918@

QLIT7  =V8  =     .951*F1    + 1.000 E8
                  .049
                19.555@

RSES1  =V9  =    1.000 F2    + 1.000 E9

RSES2  =V10 =    1.310*F2    + 1.000 E10
                  .605
                 2.163@

RSES3  =V11 =    1.566*F2    + 1.000 E11
                  .698
                 2.245@

RSES4  =V12 =    2.333*F2    + 1.000 E12
                 1.015
                 2.299@

RSES5  =V13 =    1.000 F3    + 1.000 E13

RSES6  =V14 =    1.524*F3    + 1.000 E14
                  .391
                 3.896@
```

VARIANCES OF INDEPENDENT VARIABLES

```
                V                               F
              ---                             ---
                          I  F1 -  F1          16.366*I
                          I                     3.445 I
                          I                     4.750@I
                          I                           I
                          I  F2 -  F2            .003*I
                          I                      .003 I
                          I                     1.124 I
                          I                           I
                          I  F3 -  F3            .014*I
                          I                      .008 I
                          I                     1.904 I
                          I                           I
```

(Continued)

TABLE 13.12
(Continued)

COVARIANCES AMONG INDEPENDENT VARIABLES

V			F	
I F2 -	F2			-.080*I
I F1 -	F1			.057 I
I				-1.387 I
I				I
I F3 -	F3			-.381*I
I F1 -	F1			.130 I
I				-2.921@I
I				I
I F3 -	F3			.005*I
I F2 -	F2			.003 I
I				1.716 I

CORRELATIONS AMONG INDEPENDENT VARIABLES

V			F	
I F2 -	F2			-.360*I
I F1 -	F1			I
I				I
I F3 -	F3			-.786*I
I F1 -	F1			I
I				I
I F3 -	F3			.842*I
I F2 -	F2			I
I				I

TABLE 13.13
Selected EQS Output for Hypothesized Multilevel Model: Goodness-of-Fit Statistics

*** WARNING *** TEST RESULTS MAY NOT BE APPROPRIATE DUE TO CONDITION CODE

GOODNESS OF FIT SUMMARY FOR METHOD = ML

BENTLER-LIANG LIKELIHOOD RATIO STATISTIC =   131.119 BASED ON   64 D.F.
PROBABILITY VALUE FOR THE CHI-SQUARE STATISTIC IS   .00000

FIT INDICES

BENTLER-BONETT   NORMED FIT INDEX =   .980
BENTLER-BONETT NON-NORMED FIT INDEX =   .987
COMPARATIVE FIT INDEX (CFI)   =   .991
ROOT MEAN-SQUARE RESIDUAL (RMR)   =   .328
STANDARDIZED RMR   =   .020
ROOT MEAN-SQUARE ERROR OF APPROXIMATION (RMSEA)   =   .020
90% CONFIDENCE INTERVAL OF RMSEA (.015,   .025)

TABLE 13.14

Selected EQS Input for Multilevel Model 2: Between-Level Specification

```
/TITLE
Testing for Validity of Multilevel Model 2 "MLEVEL2"
Within-Level - 3-Factor Model; Between Level - 1 Factor Model
/LABELS
V1=CHILDID; V2=SCHOOLID; V3=FEMALE; V4=ETHNIC; V5=BAS7;
V6=ALG7; V7=GEO7; V8=QLIT7; V9=RSES1; V10=RSES2;
V11=RSES3; V12=RSES4; V13=RSES5; V14=RSES6;
/EQUATIONS
V5  =    1F1 + E5;
V6  =    *F1 + E6;
V7  =    *F1 + E7;
V8  =    *F1 + E8;
V9  =    E9;
V10 =    E10;
V11 =    E11;
V12 =    E12;
V13 =    E13;
V14 =    E14;
/VARIANCES
 F1 = *;
 E5 = *;
 E6 = *;
 E7 = *;
 E8 = *;
 E9 = *;
 E10 = *;
 E11 = *;
 E12 = *;
 E13 = *;
 E14 = *;
/PRINT
FIT=ALL;
/END
```

It is surprising that one error variance associated with Self-Derogation was also found to be significant, but all other Self-Derogation variables have no significant between-school variance. The fit statistics in Table 13.16 show that overall fit of the model remained virtually unchanged.

In summary, multilevel modeling has the potential to impart answers to a variety of research questions in the social and behavioral sciences that bear on individual processes, group processes, and outcomes (Heck, 2001). In particular, it serves well in untangling and delineating effects that are typically lost when the sample of individuals under study is nested within a hierarchical structure. Furthermore, there are many different ways to model multilevel structures (see, e.g., Heck, 2001; Hox, 2002; Reise & Duan, 2003; and Tomarken & Waller, 2005), thereby

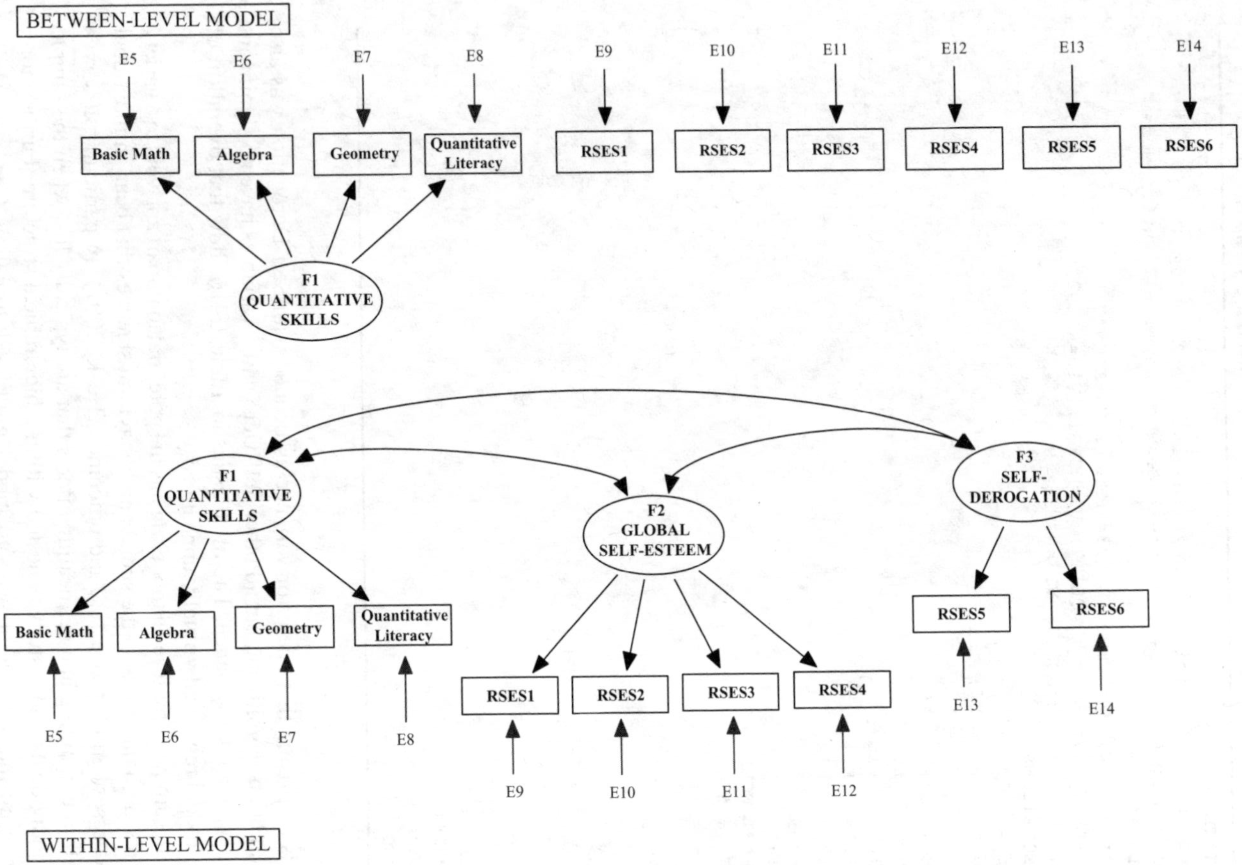

FIG. 13.14. Modified multilevel model.

BETWEEN-LEVEL MODEL

WITHIN-LEVEL MODEL

TABLE 13.15

Selected EQS Output for Multilevel Model 2: Between-Level Parameter Estimates

PARAMETER	CONDITION CODE
E5,E5	CONSTRAINED AT LOWER BOUND

MEASUREMENT EQUATIONS WITH STANDARD ERRORS AND TEST STATISTICS
STATISTICS SIGNIFICANT AT THE 5% LEVEL ARE MARKED WITH @.

```
BAS7   =V5  =    1.000 F1     + 1.000 E5

ALG7   =V6  =     .639*F1     + 1.000 E6
                  .052
                12.279@

GEO7   =V7  =     .808*F1     + 1.000 E7
                  .066
                12.275@

QLIT7  =V8  =     .952*F1     + 1.000 E8
                  .052
                18.369@

RSES1  =V9  =    1.000 E9

RSES2  =V10 =    1.000 E10

RSES3  =V11 =    1.000 E11

RSES4  =V12 =    1.000 E12

RSES5  =V13 =    1.000 E13

RSES6  =V14 =    1.000 E14
```

VARIANCES OF INDEPENDENT VARIABLES

STATISTICS SIGNIFICANT AT THE 5% LEVEL ARE MARKED WITH @.

```
            V                                  F
            ---                                ---
                       I F1  -  F1         14.698*I
                       I                    3.115 I
                       I                    4.718@I
```

VARIANCES OF INDEPENDENT VARIABLES

STATISTICS SIGNIFICANT AT THE 5% LEVEL ARE MARKED WITH @.

```
                  E                               D
                  ---                             ---
E5  -  BAS7          .000*I                          I
                     .002 I                          I
                     .000I                           I
                         I                           I
E6  -  ALG7          .360*I                          I
                     .363 I                          I
                     .991 I                          I
                         I                           I
```

(Continued)

TABLE 13.15
(Continued)

E7 - GEO7	1.639*I		I
	.588 I		I
	2.789@I		I
	I		I
E8 -QLIT7	.752*I		I
	.356 I		I
	2.114@I		I
	I		I
E9 -RSES1	.003*I		I
	.003 I		I
	1.018 I		I
	I		I
E10 -RSES2	.003*I		I
	.003 I		I
	.892 I		I
	I		I
E11 -RSES3	.004*I		I
	.003 I		I
	1.146 I		I
	I		I
E12 -RSES4	.008*I		I
	.005 I		I
	1.731 I		I
	I		I
E13 -RSES5	.008*I		I
	.007 I		I
	1.250 I		I
	I		I
E14 -RSES6	.022*I		I
	.009 I		I
	2.503@I		I
	I		I

TABLE 13.16
Selected EQS Output for Multilevel Model 2: Goodness-of-Fit Statistics

*** WARNING *** TEST RESULTS MAY NOT BE APPROPRIATE DUE TO CONDITION CODE

GOODNESS OF FIT SUMMARY FOR METHOD = ML

BENTLER-LIANG LIKELIHOOD RATIO STATISTIC =   183.605 BASED ON   73 D.F.
PROBABILITY VALUE FOR THE CHI-SQUARE STATISTIC IS   .00000

FIT INDICES

BENTLER-BONETT   NORMED FIT INDEX =   .979
BENTLER-BONETT NON-NORMED FIT INDEX =   .989
COMPARATIVE FIT INDEX (CFI)   =   .991
ROOT MEAN-SQUARE RESIDUAL (RMR)   =   .330
STANDARDIZED RMR   =   .075
ROOT MEAN-SQUARE ERROR OF APPROXIMATION (RMSEA)   =   .024
90% CONFIDENCE INTERVAL OF RMSEA (.020,   .028)

serving a wide variety of needs. Nonetheless, although the advantages of multilevel modeling are many, the procedure is not without its problems, not the least of which are adequate sample sizes at the between-level of the model and software that can handle its more complex applications. Also, as we found previously, multigroup models often can be hard to fit in practice, and this aspect can be expected to occur in multilevel modeling as well. However, given the surge of interest in multilevel modeling in recent years, it seems likely that these difficulties will be resolved in the not-too-distant future.

References

Aiken, L. S., Stein, J. A., & Bentler, P. M. (1994). Structural equation analyses of clinical sub-population differences and comparative treatment outcomes: Characterizing the daily lives of drug addicts. *Journal of Consulting and Clinical Psychology, 62,* 488–499.

Aiken, L., West, S., & Pitts, S. C. (2003). Multiple regression analysis. In John A. Schinka & Wayne F. Velicer (Eds.), *Comprehensive handbook of psychology. Volume 2. Research methods in psychology* (pp. 483–507). New York: Wiley.

Aish, A. M., & Jöreskog, K. G. (1990). A panel model for political efficacy and responsiveness: An application of LISREL 7 with weighted least squares. *Quality and Quantity, 19,* 716–723.

Akaike, H. (1987). Factor analysis and AIC. *Psychometrika, 52,* 317–332.

American Psychiatric Association. (1994). *Diagnostic and statistical manual of mental disorders* (4th ed.). Washington, DC: Author.

Anderson, J. C., & Gerbing, D. W. (1988). Structural equation modeling in practice: A review and recommended two-step approach. *Psychological Bulletin, 103,* 411–423.

Arbuckle, J. L. (1996). Full information estimation in the presence of incomplete data. In G. A. Marcoulides & R. E. Schumacker (Eds.), *Advanced structural equation modeling: Issues and techniques* (pp. 243–277). Mahwah, NJ: Lawrence Erlbaum & Associates.

Arbuckle, J. L. (2003). *Amos 5.0* [Computer software]. Chicago, IL: SPSS.

Atkinson, L. (1988). The measurement-statistics controversy: Factor analysis and subinterval data. *Bulletin of the Psychonomic Society, 26,* 361–364.

Austin, J. T., & Calderón, R. F. (1996). Theoretical and technical contributions to structural equation modeling: An updated bibliography. *Structural Equation Modeling: A Multidisciplinary Journal, 3,* 105–175.

Babakus, E., Ferguson, C. E., Jr., & Jöreskog, K. G. (1987). The sensitivity of confirmatory maximum likelihood factor analysis to violations of measurement scale and distributional assumptions. *Journal of Marketing Research, 24,* 222–228.

Bacharach, S. B., Bauer, S. C., & Conley, S. (1986). Organizational analysis of stress: The case of elementary and secondary schools. *Work and Occupations, 13,* 7–32.

Bagozzi, R. P. (1993). Assessing construct validity in personality research: Applications to measures of self-esteem. *Journal of Research in Personality, 27,* 49–87.

Bagozzi, R. P., & Yi, Y. (1990). Assessing method variance in multitrait-multimethod matrices: The case of self-reported affect and perceptions at work. *Journal of Applied Psychology, 75,* 547–560.

Bagozzi, R. P., & Yi, Y. (1993). Multitrait-multimethod matrices in consumer research: Critique and new developments. *Journal of Consumer Psychology, 2,* 143–170.

Bandalos, D. L. (1993). Factors influencing cross-validation of confirmatory factor analysis models. *Multivariate Behavioral Research, 28,* 351–374.

Bandalos, D. L. (2002). The effects of item parceling on goodness-of-fit and parameter estimate bias in structural equation modeling. *Structural Equation Modeling: A Multidisciplinary Journal, 9,* 78–102.

411

Bandalos, D. L., & Finney, S. J. (2001). Item parceling issues in structural equation modeling. In G. A. Marcoulides & R. E. Schumacker (Eds.), *New developments and techniques in structural equation modeling* (pp. 269–296). Mahwah, NJ: Lawrence Erlbaum & Associates.

Beck, A., Steer, R., & Brown, G. (1996). *Beck Depression Inventory manual* (2nd ed.). San Antonio, TX: The Psychological Association.

Beck, A. T., Ward, C. H., Mendelson, M., Mock, J., & Erbaugh, J. (1961). An inventory for measuring depression. *Archives of General Psychiatry, 4*, 561–571.

Benson, J., & Bandalos, D. L. (1992). Second-order confirmatory factor analysis of the Reactions to Tests Scale with cross-validation. *Multivariate Behavioral Research, 27*, 459–487.

Bentler, P. M. (1980). Multivariate analysis with latent variables: Causal modeling. *Annual Review of Psychology, 31*, 419–456.

Bentler, P. M. (1988). Causal modeling via structural equation systems. In J. R. Nesselroade & R. B. Cattell (Eds.), *Handbook of multivariate experimental psychology* (2nd edition, pp. 317–335). New York: Plenum.

Bentler, P. M. (1990). Comparative fit indexes in structural models. *Psychological Bulletin, 107*, 238–246.

Bentler, P. M. (1992). On the fit of models to covariances and methodology to the *Bulletin*. *Psychological Bulletin, 112*, 400–404.

Bentler, P. M. (2005). *EQS 6 structural equations program manual*. Encino, CA: Multivariate Software (www.mvsoft.com).

Bentler, P. M., & Bonett, D. G. (1980). Significance tests and goodness of fit in the analysis of covariance structures. *Psychological Bulletin, 88*, 588–606.

Bentler, P. M., & Bonett, D. G. (1987). This week's citation classic. *Current Contents, 19*, 16.

Bentler, P. M., & Chou, C. P. (1987). Practical issues in structural modeling. *Sociological Methods & Research, 16*, 78–117.

Bentler, P. M., & Dijkstra, T. (1985). Efficient estimation via linearization in structural models. In P. R. Krishnaiah (ed.), *Multivariate analysis VI* (pp. 9–42). Amsterdam: North-Holland.

Bentler, P. M., & Liang, J. -J. (2003a). Two-level mean and covariance structures: Maximum likelihood via an EM algorithm (pp. 53–70). In S. P. Reise & N. Duan (Eds.), *Multilevel modeling: Methodological advances, issues, and applications*. Mahwah, NJ: Lawrence Erlbaum & Associates.

Bentler, P. M., & Liang, J. -J. (2003b). Simultaneous mean and covariance structure analysis for two-level structural equation models in EQS. In H. Yanai, A. Okada, K. Shigemasu, Y. Kano, & J. J. Meulman (Eds.), *New developments in psychometrics* (pp. 123–132). Tokyo: Springer-Verlah.

Bentler, P. M., & Raykov, T. (2000). On measures of explained variance in nonrecursive structural equation models. *Journal of Applied Psychology, 85*, 125–131.

Bentler, P. M., & Weeks, D. G. (1979). Interrelations among models for the analysis of moment structures. *Multivariate Behavioral Research, 14*, 169–185.

Bentler, P. M., & Weeks, D. G. (1980). Linear structural equations with latent variables. *Psychometrika, 45*, 289–308.

Bentler, P. M., & Wu, E. J. C. (2002). *EQS for Windows: User's guide*. Encino, CA: Multivariate Software, Inc.

Bentler, P. M., & Yuan, K. -H. (1999). Structural equation modeling with small samples: Test statistics. *Multivariate Behavioral Research, 34*, 181–197.

Berkane, M., & Bentler, P. M. (1988). Estimation of contamination parameters and identification of outliers in multivariate data. *Sociological Methods & Research, 17*, 55–64.

Biddle, B. J., & Marlin, M. M. (1987). Causality, confirmation, credulity, and structural equation modeling. *Child Development, 58*, 4–17.

Bollen, K. A. (1989a). *Structural equations with latent variables*. New York: Wiley.

Bollen, K. A. (1989b). A new incremental fit index for general structural models. *Sociological Methods & Research, 17*, 303–316.

Bollen, K. A., & Barb, K. H. (1981). Pearson's *r* and coarsely categorized measures. *American Sociological Review, 46*, 232–239.

Bollen, K. A., & Long, J. S. (Eds.) (1993). *Testing structural equation models.* Newbury Park, CA: Sage.

Boomsma, A. (1982). The robustness of LISREL against small sample sizes in factor analysis models. In H. Wold & K. Jöreskog (Eds.), *Systems under indirect observation* (pp. 149–173). New York: Elsevier-North Holland.

Boomsma, A. (1985). Nonconvergence, improper solutions, and starting values in LISREL maximum likelihood estimation. *Psychometrika, 50*, 229–242.

Boomsma, A., & Hoogland, J. J. (2001). The robustness of LISREL modeling revisited. In R. Cudeck, S. du Toit, & D. Sörbom (Eds.), *Structural equation modeling: A festschrift in honor of Karl Jöreskög.* Lincolnwood, IL: Scientific Software.

Bozdogan, H. (1987). Model selection and Akaike's information criteria (AIC): The general theory and its analytical extensions. *Psychometrika, 52*, 345–370.

Breckler, S. J. (1990). Applications of covariance structure modeling in psychology: Cause for concern? *Psychological Bulletin, 107*, 260–271.

Browne, M. W. (1982). Covariance structures. In D. M. Hawkins (Ed.), *Topics in applied multivariate analysis* (pp. 72–141). Cambridge: Cambridge University Press.

Browne, M. W. (1984a). Asymptotically distribution-free methods for the analysis of covariance structures. *British Journal of Mathematical and Statistical Psychology, 37*, 62–83.

Browne, M. W. (1984b). The decomposition of multitrait-multimethod matrices. *The British Journal of Mathematical and Statistical Psychology, 37*, 1–21.

Browne, M. W., & Cudeck, R. (1989). Single sample cross-validation indices for covariance structures. *Multivariate Behavioral Research, 24*, 445–455.

Browne, M. W., & Cudeck, R. (1993). Alternative ways of assessing model fit. In K. A. Bollen & J. S. Long (Eds.), *Testing structural equation models* (pp. 445–455). Newbury Park, CA: Sage.

Browne, M. W., MacCallum, R. C., Kim, C. -T., Andersen, B. L., & Glaser, R. (2002). When fit indices and residuals are incompatible. *Psychological Methods, 7*, 403–421.

Bryk, A. S., & Raudenbush, S. W. (1987). Applications of hierarchical linear models to assessing change. *Psychological Bulletin, 101*, 147–158.

Bryk, A. S. & Raudenbush, S. W. (1992). *Hierarchical linear models: Applications and data analysis methods.* Newbury Park, CA: Sage.

Buse, A. (1982). The likelihood ratio, Wald, and Lagrange multiplier tests: An expository note. *American Statistician, 36*, 153–157.

Byrne, B. M. (1988a). The Self Description Questionnaire III: Testing for equivalent factorial validity across ability. *Educational and Psychological Measurement, 48*, 397–406.

Byrne, B. M. (1988b). Adolescent self-concept, ability grouping, and social comparison: Reexamining academic track differences in high school. *Youth and Society, 20*, 46–67.

Byrne, B. M. (1989). *A primer of LISREL: Basic applications and programming for confirmatory factor analytic models.* New York, NY: Springer-Verlag.

Byrne, B. M. (1991). The Maslach Inventory: Validating factorial structure and invariance across intermediate, secondary, and university educators. *Multivariate Behavioral Research, 26*, 583–605.

Byrne, B. M. (1993). The Maslach Inventory: Testing for factorial validity and invariance across elementary, intermediate, and secondary teachers. *Journal of Occupational and Organizational Psychology, 66*, 197–212.

Byrne, B. M. (1994a). *Structural equation modeling with EQS and EQS/Windows: Basic concepts, applications, and programming.* Thousand Oaks, CA: Sage.

Byrne, B. M. (1994b). Testing for the factorial validity, replication, and invariance of a measuring instrument: A paradigmatic application based on the Maslach Burnout Inventory. *Multivariate Behavioral Research, 29*, 289–311.

Byrne, B. M. (1994c). Burnout: Testing for the validity, replication, and invariance of causal structure across elementary, intermediate, and secondary teachers. *American Educational Research Journal, 31*, 645–673.

Byrne, B. M. (1996). *Measuring self-concept across the lifespan: Issues and instrumentation.* Washington, DC: American Psychological Association.

Byrne, B. M. (1998). *Structural equation modeling with LISREL, PRELIS, and SIMPLIS: Basic concepts, applications, and programming.* Mahwah, NJ: Lawrence Erlbaum & Associates.

Byrne, B. M. (1999). The nomological network of teacher burnout: A literature review and empirically validated model. In M. Huberman & R. Vandenberghe (Eds.), *Understanding and preventing teacher burnout: A sourcebook of international research and practice* (pp. 15–37). London: Cambridge Press.

Byrne, B. M. (2001). *Structural equation modeling with AMOS: Basic concepts, applications, and programming.* Mahwah, NJ: Lawrence Erlbaum & Associates.

Byrne, B. M. (2003). Testing for equivalent self-concept measurement across culture: Issues, caveats, and application. In H. W. Marsh, R. Craven, & D. M. McInerney (Eds.), *International advances in self-research* (pp. 291–313). Greenwich, CT: Information Age Publishing.

Byrne, B. M. (2005a). Factor analytic models: Viewing the structure of an assessment instrument from three perspectives. *Journal of Personality Assessment, 85*, 17–30.

Byrne, B. M. (2005b). Factor analysis: Confirmatory. In B. S. Everitt & D. C. Howell (Eds.), *Encyclopedia of Statistics in Behavioural Science* (pp. 599–606). London, UK: Wiley.

Byrne, B. M. (in press). Testing for time-invariant and time-varying predictors of self-perceived ability in math, language and science: A look at the gender factor. In H. M. G. Watts & J. S. Eccles, (eds.), *Explaining gendered occupational outcomes.* Washington, DC: American psychological association.

Byrne, B. M., & Baron, P. (1993). The Beck Depression Inventory: Testing and cross-validating an hierarchical factor structure for nonclinical adolescents. *Measurement and Evaluation in Counseling and Development, 26*, 164–178.

Byrne, B. M., & Baron, P. (1994). Measuring adolescent depression: Tests of equivalent factorial structure for English and French versions of the Beck Depression Inventory. *Applied Psychology: An International Review, 43*, 33–47.

Byrne, B. M., Baron, P., & Balev, J. (1996). The Beck Depression Inventory: Testing for its factorial validity and invariance across gender for Bulgarian adolescents. *Personality and Individual Differences, 21*, 641–651.

Byrne, B.M., Baron, P., & Balev, J. (1998). The Beck Depression Inventory: A cross-validated test of second-order structure for Bulgarian adolescents. *Educational and Psychological Measurement, 58*, 241–251.

Byrne, B. M., Baron, P., & Campbell, T. L. (1993). Measuring adolescent depression: Factorial validity and invariance of the Beck Depression Inventory across gender. *Journal of Research on Adolescence, 3*, 127–143.

Byrne, B. M., Baron, P., & Campbell, T. L. (1994). The Beck Depression Inventory (French Version): Testing for gender-invariant factorial structure for nonclinical adolescents. *Journal of Adolescent Research, 9*, 166–179.

Byrne, B. M., Baron, P., Larsson, B., & Melin, L. (1995). The Beck Depression Inventory: Testing and cross-validating a second-order factorial structure for Swedish nonclinical adolescents. *Behaviour Research and Therapy, 33*, 345–356.

Byrne, B. M., Baron, P., Larsson, B., & Melin, L. (1996). Measuring depression for Swedish nonclinical adolescents: Factorial validity and equivalence of the Beck Depression Inventory. *Scandinavian Journal of Psychology, 37*, 37–45.

Byrne, B. M., & Bazana, P. G. (1996). Investigating the measurement of social and academic competencies for early/late preadolescents and adolescents: A multitrait-multimethod analysis. *Applied Measurement in Education, 9*, 113–132.

Byrne, B. M., & Campbell, T. L. (1999). Cross-cultural comparisons and the presumption of equivalent measurement and theoretical structure: A look beneath the surface. *Journal of Cross-cultural Psychology, 30*, 557–576.

Byrne, B. M., & Crombie, G. (2003). Modeling and testing change over time: An introduction to the latent growth curve model. *Understanding Statistics: Statistical Issues in Psychology, Education, and the Social Sciences, 2*, 177–203.

Byrne, B. M., & Goffin, R. D. (1993). Modeling MTMM data from additive and multiplicative covariance structures: An audit of construct validity concordance. *Multivariate Behavioral Research, 28*, 67–96.

Byrne, B. M., & Shavelson, R. J. (1986). On the structure of adolescent self-concept. *Journal of Educational Psychology, 78*, 474–481.

Byrne, B. M., & Shavelson, R. J. (1987). Adolescent self-concept: Testing the assumption of equivalent structure across gender. *American Educational Research Journal, 24*, 365–385.

Byrne, B. M., & Shavelson, R. J. (1996). On the structure of social self-concept for pre-, early, and late adolescents. *Journal of Personality and Social Psychology, 70*, 599–613.

Byrne, B. M., Shavelson, R. J., & Muthen, B. (1989). Testing for the equivalence of factor covariance and mean structures: The issue of partial measurement invariance. *Psychological Bulletin, 105*, 456–466.

Byrne, B.M., & Stewart, S. M. (in press). The MACS approach to testing for multigroup invariance of a second-order structure: A walk through the process. *Structural Equation Modeling: A Multidisciplinary Journal.*

Byrne, B. M., Stewart, S. M., & Lee, P. W. H. (2004). Validating the Beck Depression Inventory-II for Hong Kong Community Adolescents. *International Journal of Testing, 4*, 199–216.

Byrne, B. M., & Watkins, D. (2003). The issue of measurement invariance revisited. *Journal of Cross-cultural Psychology, 34*, 155–175.

Byrne, B. M., & Worth Gavin, D. A. (1996). The Shavelson model revisited: Testing for the structure of academic self-concept across pre-, early, and late adolescents. *Journal of Educational Psychology, 88*, 215–228.

Campbell, D. T., & Fiske, D. W. (1959). Convergent and discriminant validation by the multitrait-multimethod matrix. *Psychological Bulletin, 56*, 81–105.

Chan, D. (2000). Detection of differential item functioning on the Kirton Adaptation-Innovation Inventory using multiple-group mean and covariance structure analysis. *Multivariate Behavioral Research, 35*, 169–199.

Cheong, J. W., MacKinnon, D. P., & Khoo, S. T. (2003). Investigation of mediational processes using parallel process latent growth curve modeling. *Structural Equation Modeling: A Multidisciplinary Journal, 10*, 238–262.

Cheung, G. W., & Rensvold, R. B. (2002). Evaluating goodness-of-fit indexes for testing measurement invariance. *Structural Equation Modeling: A Multidisciplinary Journal, 9*, 233–255.

Chinese Behavioral Sciences Society (2000). *The Chinese version of the Beck Depression Inventory, Second Edition. Licensed Chinese translation*, The Psychological Corporation, New York: Harcourt Brace.

Chou, C. -P., & Bentler, P. M. (1990). Model modification in covariance structure modeling: A comparison among likelihood ratio, Lagrange multiplier, and Wald tests. *Multivariate Behavioral Research, 25*, 115–136.

Chou, C. -P., Bentler, P. M., & Pentz, M. A. (1998). Comparisons of two approaches to study growth curves: The multilevel model and the latent curve analysis. *Structural Equation Modeling: A Multidisciplinary Journal, 5*, 247–266.

Chou, C. -P., Bentler, P. M., & Pentz, M. A. (2000). A two-stage approach to multilevel structural equation models: Application to longitudinal data (pp. 33–49). In T. D. Little, K. U. Schnabel, & J. Baumert (Eds.), *Modeling longitudinal and multilevel data: Practical issues, applied approaches, and specific examples.* Mahwah, NJ: Lawrence Erlbaum & Associates.

Chou, C. -P., Bentler, P. M., & Satorra, A. (1991). Scaled test statistics and robust standard errors for nonnormal data in covariance structure analysis. *British Journal of Mathematical and Statistical Psychology, 44*, 347–357.

Cliff, N. (1983). Some cautions concerning the application of causal modeling methods. *Multivariate Behavioral Research, 18*, 115–126.

Coenders, G., & Saris, W. E. (2000). Testing nested additive, multiplicative, and general multitrait-multimethod models. *Structural Equation Modeling: A Multidisciplinary Journal, 7*, 219–250.

Coenders, G., Satorra, A., & Saris, W. E. (1997). Alternative approaches to structural modeling of ordinal data: A Monte Carlo study. *Structural Equation Modeling: A Multidisciplinary Journal, 4*, 261–282.

Cohen, J. (1994). The earth is round ($p < .05$). *American Psychologist, 49*, 997–1003.

Comrey, A. L. (1992). *A First Course in Factor Analysis*. Hillsdale, NJ: Lawrence Erlbaum & Associates.

Conway, J. M., Scullen, S. E., Lievens, F., & Lance, C. E. (2004). Bias in the correlated uniqueness model for MTMM data. *Structural Equation Modeling: A Multidisciplinary Journal, 11*, 535–559.

Cooke, D. J., Kosson, D. S., & Michie, C. (2001). Psychopathy and ethnicity: Structural, item, and test generalizability of the Psychopathy Checklist-Revised (PCL-R) in Caucasian and African American participants. *Psychological Assessment, 13*, 531–542.

Corten, I. W., Saris, W. E., Coenders, G., van der Veld, W., Aalberts, C. E., & Kornelis, C. (2002). Fit of different models for multitrait-multimethod experiments. *Structural Equation Modeling: A Multidisciplinary Journal, 9*, 213–232.

Cronbach, L. J. (1951). Coefficient alpha and the internal structure of tests. *Psychometrika, 16*, 297.

Cudeck, R. (1989). Analysis of correlation matrices using covariance structure models. *Psychological Bulletin, 105*, 317–327.

Cudeck, R., & Browne, M. W. (1983). Cross-validation of covariance structures. *Multivariate Behavioral Research, 18*, 147–167.

Cudeck, R., & Henly, S. J. (1991). Model selection in covariance structures analysis and the "problem" of sample size: A clarification. *Psychological Bulletin, 109*, 512–519.

Curran, P. J., West, S. G., & Finch, J. F. (1996). The robustness of test statistics to nonnormality and specification error in confirmatory factor analysis. *Psychological Methods, 1*, 16–29.

Dillon, W. R., Kumar, A., & Mulani, N. (1987). Offending estimates in covariance structure analysis: Comments on causes of and solutions to Heywood cases. *Psychological Bulletin, 101*, 126–135.

DiStefano, C. (2002). The impact of categorization with confirmatory factor analysis. *Structural Equation Modeling: A Multidisciplinary Journal, 9*, 327–346.

Dolan, C. V. (1994). Factor analysis of variables with 2, 3, 5, and 7 response categories: A comparison of categorical variable estimators using simulated data. *British Journal of Mathematical and Statistical Psychology, 47*, 309–326.

Dozois, D. J. A., Dobson, K. S., & Ahnberg, J. L. (1998). A psychometric evaluation of the Beck Depression Inventory-II. *Psychological Assessment, 10*, 83–89.

Duncan, T. E., & Duncan, S. C. (1994). Modeling incomplete longitudinal substance use data using latent variable growth curve methodology. *Multivariate Behavioral Research, 29*, 313–338.

Duncan, T. E., & Duncan, S. C. (1995). Modeling the processes of development via latent growth curve methodology. *Structural Equation Modeling: A Multidisciplinary Journal, 3*, 187–205.

Duncan, T. E., Duncan, S. C., Okut, H., Stryker, L. A., & Li, F. (2002). An extension of the general latent variable growth modeling framework to four levels of the hierarchy. *Structural Equation Modeling: A Multidisciplinary Journal, 9*, 303–326.

Duncan, T. E., Duncan, S. C., Stryker, L. A., Li, F., & Alpert, A. (1999). *An introduction to latent variable growth curve modeling*. Mahwah, NJ: Lawrence Erlbaum & Associates.

Eid, M., Lischetzke, T., Nussbeck, F. W., & Trierweiler, L. I. (2003). Separating trait effects from trait-specific method effects in multitrait-multimethod models: A multiple-indicator CT-C(M-1) model. *Psychological Methods, 8*, 38–60.

Enders, C. K. (2001). A primer on maximum likelihood algorithms available for use with missing data. *Structural Equation Modeling: A Multidisciplinary Journal, 8*, 128–141.

Enders, C. K., & Bandalos, D. L. (2001). The relative performance of full information likelihood estimation for missing data in structural equation models. *Structural Equation Modeling: A Multidisciplinary Journal, 8*, 430–457.

Fabrigar, L. R., Wegener, D. T., MacCallum, R. C., & Strahan, E. J. (1999). Evaluating the use of exploratory factor analysis in psychological research. *Psychological Methods, 4*, 272–299.

Fan, X., Thompson, B., & Wang, L. (1999). Effects of sample size, estimation methods, and model specification on structural equation modeling fit indexes. *Structural Equation Modeling: A Multidisciplinary Journal, 6*, 56–83.

Ferrando, P. J. (1996). Calibration of invariant item parameters in a continuous item response model using the extended LISREL measurement submodel. *Multivariate Behavioral Research, 31*, 419–439.

Finch, J. F., West, S. G., & MacKinnon, D. P. (1997). Effects of sample size and nonnormality on the estimation of mediated effects in latent variable models. *Structural Equation Modeling: A Multidisciplinary Journal, 4*, 87–107.

Francis, D. J., Fletcher, J. M., & Rourke, B. P. (1988). Discriminant validity of lateral sensorimotor tests in children. *Journal of Clinical and Experimental Neuropsychology, 10*, 779–799.

Gerbing, D. W., & Anderson, J. C. (1984). On the meaning of within-factor correlated measurement errors. *Journal of Consumer Research, 11*, 572–580.

Gerbing, D. W., & Anderson, J. C. (1993). Monte Carlo evaluations of goodness-of-fit indices for structural equation models. In K. A. Bollen & J. S. Long (Eds.), *Testing structural equation models* (pp. 40–65). Newbury Park, CA: Sage.

Goffin, R. D. (1987). *The analysis of multitrait-multimethod matrices: An empirical and Monte Carlo comparison of two procedures.* Unpublished doctoral dissertation. University of Western Ontario, London, Canada.

Goffin, R. D. (1993). A comparison of two new indices for the assessment of fit of structural equation models. *Multivariate Behavioral Research, 28*, 205–214.

Goffin, R. D., & Jackson, D. N. (1992). Analysis of multitrait-multirater performance appraisal data: Composite direct product method versus confirmatory factor analysis. *Multivariate Behavioral Research, 27*, 363–385.

Gold, M. S., & Bentler, P. M. (2000). Treatments of missing data: A Monte Carlo comparison of RBHDI, iterative stochastic regression imputation, and expectation-maximization. *Structural Equation Modeling: A Multidisciplinary Journal, 7*, 319–355.

Gorsuch, R. L. (1983). *Factor Analysis.* Hillsdale, NJ: Lawrence Erlbaum & Associates.

Green, S. B., Akey, T. M., Fleming, K. K., Hershberger, S. L., & Marquis, J. G. (1997). Effect of the number of scale points on chi square fit indices in confirmatory factor analysis. *Structural Equation Modeling: A Multidisciplinary Journal, 4*, 108–120.

Green, S. B., & Babyak, M. A. (1997). Control of Type I errors with multiple tests of constraints in structural equation modeling. *Multivariate Behavioral Research, 32*, 39–51.

Green, S. B., Thompson, M. S., & Poirier, J. (1999). Exploratory analyses to improve fit: Errors due to misspecification and a strategy to reduce their occurrence. *Structural Equation Modeling: A Multidisciplinary Journal, 6*, 113–126.

Green, S. B., Thompson, M. S., & Poirier, J. (2001). An adjusted Bonferroni method for elimination of parameters in specification addition searches. *Structural Equation Modeling: A Multidisciplinary Journal, 8*, 18–39.

Hagtvet, K. A., & Nasser, F. M. (2004). How well do item parcels represent conceptually defined latent constructs?: A two-facet approach. *Structural Equation Modeling: A Multidisciplinary Journal, 11*, 168–193.

Hancock, G. R. (1999). A sequential Sheffé-type respecification for controling Type I error in exploratory structural equation model modification. *Structural Equation Modeling: A Multidisciplinary Journal, 6*, 158–168.

Hancock, G. R., Kuo, W. -L., & Lawrence, F. R. (2001). An illustration of second-order latent growth models. *Structural Equation Modeling: A Multidisciplinary Journal, 8,* 470–489.

Harter, S. (1990). Causes, correlates, and the functional role of global self-worth: A lifespan perspective. In R. J. Sternberg & J. Kolligian (Eds.), *Competence considered* (pp. 67–97). New Haven, CT: Yale University Press.

Heck, R. H. (2001). Multilevel modeling with SEM. In G. A. Marcoulides & R. E. Schumacker (Eds.), *New developments and techniques in structural equation modeling.* Mahwah, NJ: Lawrence Erlbaum & Associates.

Hernández, A., & González-Romá, V. (2002). Analysis of multitrait-multioccasion data: Additive versus multiplicative models. *Multivariate Behavioral Research, 37,* 59–87.

Hox, J. (2002). *Multilevel analysis: Techniques and applications.* Mahwah, NJ: Lawrence Erlbaum & Associates.

Hoyle, R. H. (Ed.) (1995a). *Structural equation modeling: Concepts, issues, and applications.* Thousand Oaks, CA: Sage.

Hu, L. -T., & Bentler, P. M. (1995). Evaluating model fit. In R. H. Hoyle, (Ed.), *Structural equation modeling: Concepts, issues, and applications* (pp. 76–99). Thousand Oaks, CA: Sage.

Hu, L. -T., & Bentler, P. M. (1998). Fit indices in covariance structure modeling: Sensitivity to underparameterized model misspecification. *Psychological Methods, 3,* 424–453.

Hu, L. -T., & Bentler, P. M. (1999). Cutoff criteria for fit indexes in covariance structure analysis: Conventional criteria versus new alternatives. *Structural Equation Modeling: A Multidisciplinary Journal, 6,* 1–55.

Hu, L. -T., Bentler, P. M., & Kano, Y. (1992). Can test statistics in covariance structure analysis be trusted? *Psychological Bulletin, 112,* 351–362.

Hutchinson, S. R., & Olmos, A. (1998). Behavior of descriptive fit indexes in confirmatory factor analysis using ordered categorical data. *Structural Equation Modeling: A Multidisciplinary Journal, 5,* 344–364.

Jamshidian, M., & Bentler, P. M. (1999). ML estimation of mean and covariance structures with missing data using complete data routines. *Journal of Educational and Behavioural Statistics, 24,* 21–41.

Jöreskog, K. G. (1971a). Statistical analysis of sets of congeneric tests. *Psychometrika, 36,* 109–133.

Jöreskog, K. G. (1971b). Simultaneous factor analysis in several populations. *Psychometrika, 36,* 409–426.

Jöreskog, K. G. (1990). New developments in LISREL: Analysis of ordinal variables using polychoric correlations and weighted least squares. *Quality and Quantity, 24,* 387–404.

Jöreskog, K. G. (1993). Testing structural equation models. In K. A. Bollen & J. S. Long (Eds.), *Testing structural equation models* (pp. 294–316). Newbury Park, CA: Sage.

Jöreskog, K. G. (1994). On the estimation of polychoric correlations and their asymptotic covariance matrix. *Psychometrika, 59,* 381–389.

Jöreskog, K. G., & Sörbom, D. (1984). *LISREL VI: User's guide* (3rd ed.). Mooresville, IN: Scientific Software, Inc.

Jöreskog, K. G., & Sörbom, D. (1988). *LISREL 7: A guide to the program and applications.* Chicago, IL: SPSS Inc.

Jöreskog, K. G., & Sörbom, D. (1989). *LISREL 7: User's reference guide.* Chicago, IL: Scientific Software Inc.

Jöreskog, K. G., & Sörbom, D. (1993). *LISREL 8: Structural equation modeling with the SIMPLIS command language.* Chicago, IL: Scientific Software International.

Jöreskog, K. G., & Sörbom, D. (1996). *LISREL 8: User's reference guide.* Chicago, IL: Scientific Software International.

Kaplan, D. (1998). Methods for multilevel data analysis. In G. A. Marcoulides (Ed.), *Modern methods for business research* (pp. 337–358). Mahwah, NJ: Lawrence Erlbaum & Associates.

Kaplan, D. (2000). *Structural equation modeling: Foundations and extensions.* Thousand Oaks, CA: Sage.

Kaplan, D., & Elliott, P. R. (1997). A didactic example of multilevel structural equation modeling applicable to the study of organizations. *Structural Equation Modeling: A Multidisciplinary Journal, 4,* 1–23.

Kaplan, D., & George, R. (1995). A study of power associated with testing factor mean differences under violations of factorial invariance. *Structural Equation Modeling: A Multidisciplinary Journal, 2,* 101–118.

Kenny, D. A. (1976). An empirical application of confirmatory factor analysis to the multitrait-multimethod matrix. *Journal of Experimental Social Psychology, 12,* 247–252.

Kenny, D. A. (1979). *Correlation and causality.* New York: Wiley.

Kenny, D. A. & Kashy, D. A. (1992). Analysis of the multitrait-multimethod matrix by confirmatory factor analysis. *Psychological Bulletin, 112,* 165–172.

Kim, K. H., & Bentler, P. M. (2002). Tests of homogeneity of means a and covariance matrices for multivariate incomplete data. *Psychometrika, 67,* 609–624.

Kim, S., & Hagtvet, K. A. (2003). The impact of misspecified item parceling on representing latent variables in covariance structure modeling: A simulation study. *Structural Equation Modeling: A Multidisciplinary Journal, 10,* 101–127.

Kirk, R. E. (1996). Practical significance: A concept whose time has come. *Educational and Psychological Measurement, 56,* 746–759.

Kishton, J. M., & Widaman, K. F. (1994). Unidimensional versus domain representative parceling of questionnaire items: An empirical example. *Educational and Psychological Measurement, 54,* 757–765.

Kline, R. B. (1998). *Principles and practice of structural equation modeling.* New York: The Guildford Press.

Kreft, I., & de Leeuw, J. (1998). *Introducing multilevel modeling.* Newbury Park, CA: Sage.

La Du, T. J., & Tanaka, J. S. (1989). Influence of sample size, estimation method, and model specification on goodness-of-fit assessments in structural equation modeling. *Journal of Applied Psychology, 74,* 625–636.

Lance, C. E., Noble, C. L., & Scullen, S. E. (2002). A critique of the correlated trait-correlated method and correlated uniqueness models for multitrait-multimethod data. *Psychological Methods, 7,* 228–244.

Lee, S. -Y. (1985). On testing functional constraints in structural equation models. *Biometrika, 72,* 125–131.

Lee, S. -Y., Poon, W. -Y., & Bentler, P. M. (1990). Full maximum likelihood analysis of structural equation models with polytomous variables. *Statistics and Probability Letters, 9,* 91–97.

Lee, S. -Y., Poon, W. -Y., & Bentler, P. M. (1992). Structural equation models with continuous and polytomous variables. *Psychometrika, 57,* 89–105.

Lee, S. -Y., Poon, W. -Y., & Bentler, P. M. (1995). A two-stage estimation of structural equation models with continuous and polytomous variables. *British Journal of Mathematical and Statistical Psychology, 48,* 339–358.

Leiter, M. P. (1991). Coping patterns as predictors of burnout: The function of control and escapist coping patterns. *Journal of Organizational Behavior, 12,* 123–144.

Li, F., Duncan, T. E., & Duncan, S. C. (2001). Latent growth modeling of longitudinal data: A finite growth mixture modeling approach. *Structural Equation Modeling: A Multidisciplinary Journal, 8,* 493–530.

Li, F., Duncan, T. E., Duncan, S. C., McAuley, E., Chaumeton, N. R., & Harmer, P. (2001). Enhancing the psychological well-being of elderly individuals through Tai Chi exercise: A latent growth curve analysis. *Structural Equation Modeling: A Multidisciplinary Journal, 8,* 493–530.

Liang, J. -J. & Bentler, P. M. (2004). An EM algorithm for fitting two-level structural equation models. *Psychometrika, 69,* 101–122.

Little, T. D. (1997). Mean and covariance structures (MACS) analyses of cross-cultural data: Practical and theoretical issues. *Multivariate Behavioral Research, 32,* 53–76.

Little, T. D., Cunningham, W. A., Shahar, G., & Widaman, K. F. (2002). To parcel or not to parcel: Exploring the question, weighing the merits. *Structural Equation Modeling: A Multidisciplinary Journal, 9*, 151–173.

Little, T. D., Lindenberger, U., & Nesselroade, J. R. (1999). On selecting indicators for multivariate measurement and modeling with latent variables: When "good" indicators are bad and "bad" indicators are good. *Psychological Methods, 4*, 192–211.

Little, R. J. A., & Rubin, D. B. (1987). *Statistical analysis with missing data.* New York: Wiley.

Loehlin, J. C. (1992). *Latent variable models: An introduction to factor, path, & structural analyses.* Hillsdale, NJ: Lawrence Erlbaum & Associates.

Long, J. S. (1983a). *Confirmatory factor analysis.* Beverly Hills, CA: Sage.

Long, J. S. (1983b). *Covariance structure models: An introduction to LISREL.* Beverly Hills, CA: Sage.

Lubke, G. H., Dolan, C. V., & Kelderman, H. (2001). Investigating group differences on cognitive tests using Spearman's hypothesis: An evaluation of Jensen's Method. *Multivariate Behavioural Research, 36*, 299–324.

MacCallum, R. C. (1986). Specification searches in covariance structure modeling. *Psychological Bulletin, 100*, 107–120.

MacCallum, R. C. (1995). Model specification: Procedures, strategies, and related issues. In R. H. Hoyle (Ed.), *Structural equation modeling: Concepts, issues, and applications* (pp. 76–99). Newbury Park, CA: Sage.

MacCallum, R. C., & Austin, J. T. (2000). Applications of structural equation modeling in psychological research. *Annual Review of Psychology, 51*, 201–226.

MacCallum, R. C., Browne, M. W., & Sugawara, H. M. (1996). Power analysis and determination of sample size for covariance structure modeling. *Psychological Methods, 1*, 130–149.

MacCallum, R. C., Roznowski, M., Mar, M., & Reith, J. V. (1994). Alternative strategies for cross-validation of covariance structure models. *Multivariate Behavioral Research, 29*, 1–32.

MacCallum, R. C., Roznowski, M., & Necowitz, L. B. (1992). Model modifications in covariance structure analysis: The problem of capitalization on chance. *Psychological Bulletin, 111*, 490–504.

MacCallum, R. C., Wegener, D. T., Uchino, B. N., & Fabrigar, L. R. (1993). The problem of equivalent models in applications of covariance structure analysis. *Psychological Bulletin, 114*, 185–199.

MacCallum, R. C., Widaman, K. F., Zhang, S., & Hong, S. (1999). Sample size in factor analysis. *Psychological Methods, 4*, 84–99.

Marcoulides, G. A., & Moustaki, I. (Eds.) (2002). *Latent variable and latent structure models.* Mahwah, NJ: Lawrence Erlbaum & Associates.

Marcoulides, G. A., & Schumacker, R. E. (Eds.) (1996). *Advanced structural equation modeling: Issues and techniques.* Mahwah, NJ: Lawrence Erlbaum & Associates.

Mardia, K. V. (1970). Measures of multivariate skewness and kurtosis with applications. *Biometrika, 57*, 519–530.

Mardia, K. V. (1974). Applications of some measures of multivariate skewness and kurtosis in testing normality and robustness studies. *Sankhya, B36*, 115–128.

Marsh, H. W. (1988). Multitrait-multimethod analyses. In J. P. Keeves (Ed.), *Educational research methodology, measurement, and evaluation: An international handbook* (pp. 570–578). Oxford: Pergamon.

Marsh, H. W. (1989). Confirmatory factor analyses of multitrait-multimethod data: Many problems and a few solutions. *Applied Psychological Measurement, 15*, 47–70.

Marsh, H. W. (1992). *Self Description Questionnaire (SDQ) II: A theoretical and empirical basis for the measurement of multiple dimensions of adolescent self-concept: An interim test manual and research monograph.* Macarthur, NSW Australia: Faculty of Education, University of Western Sydney.

Marsh, H. W., & Bailey, M. (1991). Confirmatory factor analyses of multitrait-multimethod data: A comparison of alternative models. *Applied Psychological Measurement, 15*, 47–70.

Marsh, H. W., Balla, J. R., & McDonald, R. P. (1988). Goodness-of-fit indexes in confirmatory factor analysis: The effect of sample size. *Psychological Bulletin, 103*, 391–410.

Marsh, H. W., Byrne, B. M., & Craven, R. (1992). Overcoming problems in confirmatory factor analyses of MTMM data: The correlated uniqueness model and factorial invariance. *Multivariate Behavioral Research, 27*, 489–507.

Marsh, H. W., & Grayson, D. (1994). Longitudinal stability of means and individual differences: A unified approach. *Structural Equation Modeling, 1*, 317–359.

Marsh, H. W., & Grayson, D. (1995). Latent variable models of multitrait-multimethod data. In R. H. Hoyle (Ed.), *Structural equation modeling: Concepts, issues, and applications* (pp. 177–198). Thousand Oaks, CA: Sage.

Marsh, H. W., Hau, K. -T., Balla, J. R., & Grayson, D. (1998). Is more ever too much? The number of indicators per factor in confirmatory factor analysis. *Multivariate Behavioral Research, 33*, 181–220.

Marsh, H.W., Hey, J., & Roche, L. A. (1997). Structure of physical self-concept: Elite athletes and physical education students. *Journal of Educational Psychology, 89*, 369–380.

Maruyama, G. M. (1998). *Basics of structural equation modeling.* Thousand Oaks, CA: Sage.

Maslach, C., & Jackson, S. E. (1981). *Maslach Burnout Inventory Manual.* Palo Alto, CA: Consulting Psychologists Press.

Maslach, C., & Jackson, S. E. (1986). *Maslach Burnout Inventory Manual* (2nd ed.). Palo Alto, CA: Consulting Psychologists Press.

McArdle, J. J., & Epstein, D. (1987). Latent growth curves within developmental structural equation models. *Child Development, 58*, 110–133.

McArdle, J. J., & Hamagami, F. (1996). Multilevel models from a multiple group structural equation perspective. In G. A. Marcoulides & R. E. Schumaker (Eds.), *Advanced structural equation modeling* (pp. 89–124). Mahwah, NJ: Lawrence Erlbaum & Associates.

McDonald, R. P. (1985). *Factor analysis and related methods.* Hillsdale, NJ: Lawrence Erlbaum & Associates.

McDonald, R. P. (1989). An index of goodness-of-fit based on noncentrality. *Journal of Classification, 6*, 97–103.

McGaw, B., & Jöreskog, K. G. (1971). Factorial invariance of ability measures in groups differing in intelligence and socioeconomic status. *British Journal of Mathematical and Statistical Psychology, 24*, 154–168.

Meredith, W. (1993). Measurement invariance, factor analysis, and factorial invariance. *Psychometrika, 58*, 525–543.

Meredith, W., & Tisak, J. (1990). Latent curve analysis. *Psychometrika, 55*, 107–122.

Miller, J. D., Kimmel, L., Hoffer, T. B., & Nelson, C. (1999). *Longitudinal Study of American Youth: CD-ROM and user's manual.* Chicago, IL: International Center for the Advancement of Scientific Literacy, The Chicago Academy of Sciences.

Millsap, R. E., & Kwok, O. -M. (2004). Evaluating the impact of partial factorial invariance on selection in two populations. *Psychological Methods, 9*, 93–115.

Moustaki, I. (2001). A review of exploratory factor analysis for ordinal categorical data. In R. Cudeck, S. du Toit, & D. Sörbom (Eds.), *Structural equation modeling: Present and future* (pp. 461–480). Lincolnwood, IL: Scientific Software.

Mulaik, S. A. (1972). *The foundations of factor analysis.* New York: McGraw-Hill.

Mulaik, S. A., James, L. R., van Altine, J., Bennett, N., Lind, S., & Stilwell, C. D. (1989). Evaluation of goodness-of-fit indices for structural equation models. *Psychological Bulletin, 105*, 430–445.

Muthén, B. O. (1984). A general structural equation model with dichotomous, ordered categorical, and continuous latent variable indicators. *Psychometrika, 49*, 115–132.

Muthén, B.O. (1994). Multilevel covariance structure analysis. *Sociological Methods & Research, 22*, 376–398.

Muthén, B. O. (1997). Latent variable modeling of longitudinal and multilevel data. In A. E. Raftery (Ed.), *Sociological Methodology 1997* (pp. 453–481). Washington, DC: American Sociological Association.

Muthén, B. O., & Christoffersson, A. (1981). Simultaneous factor analysis of dichotomous variables in several groups. *Psychometrika, 46*, 407–419.

Muthén, B. O., & Kaplan, D. (1985). A comparison of some methodologies for the factor analysis of non-normal Likert variables. *British Journal of Mathematical and Statistical Psychology, 38*, 171–189.

Muthén, B. O., Kaplan, D., & Hollis, M. (1987). On structural equation modeling with data that are not missing completely at random. *Psychometrika, 52*, 431–462.

Muthén, B. O., & Muthén, L. K. (2004). *Mplus user's guide.*

Muthén, B. O., & Satorra, A. (1995). Complex sample data in structural equation modeling. In P. Marsden (Ed.), *Sociological Methodology 1995* (pp. 267–316). Washington, DC: American Sociological Association.

O'Brien, R. M. (1985). The relationship between ordinal measures and their underlying values: Why all the disagreement? *Quality and Quantity, 19*, 265–277.

Pettegrew, L. S., & Wolf, G. E. (1982). Validating measures of teacher stress. *American Educational Research Journal, 19*, 373–396.

Preacher, K. J., & MacCallum, R. C. (2003). Repairing Tom Swift's electric factor analysis machine. *Understanding Statistics, 2*, 13–43.

Raykov, T., & Marcoulides, G. A. (2000). *A first course in structural equation modeling.* Mahwah, NJ: Lawrence Erlbaum & Associates.

Raykov, T., & Widaman, K. F. (1995). Issues in structural equation modeling research. *Structural Equation Modeling: A Multidisciplinary Journal, 2*, 289–318.

Reise, S. P., & Duan, N. (2003). *Multilevel modeling: Methodological advances, issues, and applications.* Mahwah, NJ: Lawrence Erlbaum & Associates.

Reise, S .P., Widaman, K. F., & Pugh, R. H. (1993). Confirmatory factor analysis and item response theory: Two approaches for exploring measurement invariance. *Psychological Bulletin, 114*, 552–566.

Rigdon, E. E. (1996). CFI versus RMSEA: A comparison of two fit indexes for structural equation modeling. *Structural Equation Modeling: A Multidisciplinary Journal, 3*, 369–379.

Rindskopf, D. (1984). Structural equation models: Empirical identification, Heywood cases, and related problems. *Sociological Methods and Research, 13*, 109–119.

Rindskopf, D., & Rose, T. (1988). Some theory and applications of confirmatory second-order factor analysis. *Multivariate Behavioral Research, 23*, 51–67.

Rogers, W. M., & Schmitt, N. (2004). Parameter recovery and model fit using multidimensional composites: A comparison of four empirical parceling algorithms. *Multivariate Behavioral Research, 39*, 379–412.

Rogosa, D. R., Brandt, D., & Zimowski, M. (1982). A growth curve approach to the measurement of change. *Psychological Bulletin, 90*, 726–748.

Rogosa, D. R., & Willett, J. B. (1985). Understanding correlates of change by modeling individual differences in growth. *Psychometrika, 50*, 203–228.

Rosenberg, M. (1965). *Society and the adolescent self-image.* Princeton, NJ: University Press.

Rosenberg, M. (1989). *Society and the adolescent self-image* (revised edition). Middletown, CT: Wesleyan University Press.

Rozeboom, W. W. (1960). The fallacy of the null hypothesis significance test. *Psychological Bulletin, 57*, 416–428.

Saris, W. E., & Aalberts, C. (2003). Different explanations for correlated disturbance terms in MTMM studies. *Structural Equation Modeling: A Multidisciplinary Journal, 10*, 193–213.

Saris, W., & Stronkhorst, H. (1984). *Causal modeling: nonexperimental research: An introduction to the LISREL approach.* Amsterdam: Sociometric Research Foundation.

Satorra, A. (1989). Alternative test criteria in covariance structure analysis: A unified approach. *Psychometrika, 54*, 131–151.

Satorra, A., & Bentler, P. M. (1988). Scaling corrections for chi square statistics in covariance structure analysis. *American Statistical Association 1988 Proceedings of the Business and Economic Sections* (pp. 308–313). Alexandria, VA: American Statistical Association.

Satorra, A.; & Bentler, P. M. (1994). Corrections to test statistics and standard errors in covariance structure analysis. In A. von Eye & C. C. Clogg (Eds.). *Latent variables analysis: Applications for developmental research* (pp. 399–419). Thousand Oaks, CA: Sage.

Satorra, A., & Bentler, P. M. (2001). A scaled difference chi-square test statistic for moment structure analysis. *Psychometrika, 66*, 507–514.

Schafer, J. L., & Graham, J. W. (2002). Missing data: Our view of the state of the art. *Psychological Methods, 7*, 147–177.

Scheffé, H. (1953). A method for judging all contrasts in the analysis of variance. *Biometrika, 40*, 87–104.

Schmidt, F. L. (1996). Statistical significance testing and cumulative knowledge in psychology: Implications for training of researchers. *Psychological Methods, 1*, 115–129.

Schmitt, N., & Stults, D. M. (1986). Methodology review: Analysis of multitrait-multimethod matrices. *Applied Psychological Measurement, 10*, 1–22.

Schumacker, R. E., & Lomax, R. G. (1996). *A beginner's guide to structural equation modeling.* Mahwah, NJ: Lawrence Erlbaum & Associates.

Shavelson, R. J., Hubner, J. J., & Stanton, G. C. (1976). Self-concept: Validation of construct interpretations. *Review of Educational Research, 46*, 407–441.

Singer, J. D., & Willett, J. D. (2003). *Applied longitudinal data analysis: Modeling change and event occurrence.* New York: Oxford.

Sobel, M. E., & Bohrnstedt, G. W. (1985). Use of null models in evaluating the fit of covariance structure models. In N. B. Tuma (Ed.), *Sociological Methodology* (pp. 152–178). San Francisco: Jossey-Bass.

Sörbom, D. (1974). A general method for studying differences in factor means and factor structures between groups. *British Journal of Mathematical and Statistical Psychology, 27*, 229–239.

Steiger, J. H. (1990). Structural model evaluation and modification: An interval estimation approach. *Multivariate Behavioral Research, 25*, 173–180.

Steiger, J. H. (1998). A note on multiple sample extensions of the RMSEA fit index. *Structural Equation Modeling: A Multidisciplinary Journal, 5*, 411–419.

Steiger, J. H., & Lind, J. C. (1980, June). *Statistically based tests for the number of common factors.* Paper presented at the Psychometric Society Annual Meeting, Iowa City, IA.

Steiger, J. H., Shapiro, A., & Browne, M. W. (1985). On the multivariate asymptotic distribution of sequential chi-square statistics. *Psychometrika, 50*, 253–264.

Sugawara, H. M., & MacCallum, R. C. (1993). Effect of estimation method on incremental fit indexes for covariance structure models. *Applied Psychological Measurement, 17*, 365–377.

Tanaka, J. S. (1993). Multifaceted conceptions of fit in structural equation models. In J. A. Bollen & J. S. Long (Eds.), *Testing structural equation models* (pp. 10–39). Newbury Park, CA: Sage.

Tanaka, J. S., & Huba, G. J. (1984). Confirmatory hierarchical factor analyses of psychological distress measures. *Journal of Personality and Social Psychology, 46*, 621–635.

Thompson, B. (1996). AERA editorial policies regarding statistical significance testing: Three suggested reforms. *Educational Researcher, 25*, 26–30.

Tomarken, A. J., & Waller, N. G. (2005). Structural equation modeling: Strengths, limitations, and misconceptions. *Annual Review of Clinical Psychology, 1*, 2.1–2.35.

Tomás, J. M., Hontangas, P. M., & Oliver, A. (2000). *Multivariate Behavioral Research, 35*, 469–499.

Tucker, L. R., & Lewis, C. (1973). A reliability coefficient for maximum likelihood factor analysis. *Psychometrika, 38*, 1–10.

Wald, A. (1943). Tests of statistical hypotheses concerning several parameters when the number of observations is large. *Transactions of the American Mathematical Society, 54*, 426–482.

Weng, L. -J., & Cheng, C. -P. (1997). Why might relative fit indices differ between estimators? *Structural Equation Modeling: A Multidisciplinary Journal, 4*, 121–128.

West, S. G., Finch, J. F., & Curran, P. J. (1995). Structural equation models with nonnormal variables: Problems and remedies. In R. H. Hoyle (Ed.), *Structural equation modeling: Concepts, issues, and applications* (pp. 56–75). Thousand Oaks, CA: Sage.

Wheaton, B. (1987). Assessment of fit in overidentified models with latent variables. *Sociological Methods & Research, 16,* 118–154.

Widaman, K. F. (1985). Hierarchically tested covariance structure models for multitrait-multimethod data. *Applied Psychological Measurement, 9,* 1–26.

Widaman, K. F., & Reise, S. P. (1997). Exploring the measurement invariance of psychological instruments: Applications in the substance use domain. In K. J. Bryant, M. Windle, & S. G. West (Eds.), *The science of prevention* (pp. 281–324). Washington, DC: American Psychological Association.

Willett, J. B. (1988). Questions and answers in the measurement of change. In E. Z. Rothkopf (Ed.), *Review of research in education* (Vol. 15, pp. 345–422). Washington, DC: American Educational Research Association.

Willett, J. B. (1989). Some results on reliability for the longitudinal measurement of change: Implications for the design of studies of individual growth. *Educational and Psychological Measurement, 49,* 587–602.

Willett, J. B., & Keiley, M. K. (2000). Using covariance structure analysis to model change over time. In H. E. A. Tinsley & S. D. Brown (Eds.), *Handbook of applied multivariate statistics and mathematical modeling* (pp. 665–694). San Diego, CA: Academic Press.

Willett, J. B., & Sayer, A. G. (1994). Using covariance structure analysis to detect correlates and predictors of individual change over time. *Psychological Bulletin, 116,* 363–381.

Willett, J. B., & Sayer, A. G. (1996). Cross-domain analyses of change over time: Combining growth modeling and covariance structure analysis. In G. A. Marcoulides & R. E. Schumacker (Eds.), *Advanced structural equation modeling: Issues and techniques* (pp. 125–157). Mahwah, NJ: Lawrence Erlbaum & Associates.

Williams, L. J., & Holahan, P. J. (1994). Parsimony-based fit indices for multiple-indicator models: Do they work? *Structural Equation Modeling: A Multidisciplinary Journal, 1,* 161–189.

Wood, J. M., Tataryn, D. J., & Gorsuch, R. L. (1996). Effects of under- and overextraction on principal axis factor analysis with varimax rotation. *Psychological Methods, 1,* 354–365.

Wothke, W. (1993). Nonpositive definite matrices in structural modeling. In K. A. Bollen & J. S. Long (Eds.), *Testing structural equation models* (pp. 256–293). Newbury Park, CA: Sage.

Wothke, W. (1996). Models for multitrait-multimethod matrix analysis. In G. A. Marcoulides & R. E. Schumacker (Eds.), *Advanced structural equation modeling: Issues and techniques* (pp. 7–56). Mahwah, NJ: Lawrence Erlbaum & Associates.

Yuan, K. -H., & Bentler, P. M. (1998). Normal theory based test statistics in structural equation modeling. *British Journal of Mathematical and Statistical Psychology, 51,* 289–309.

Yuan, K. -H., & Bentler, P. M. (2000). Three likelihood-based methods for mean and covariance structure analysis with nonnormal missing data. *Sociological Methodology* (pp. 165–200). Washington, DC: American Sociological Association.

Yuan, K. -H., & Bentler, P. M. (2002). On normal theory based inference for multilevel models with distributional violations. *Psychometrika, 67,* 539–562.

Yuan, K. -H., & Bentler, P. M. (2004a). On chi square difference and z-tests in mean and covariance structure analysis when the base model is misspecified. *Educational and Psychological Measurement, 64,* 737–757.

Yuan, K. -H., & Bentler, P. M. (2004b). On the asymptotic distributions of two statistics for two-level covariance structure models within the class of elliptical distributions. *Psychometrika, 69,* 437–457.

Yuan, K. -H., Lambert, P. L., & Fouladi, R. T. (2004). Mardia's multivariate kurtosis with missing data. *Multivariate Behavioral Research, 39,* 413–437.

Author Index

Subject Index